CLINICAL ATLAS OF CANINE AND FELINE OPHTHALMIC DISEASE

CLINICAL ATLAS OF CANINE AND FELINE OPHTHALMIC DISEASE

DOUGLAS W. ESSON, BVSC, MRCVS, DVM, DACVO,

Veterinary ophthalmologist and clinical director of Eye Care for Animals, Tustin, California, USA

WILEY Blackwell

Editorial Offices: 1606 Golden Aspen Drive, Suites 103 and 104, Ames, Iowa 50010, USA
The Atrium, Southern Gate, Chichester, West Sussex, PO19 8SQ, UK
9600 Garsington Road, Oxford, OX4 2DQ, UK

For details of our global editorial offices, for customer services and for information about how to apply for permission to reuse the copyright material in this book please see our website at www.wiley.com/wiley-blackwell.

Library of Congress Cataloging-in-Publication Data

Esson, Douglas W., author.
Clinical atlas of canine and feline ophthalmic disease / Douglas W. Esson.
p. ; cm.
Includes index.
ISBN 978-1-118-84077-1 (cloth)
1. Dogs–Diseases–Atlases. 2. Cats–Diseases–Atlases. 3. Eye–Diseases–Atlases. 4. Veterinary ophthalmology–Atlases. I. Title.
[DNLM: 1. Dog Diseases–Atlases. 2. Eye Diseases–veterinary–Atlases. 3. Cat Diseases–Atlases. 4. Ophthalmologic Surgical Procedures–Atlases. SF 992.E92]

SF992.E92 E87 2015
636.089′77–dc23

2015006624

A catalogue record for this book is available from the British Library.

Wiley also publishes its books in a variety of electronic formats. Some content that appears in print may not be available in electronic books.

Set in 10/12pt Minion by Laserwords Private Limited, Chennai, India
Printed and bound in Singapore by Markono Print Media Pte Ltd

1 2015

CONTENTS

PREFACE

It is some years since I made the conscious decision to further my postgraduate knowledge of the complex and fascinating world of veterinary ophthalmology. With the passing of the intervening years, I have had the immense good fortune to interact with a number of clinician-scientists, all of whom have generously shared their time, experience, and knowledge with me. In particular, I am indebted in this regard to Drs. Peter Bedford, Randy Scagliotti, Kirk Gelatt, Paul Miller, Dick Dubielzig, Bill Dawson, and Mark Sherwood. I am frequently asked to give lectures about various ophthalmic topics to audiences ranging from students to experienced ophthalmologists, and it is most commonly through photographic images that I am able to share my own thoughts and experience. The field of veterinary ophthalmology, detailed ophthalmic texts, and the peer-reviewed ophthalmic literature represent a sometimes challenging and potentially confusing arena and, as a consequence, I have sought here to provide the busy general practitioner with a clear, systematic, repeatable clinical picture of the most frequently encountered ophthalmic conditions in small animal practice. Images are intentionally presented in the same way as cases would be encountered in practice. In order to expand this project beyond that of simply an image atlas, I have also tried to provide clear, concise, updated, and clinically relevant information as it pertains to each of these conditions. This information has been supported with a small number of relevant references for those who to wish to read further.

Any potential drug side effects are identified by this shaded colored box.

ACKNOWLEDGMENTS

Many individuals have contributed to the development of this book. The project, from its inception, has been shaped by my editors and publishers at Wiley, with special thanks to Erica Judisch, Nancy Turner, and Catriona Cooper. The images within this volume have mostly been sourced from my own collection; however, I have relied on friends and colleagues to discuss clinical presentations, help source cases (and in some instances provide images) in order to achieve completeness. In this regard, I acknowledge Drs. Dustin Dees, Anne-Michelle Armour, Nicole McClaren, Randy Scagliotti, Al MacMillan, Christin Chapman, David Wilkie, Matthew Fife, Nancy Park, Anastasia Komenou, Jennifer Urbanz, Peter Bedford, David Williams, David Donaldson, Julius Brinkis, Dilip Bhalerao, Emily Moeller, Francesca Venturi, Neal Wasserman, Joanna Norman, Keith Collins, Steve Sissler, Melanie Church. Ashley Stich, Laura Wilson, Rudayna Gubash, Allison Kirby, Nick Millichamp, Mark Haskins, Gwen Lynch, and Kristina Narfstrom. I am additionally grateful to a number of the affiliated specialists with whom I work, for their willingness to source and discuss cases commonly presented to the services of internal medicine, dermatology, and oncology. In this regard, I particularly acknowledge Drs. Wayne Rosenkrantz, Colleen Mendelsohn, Melissa Hall, Julie Bulman-Fleming, and David Bommarito. The time taken to collate and describe these conditions was allocated by Karen Webster and sponsored by Eye Care for Animals as part of its ongoing commitment to advancing the field of veterinary ophthalmology. Finally but most importantly I am endlessly grateful to my wife Sara, herself a gifted and passionate veterinary ophthalmologist. Without her endless assistance, clinical expertise, and patient advice, this book would simply not have been possible.

For Sara and Justin With all my love Doug Esson Tustin, California, 2014

Section 1
Anatomy and Diagnostics

CHAPTER 1
NORMAL OCULAR ANATOMY

Normal canine and feline orbital anatomy comprises the following;

The orbit, made up of bones, connective tissue, lacrimal and salivary glandular tissue, adipose tissue, blood vessels, and nerves.

The eyelids, comprising skin, orbicularis oculi muscles, deep tarsal, and superficial conjunctival tissue. These tissues also contain mucus-producing goblet cells, lipid-producing meibomian glands, and the openings of the nasolacrimal drainage system.

The third eyelid, comprising a T-shaped cartilaginous structure, which surrounds the lacrimal gland of the third eyelid and is covered with conjunctival tissue.

The external shell of the eye, comprising the cornea anteriorly and the episcleral and scleral tissues posteriorly. The cornea is composed of an outer epithelium (with its basement membrane), central stroma, and underlying endothelial layer (with its basement or "Descemet's" membrane).

The uveal tract, composed of the anterior iris and ciliary body and the posterior choroid, which is the vascular supply to the retina.

The lens, which is suspended from the ciliary body by zonular ligaments and surrounded by the lens capsule.

The neuroretina which comprises;

- Nerve fiber layer and inner limiting membrane
- Ganglion cell layer
- Inner nuclear and inner plexiform layers
- Outer nuclear and outer plexiform layers
- Photoreceptors (rods & cones) and outer limiting membrane
- Retinal pigment epithelium.

Retinal ganglion cells coalesce to form the optic nerve which exits the globe posteriorly, through the porous lamina cribrosa.

Clinical Atlas of Canine and Feline Ophthalmic Disease, First Edition. Douglas Esson.

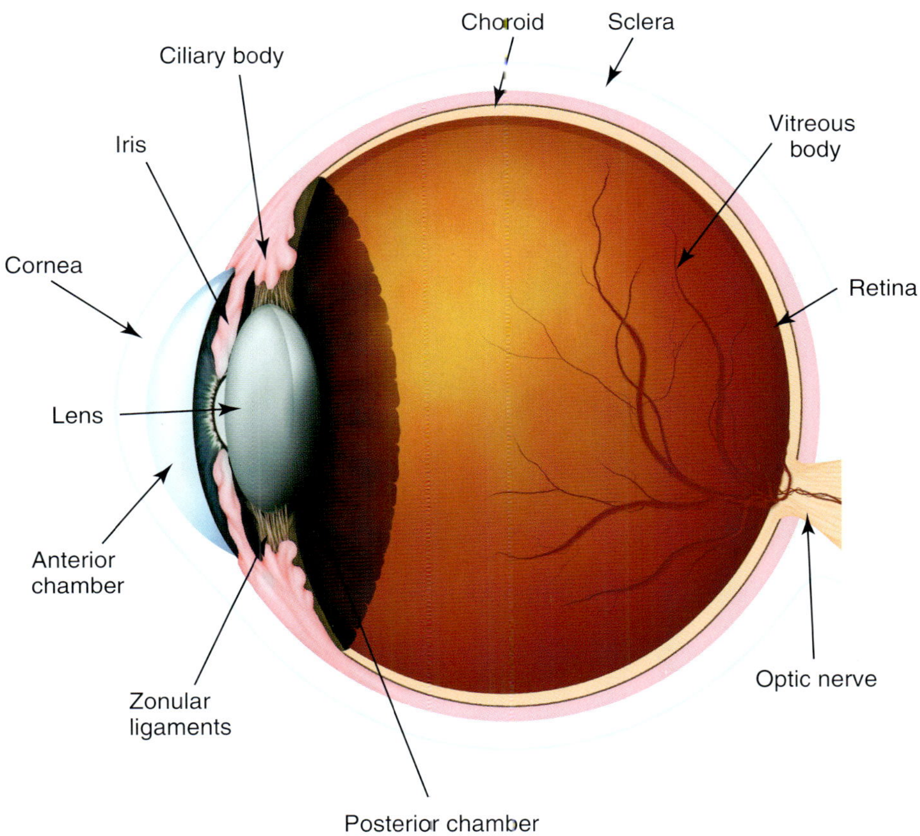

Figure 1.1 Normal ocular anatomy.

CHAPTER 2
NORMAL PIGMENTARY VARIATIONS

Both canine and feline irides may demonstrate a range of pigmentary variations. True ocular albinism (the complete lack of pigment) is rare. The term subalbinism describes pigment dilution resulting in variably grey to bluish colored iridal tissue, a finding common in animals with light hair coat colors. The term heterochromia iridis describes variable combinations of pigment within either one or both irides.

Clinical Atlas of Canine and Feline Ophthalmic Disease, First Edition. Douglas Esson.

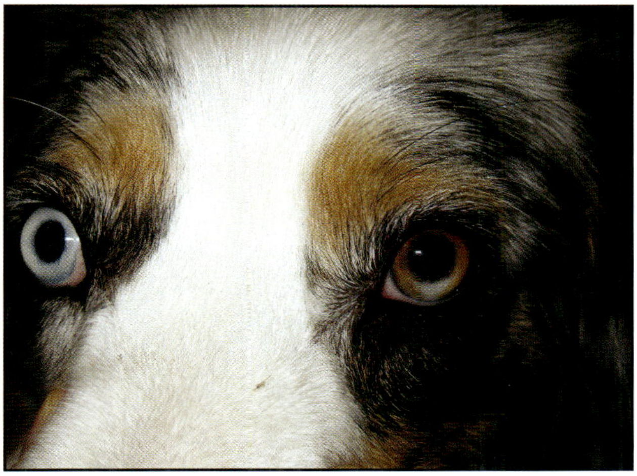

Figure 2.1 Normal variation in pigmentation between left and right eyes.

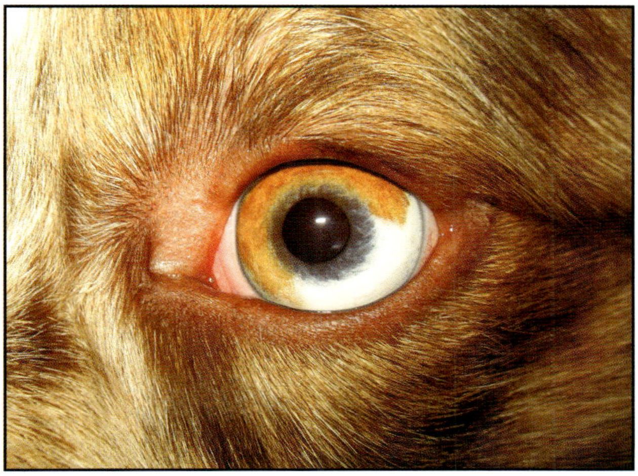

Figure 2.2 Normal heterochromic variation in pigmentation within a light colored iris.

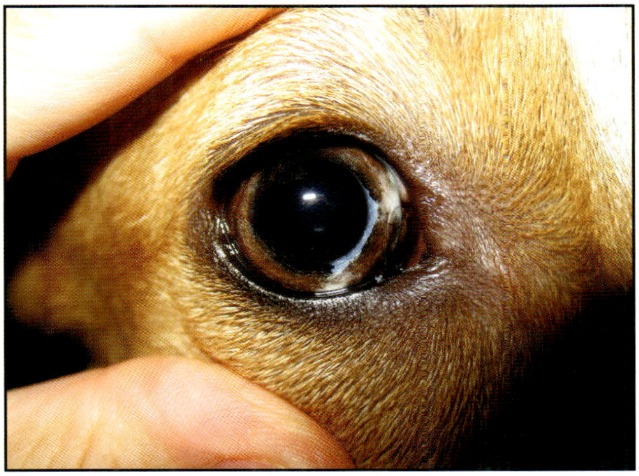

Figure 2.3 Normal heterochromic variation in pigmentation within a dark colored iris.

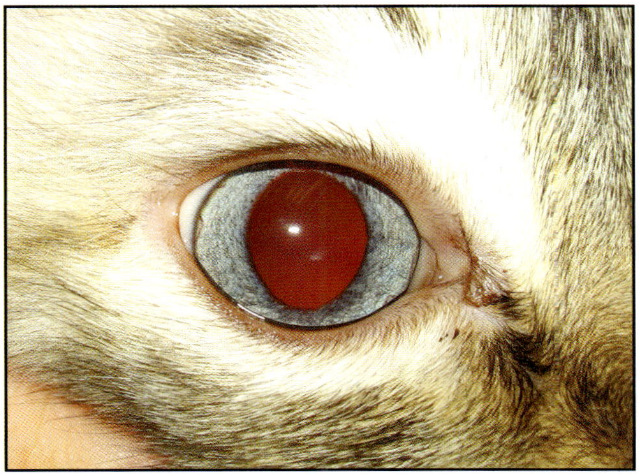

Figure 2.4 Normal blue iris (the "red reflex" of the subalbinotic fundus being visible through the pupil).

CHAPTER 3
THE NORMAL CANINE FUNDUS

The canine fundus exhibits a wide variation in normal appearance, comprising a tapetal as well as a non-tapetal region, the optic nerve head, associated vasculature, and multilayered neuroretina, all of which overlie the choroidal vascular bed. The juvenile canine fundus typically appears bluish in color until maturation within the first 3–4 months of life.

The specialized cells of the tapetal region contain reflective material comprising zinc/cysteine as well as a poorly to non-pigmented retinal pigment epithelial (RPE) layer, which facilitates low-light vision. This region is typically bright yellow to green in coloration.

The non-tapetal fundus is usually dark in color because of the presence of pigment within the RPE.

The optic nerve ("optic disc," "optic papilla") appears as a variably shaped and variably myelinated white to pink structure within the fundus, representing the accumulation of ganglion cells and displaying an incomplete vascular circle surrounding a central physiologic pit.

Radiating from the ONH are 3–4 large veins and 15–20 smaller arterioles.

Clinical Atlas of Canine and Feline Ophthalmic Disease, First Edition. Douglas Esson.

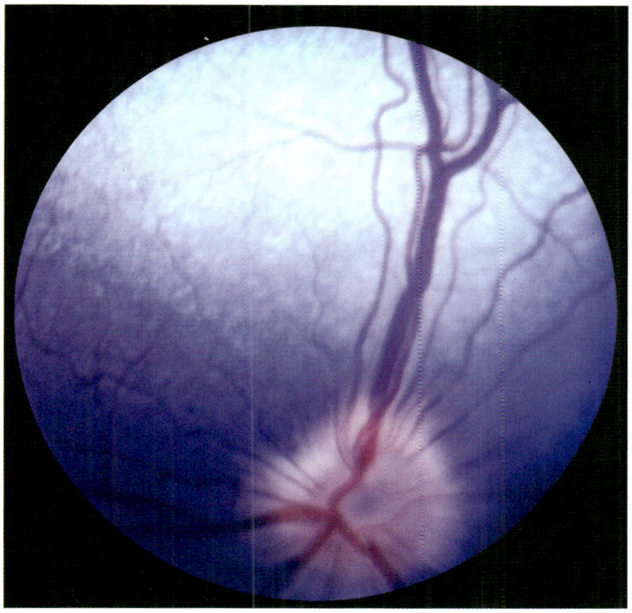

Figure 3.1 Normal pigmented canine fundus. The bluish color indicates immaturity.

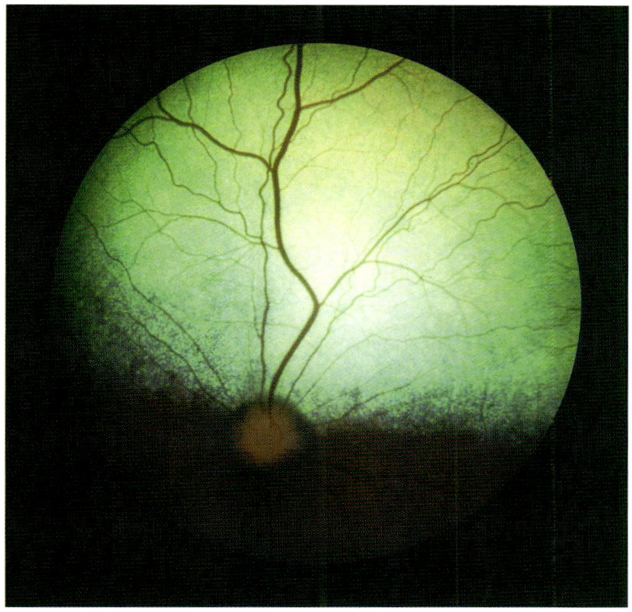

Figure 3.2 Normal pigmented canine fundus (predominantly green).

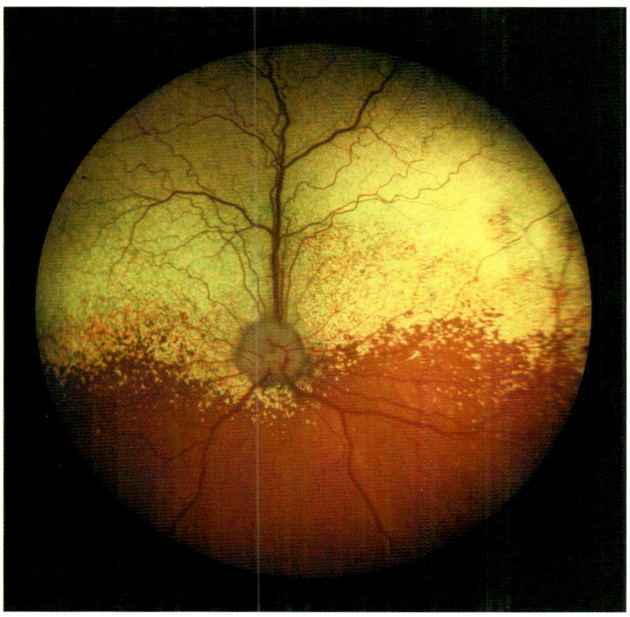

Figure 3.3 Normal pigmented canine fundus (predominantly yellow).

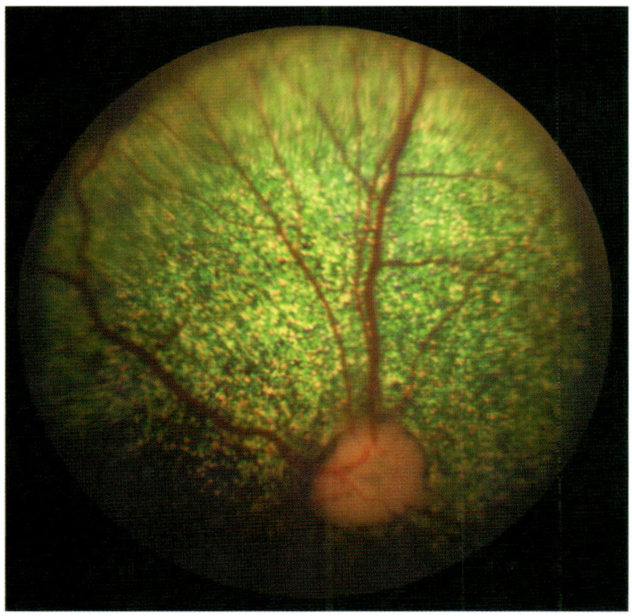

Figure 3.4 Normal pigmented canine fundus (speckled).

CHAPTER 4
THE NORMAL FELINE FUNDUS

The feline fundus exhibits a wide variation in normal appearance, comprising a relatively large tapetal as well as non-tapetal region, the optic nerve head, associated vasculature, and multilayered neuroretina, all of which overly the choroidal vascular bed.

The specialized cells of the tapetal region contain reflective material comprising zinc/riboflavin as well as a poorly to non-pigmented retinal pigment epithelial (RPE) layer, which facilitates low-light vision. This region is typically bright yellow to green in coloration.

The non-tapetal fundus is usually dark in color due to the presence of pigment within the RPE.

The optic nerve ("optic disc," "optic papilla") appears as a small, circular, unmyelinated white to grey structure within the fundus, representing the accumulation of ganglion cells.

Three major pairs of arterioles as well as larger venules radiate from the ONH.

Clinical Atlas of Canine and Feline Ophthalmic Disease, First Edition. Douglas Esson.

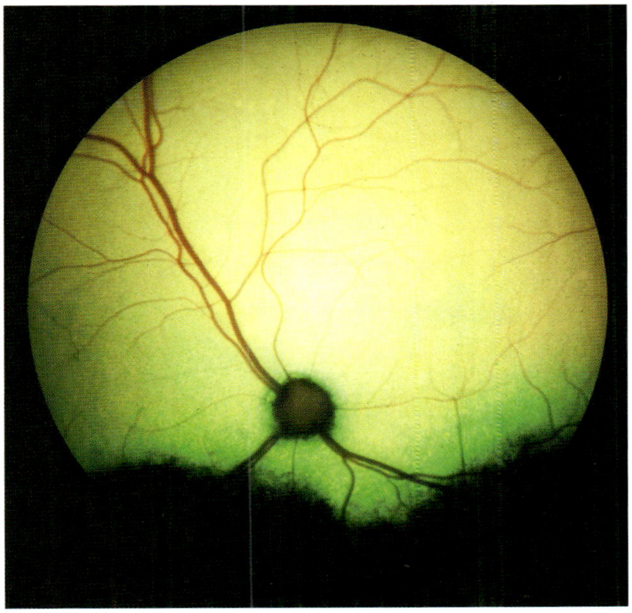

Figure 4.1 Normal pigmented feline fundus (predominantly green), note the poorly myelinated optic nerve head.

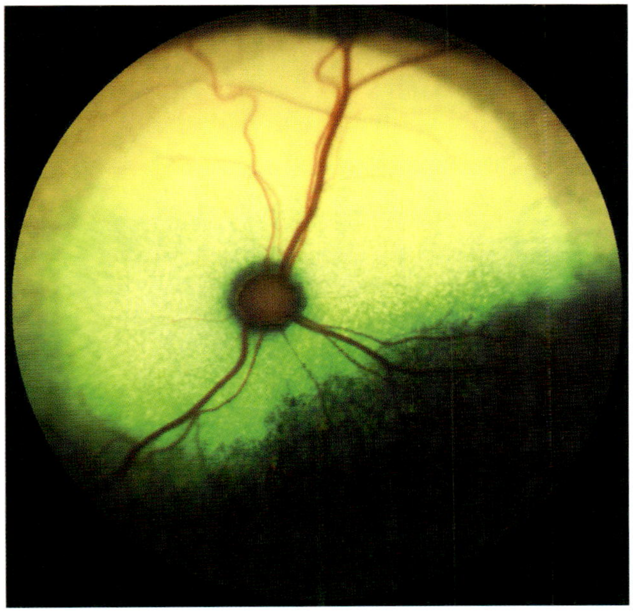

Figure 4.2 Normal pigmented feline fundus (predominantly green), note the poorly myelinated optic nerve head.

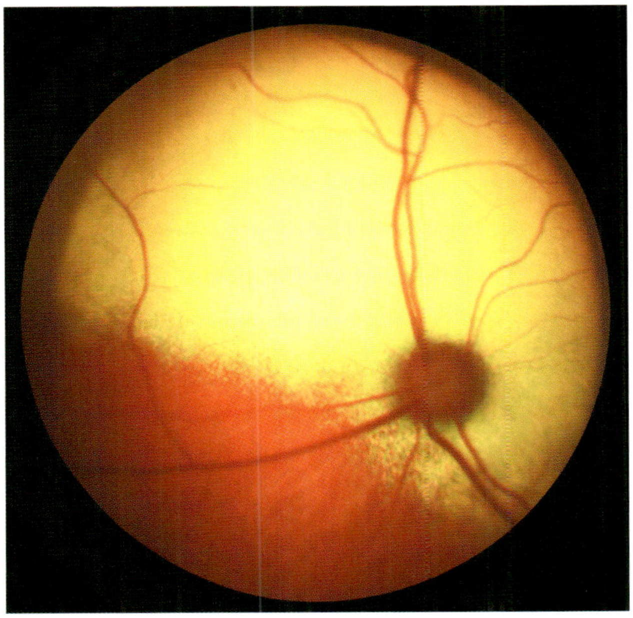

Figure 4.3 Normal pigmented feline fundus (predominantly yellow), note the poorly myelinated optic nerve head.

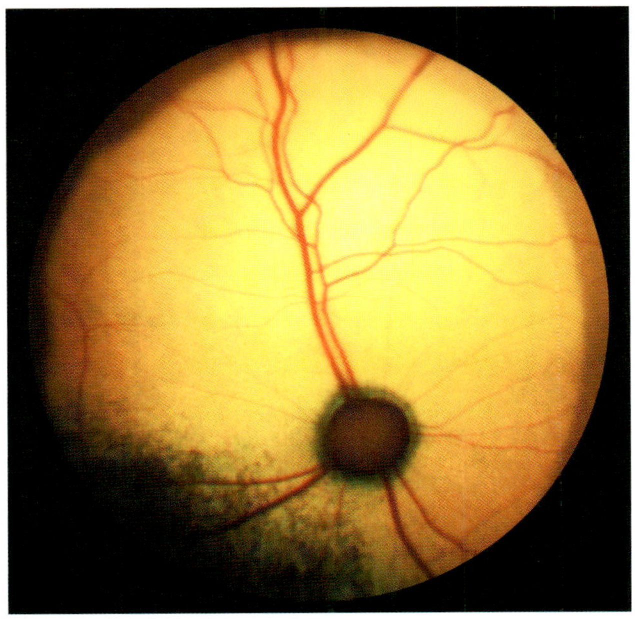

Figure 4.4 Normal pigmented feline fundus (predominantly yellow), note the poorly myelinated optic nerve head.

CHAPTER 5
THE NORMAL SUBALBINOTIC FUNDUS

Dogs or cats displaying blue irides, heterochromic irides, and/or merled coat coloration, typically display "subalbinotic" fundi. In these animals, the tapetal region may be variably reduced to absent in association with a variable to complete lack of pigment within the non-tapetal fundus. As a result, underlying choroidal vasculature is visible against the white scleral background. The subalbinotic fundus represents a normal variation in coloration.

Clinical Atlas of Canine and Feline Ophthalmic Disease, First Edition. Douglas Esson.

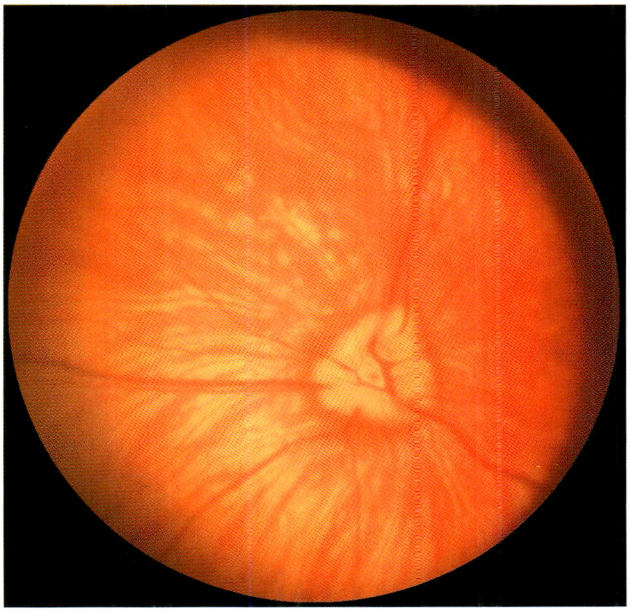

Figure 5.1 Normal (canine) subalbinotic fundus. Choroidal vessels are clearly visible against the white scleral background.

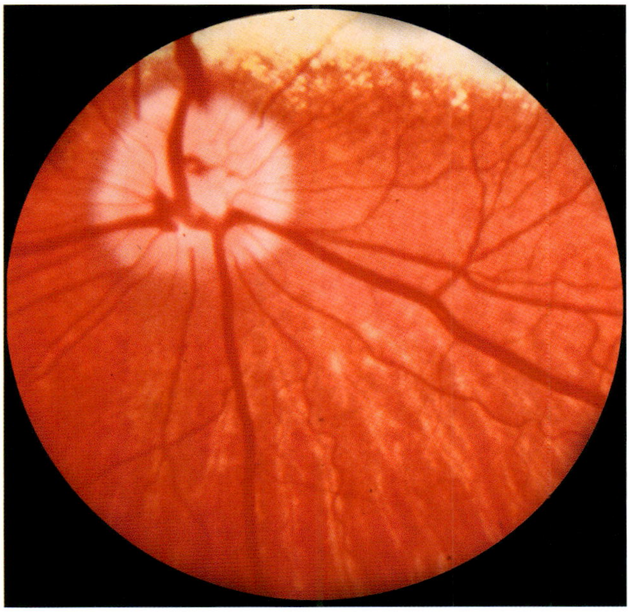

Figure 5.2 Normal (canine) subalbinotic fundus. Choroidal vessels are clearly visible against the white scleral background.

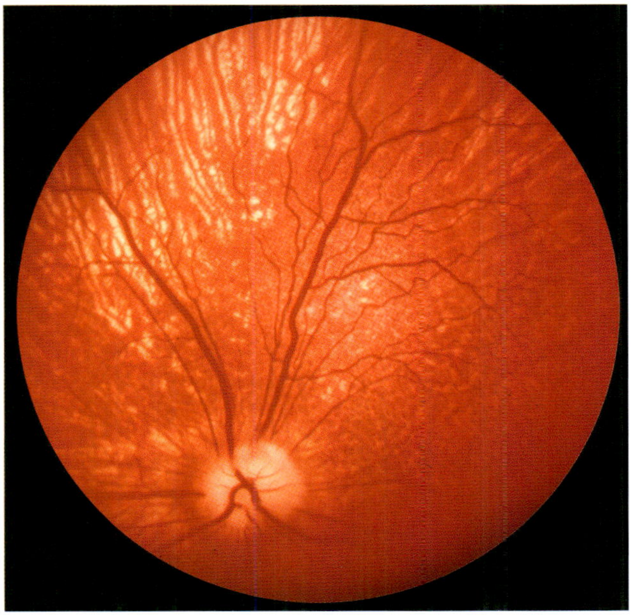

Figure 5.3 Normal (canine) subalbinotic fundus. Choroidal vessels are clearly visible against the white scleral background.

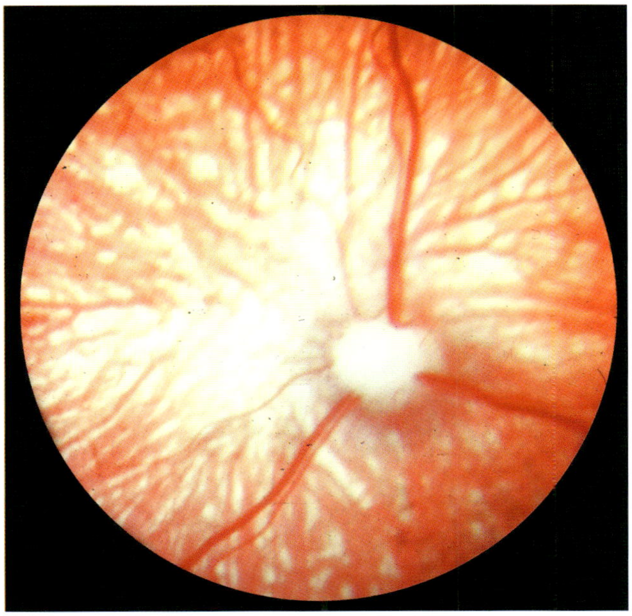

Figure 5.4 Normal (feline) subalbinotic fundus. Choroidal vessels are clearly visible against the white scleral background.

CHAPTER 6
NORMAL MYELINATION VARIATIONS

The optic nerve head (ONH) comprises coalescing ganglion cells as they converge before exiting the globe caudally through the porous lamina cribrosa. This region is variably myelinated; poorly in the cat and variably in the dog. Variations in the amount of myelin present may result in range of normal appearances when this region is visualized.

Clinical Atlas of Canine and Feline Ophthalmic Disease, First Edition. Douglas Esson.

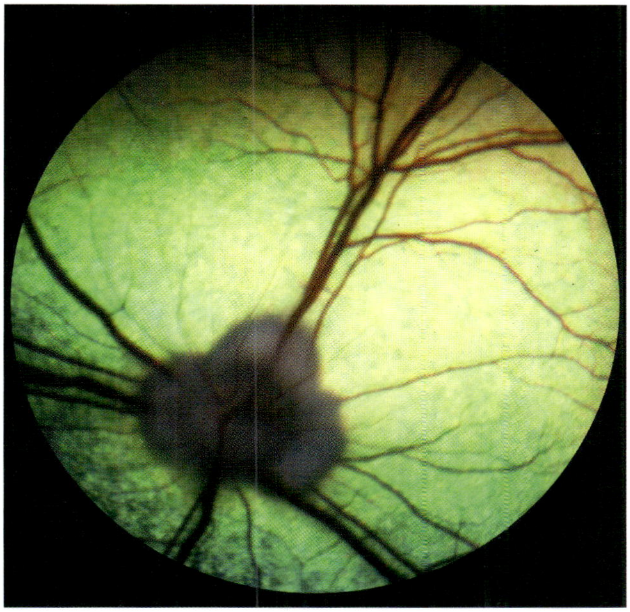

Figure 6.1 Normal moderately to heavily myelinated canine optic nerve head.

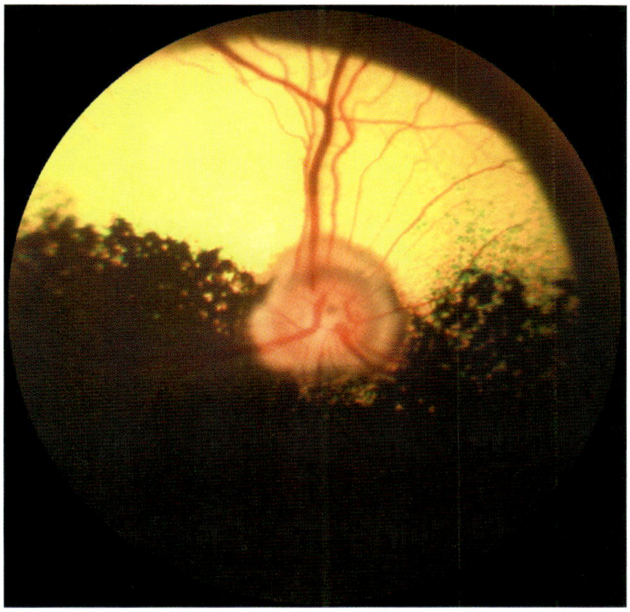

Figure 6.2 Normal moderately to heavily myelinated canine optic nerve head.

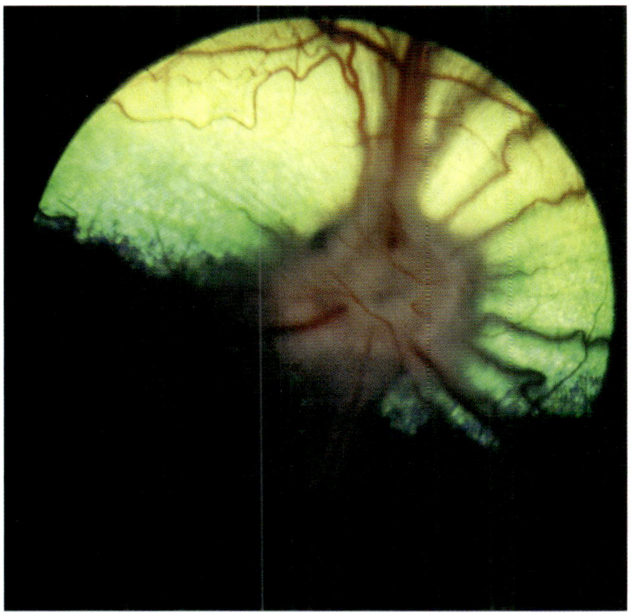

Figure 6.3 Normal moderately to heavily myelinated canine optic nerve head.

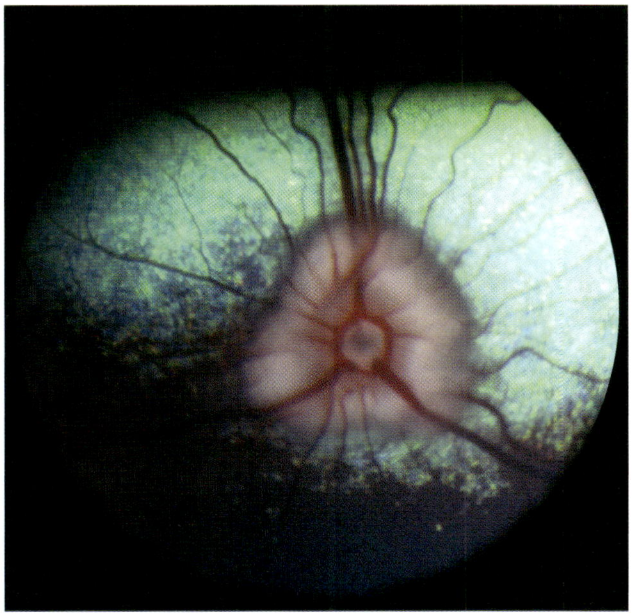

Figure 6.4 Normal moderately to heavily myelinated canine optic nerve head.

CHAPTER 7
THE OCULAR EXAMINATION

The ophthalmic examination should comprise the following components.

HISTORY

Signalment, pre-existing medical/surgical history (including travel history), and/or current medications.

PRESENTING COMPLAINT

Identification of the presenting ophthalmic complaint.

DISTANT "HANDS-OFF" EXAMINATION

Patient is allowed to move around freely—demonstrating mentation, neurological status, and visual ability.

BRIEF GENERAL PHYSICAL EXAMINATION

Includes assessment of mucous membranes, oral cavity, external ear canals, thoracic auscultation, palpation of lymph nodes and abdomen and body temperature.

CLOSE UP "HANDS-ON" EXAMINATION

Includes careful palpation of the skull and orbits, noting any deformity, asymmetry, crepitus, or discomfort.

NEURO-OPHTHALMIC EXAMINATION

- Palpebral reflex (closure of eyelids upon tactile stimulus)
- Menace response (eyelid closure and/or head withdrawal in response to menacing hand gesture)
- Dazzle reflex (closure of eyelids in response to bright focal light source being shined into eye)
- Pupillary light reflex (PLR) (direct and consensual reflex pupillary miosis in response to a focal light source).

SEGMENTAL ANTERIOR EXAMINATION

A focal light source is used to examine the eyelids, conjunctival surfaces, third eyelid, sclera, cornea, anterior chamber (AC), iris, lens, and anterior vitreous face.

FUNDIC EXAMINATION

The posterior segment is examined using either a focal light source and handheld lens or an ophthalmoscope.

ANCILLARY DIAGNOSTICS

- **Schirmer tear test I (STT1)**. Schirmer strip placed into ventral fornix for one minute, normal value = 15–20 mm/wetting/min
- **Intraocular pressure (IOP) estimation**. Using either an applanation or rebound tonometer, the probe tip is applied to the axial cornea several times in order to generate an average estimation of IOP (normal value = 15–25 mmHg)
- **Vital corneal staining.** Sodium fluorescein dye is applied to the cornea then excess carefully irrigated away to detect retention associated with epithelial defects. Fluorescein dye may also be used to assess nasolacrimal duct patency ("Jones" test) and/or aqueous leakage from the anterior chamber ("Seidel" test).

Where indicated, additional diagnostic aids may include obtaining blood samples for complete blood count (CBC), chemistry, metabolic, endocrine and/or infectious titer testing, the harvesting of microbial samples for culture and sensitivity testing as well as cytological and/or histological examination and/or advanced imaging (including radiography, B-mode ultrasonography, computed tomography, and/or magnetic resonance imaging).

Clinical Atlas of Canine and Feline Ophthalmic Disease, First Edition. Douglas Esson.

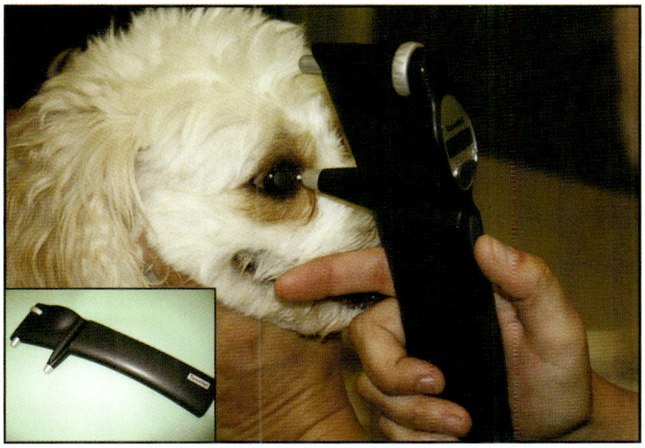

Figure 7.1 Estimation of intraocular pressure (IOP) using a rebound tonometer ("*Tonovet*"). The probe-tip is gently allowed to contact the axial corneal surface (without the use of local anesthetic) by pressing the measurement button. Several readings are taken, so that aberrant readings may be disregarded.

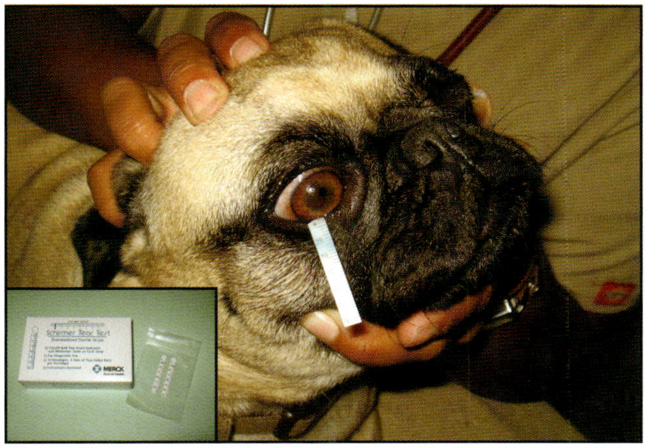

Figure 7.2 Measurement of lacrimal function using gradated ("*Schirmer*") tear strips. The tip of each strip is folded and placed into the lower medial fornix for one minute and the resultant STT1 value recorded. This test should be performed before the installation of any topical agents.

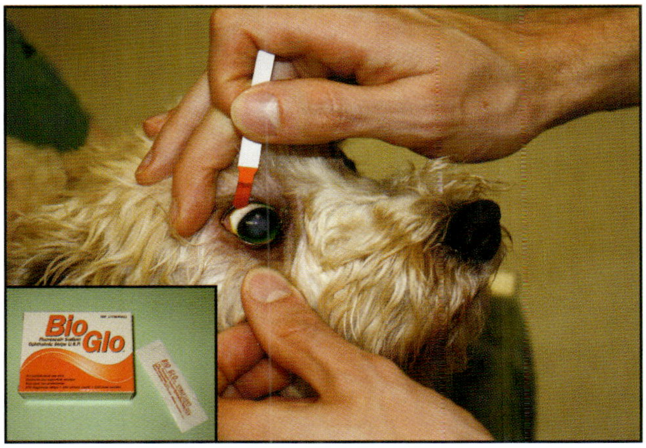

Figure 7.3 Vital staining of the corneal surface using fluorescein-impregnated strips. Strips are moistened using a physiologic solution and gently touched to the scleral limbus. Excess stain is then carefully irrigated away using eyewash to prevent "pooling" of residual stain.

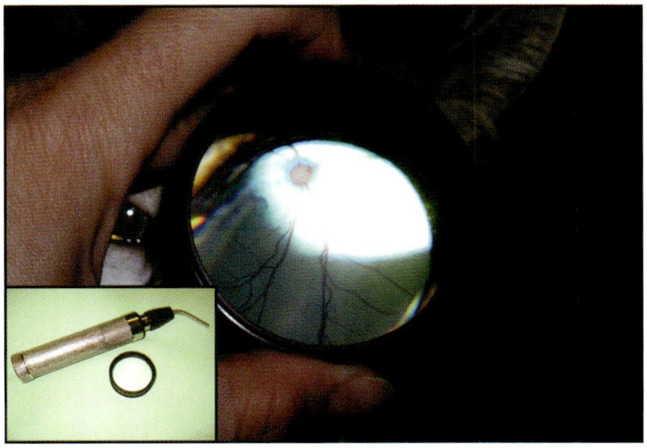

Figure 7.4 Visualization of the fundus using a simple handheld indirect lens, positioned just in front of the eye and parallel to the posterior segment. Where an indirect ophthalmoscope is unavailable, a small flashlight or transilluminator, held adjacent to the examiner's head, will suffice as a distant focal light source.

Section 2

Diseases of the Eyelids

CHAPTER 8
EYELID AGENESIS

PRESENTATION

Feline eyelid agenesis describes a congenital condition in which affected animals are born with incomplete eyelid margins. Multiple kittens from a single litter are commonly affected. Typically, the presentation is bilateral and symmetrical with the full thickness defect affecting the superotemporal eyelid margins; however, variations may occur. The size of the defect may also vary. Additional ocular abnormalities may be present, with persistent pupillary membranes (PPMs) being the most common. Eyelid agenesis commonly results in trichiasis or contact between hairs and the corneal surface. Potential sequelae include fibrosing, vascular and pigmentary keratitis, the formation of corneal sequestra, and/or corneal ulceration, which may become severe enough to result in perforation of the globe.

DIAGNOSIS AND TREATMENT

Medical management of this condition includes the frequent application of a topical lubricant to coat and protect the corneal surfaces as well as the treatment of inflammatory and/or ulcerative lesions. The use of immunosuppressive medications and/or corticosteroids should be cautiously considered as a result of their potential to facilitate herpesviral recrudescence and/or aggravate ulcerative lesions. In simple or less severe cases, offending hairs (and their follicles) may be permanently removed via cryoepilation. More elegant but complex surgical techniques to recreate a functional eyelid margin have been described (generally encompassing the transposition of skin, orbicularis muscle and conjunctival tissue), the most typically appropriate being that by Dziezyc and Millichamp. These procedures, however, may require a multistage surgical approach and limited subsequent cryoepilation may additionally be necessary. Postoperative care comprises routine systemic antimicrobial (if indicated), anti-inflammatory and analgesic care. An Elizabethan collar should be placed following eyelid surgery in order to prevent self-trauma and corneal health should be frequently monitored until eyelid healing is complete.

SELECTED REFERENCES

Dziezyc J and Millichamp NJ. Surgical correction of eyelid agenesis in a cat. *J Am Anim Hosp Assoc*. 1989;**25**, 513–516.

Glaze MB. Congenital and hereditary ocular abnormalities in cats. *Clin Tech Small Anim Pract*. 2005;**20**(2):74–82.

Reinstein SL, Gross SL, Komáromy AM. Successful treatment of distichiasis in a cat using transconjunctival electrocautery. *Vet Ophthalmol*. 2011;**14** Suppl 1:130–134. doi: 10.1111/j.1463-5224.2011.

Whittaker CJ, Wilkie DA, Simpson DJ, Deykin A, Smith JS, Robinson CL. Lip commissure to eyelid transposition for repair of feline eyelid agenesis. *Vet Ophthalmol*. 2010;**13**(3):173–178. doi: 10.1111/j.1463-5224.2010.

Clinical Atlas of Canine and Feline Ophthalmic Disease, First Edition. Douglas Esson.

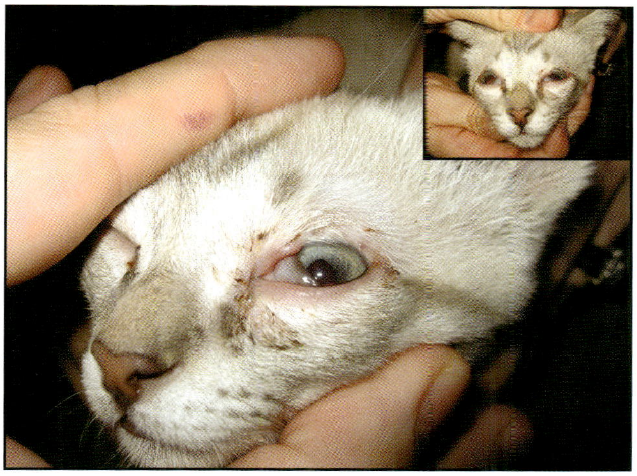

Figure 8.1 Feline upper eyelid agenesis (the inset demonstrates typical bilateral presentation).

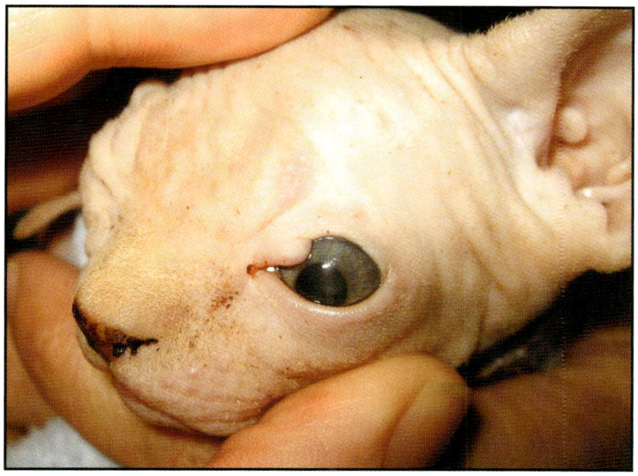

Figure 8.2 Feline upper eyelid agenesis in a hairless kitten.

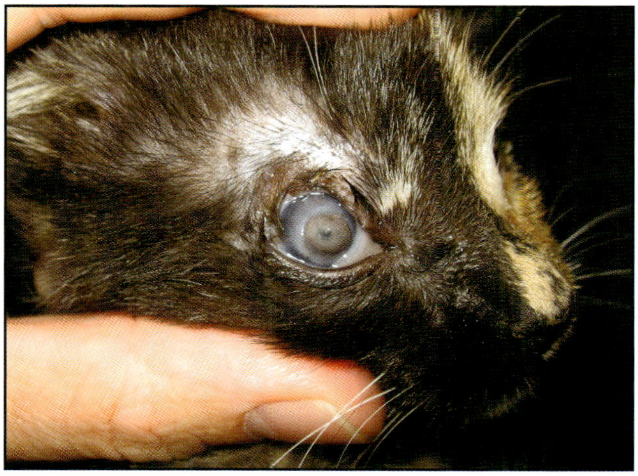

Figure 8.3 Feline upper eyelid agenesis. Notable is perforating ulcerative keratitis secondary to chronic trichiasis.

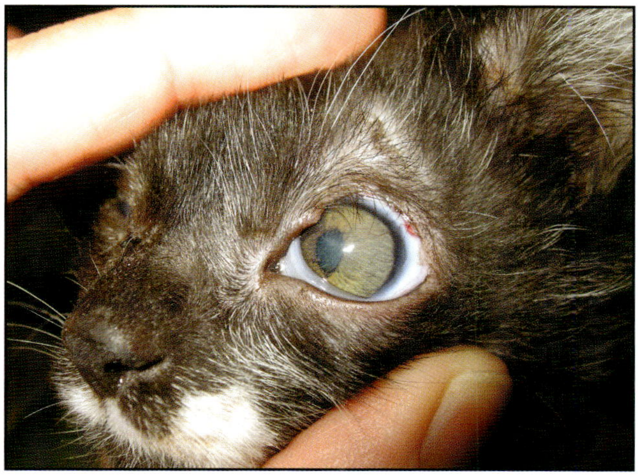

Figure 8.4 Feline upper eyelid agenesis. Notable is the presence of fine persistent pupillary membranes (PPMs) within the anterior chamber.

CHAPTER 9
EYELID LACERATION

PRESENTATION

The eyelids comprise an inner layer (made up of conjunctiva and underlying connective tissue) and an outer layer (made of up haired skin and underlying orbicularis muscle). The eyelid margins also contain the lipid-secreting meibomian glands. Eyelid lacerations are commonly encountered, as a result of trauma such as bite wounds. Full-thickness lacerations disrupt normal eyelid structure & function and require accurate reconstruction.

DIAGNOSIS AND TREATMENT

Potentially life-threatening injuries should be addressed and stabilized before treating eyelid injuries. Sedation or anesthesia may be required in order to facilitate adequate evaluation and treatment. Affected tissues should be carefully cleansed and copiously irrigated using physiologic saline and foreign material as well as accumulated mucous and blood gently removed in order to assess the extent of injury and tissue viability. Devitalized tissues should be carefully debrided, taking care to retain as much of the eyelid margin as possible as well as to preserve subcutaneous vascular structures. Fresh wounds (24–48 hrs) can usually be debrided and repaired immediately. Older wounds may require the treatment of significant inflammation and/or secondary bacterial infection before debridement and repair. Ultimately, however, full-thickness eyelid lacerations should be surgically repaired rather than being allowed to heal by second intention in order to ensure accurate apposition and long-term functionality. Full-thickness eyelid lacerations should be repaired in two layers. A continuous absorbable suture material should be used to appose deeper conjunctival and connective tissue layers. Interrupted nonabsorbable sutures should be used to close the outer skin and muscular layers. Careful and accurate apposition of the eyelid margin (ideally by placing a "figure-8" suture) is critical in order to prevent subsequent keratopathy. Where appropriate, dead space should be closed and drains placed. If laceration of the nasolacrimal duct and/or canaliculi is identified, these structures may be stented using silicone or nylon. Postoperative care comprises routine systemic antimicrobial, anti-inflammatory, and analgesic care. An Elizabethan collar should be placed pending eyelid healing in order to prevent self-trauma and corneal health should be frequently monitored until eyelid healing is complete.

SELECTED REFERENCES

Aquino SM. Surgery of the eyelids. *Top Companion Anim Med*. 2008;**23**(1):10–22. doi: 10.1053/j.ctsap.2007.12.003.

Lackner PA. Techniques for surgical correction of adnexal disease. *Clin Tech Small Anim Pract*. 2001;**16**(1):40–50.

Mandell DC, Holt E. Ophthalmic emergencies. *Vet Clin North Am Small Anim Pract*. 2005;**35**(2):455–480, vii–viii. Review.

Reifler DM. Management of canalicular laceration. *Surv Ophthalmol*. 1991;**36**(2):113–132.

Clinical Atlas of Canine and Feline Ophthalmic Disease, First Edition. Douglas Esson.

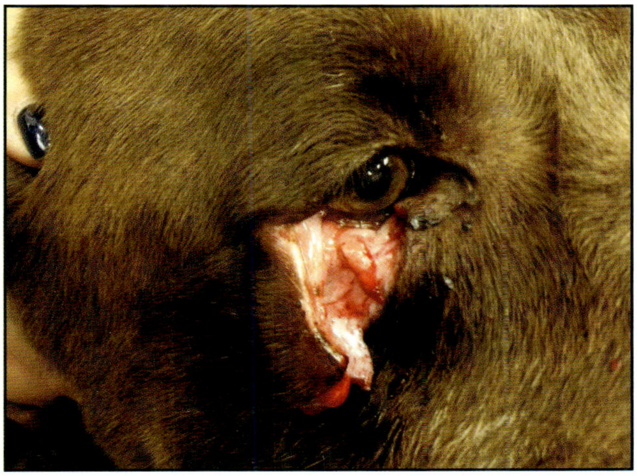

Figure 9.1 Full-thickness eyelid laceration; the fresh wound requires prompt two-layer closure.

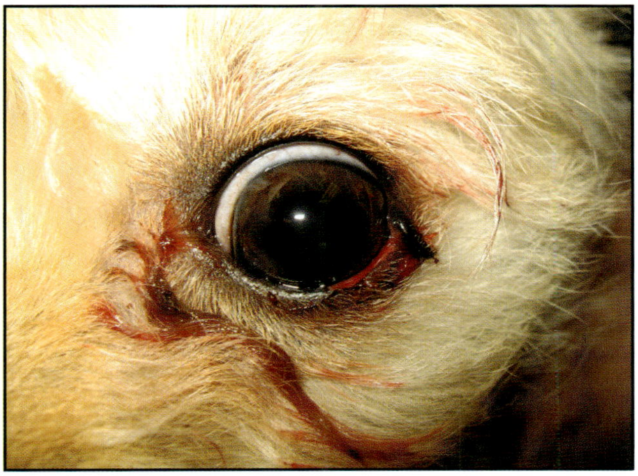

Figure 9.2 Superficial eyelid laceration.

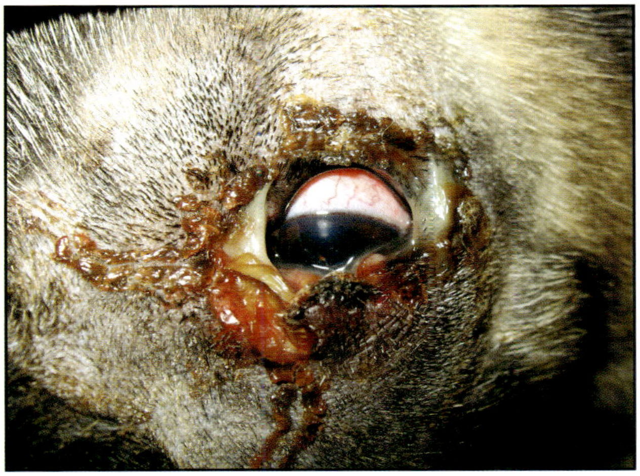

Figure 9.3 Infected eyelid laceration; the wound requires medical treatment before surgical repair.

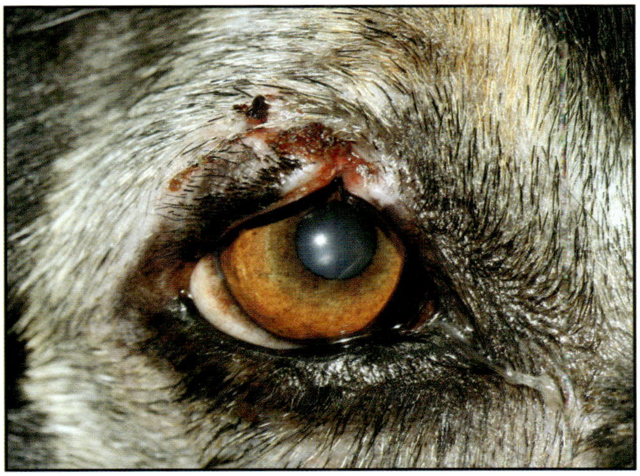

Figure 9.4 Granulating eyelid laceration; the fibrosed wound edges require resection before reconstruction.

CHAPTER 10
DISTICHIASIS

PRESENTATION

Distichiae are abnormal cilia arising from the eyelid margin at/or close to the level of the meibomian gland openings. In many cases, distichiae do not result in significant ocular pathology; however, contact between distichiae and the corneal surface may result in discomfort marked by epiphora and blepharospasm and may lead to secondary keratitis and/or corneal ulceration. Distichiae may affect one or both eyelids (upper and/or lower). Distichiae occur commonly in dogs and less commonly in cats. Commonly affected breeds include the Cocker Spaniel, Boxer, English Bulldog, Yorkshire Terrier, and Shih Tzu.

DIAGNOSIS AND TREATMENT

Where indicated, the appropriate treatment of distichiae represents removal and the permanent destruction of their associated follicle. Manual epilation alone may provide temporary relief but will result in regrowth. Permanent follicular destruction may be achieved using surgical excision, cryoepilation in a double freeze–thaw cycle and/or electroepilation. Cryoepilation should only be undertaken using an appropriate nitrous-oxide cooled unit. Focal swelling and eyelid depigmentation are common following cryoepilation; however, affected tissues typically repigment with time. Extreme care should be taken to preserve the eyelid margins and to avoid excessive eyelid tissue damage or necrosis and the generation of excessive fibrosis, which may lead to cicatricial entropion. Postoperative care comprises routine systemic antimicrobial (if indicated), anti-inflammatory, and analgesic care. An Elizabethan collar should be placed post-operatively in order to prevent self-trauma and corneal health should be frequently monitored until eyelid healing is complete.

Keratitis and/or corneal ulceration should be managed using routine topical antimicrobial therapy as well as the judicious use of a lubricating and protective agent.

SELECTED REFERENCES

Aquino SM. Surgery of the eyelids. *Top Companion Anim Med*. 2008;**23**(1):10–22. doi: 10.1053/j.ctsap.2007.12.003.

Lackner PA. Techniques for surgical correction of adnexal disease. *Clin Tech Small Anim Pract*. 2001;**16**(1):40–50.

Raymond-Letron I, Bourges-Abella N, Rousseau T, Douet JY, de Geyer G, Regnier A. Histopathologic features of canine distichiasis. *Vet Ophthalmol*. 2012;**15**(2):92–7. doi: 10.1111/j.1463-5224.2011.00946.x. Epub 2011 Sep 29.

Wheeler CA, Severin GA. Cryosurgical epilation for the treatment of distichiasis in the dog and cat. *J Am Anim Hosp Assoc* 1984;**20**:877–884.

Clinical Atlas of Canine and Feline Ophthalmic Disease, First Edition. Douglas Esson.

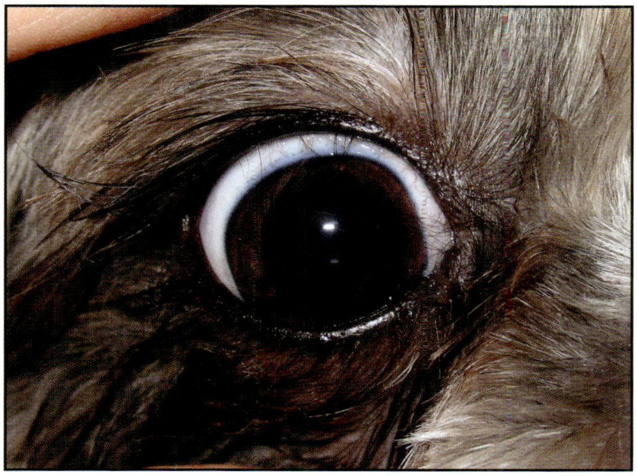

Figure 10.1 Canine distichiasis. Aberrant eyelid hairs are most readily identified against the pale conjunctival and episcleral tissues.

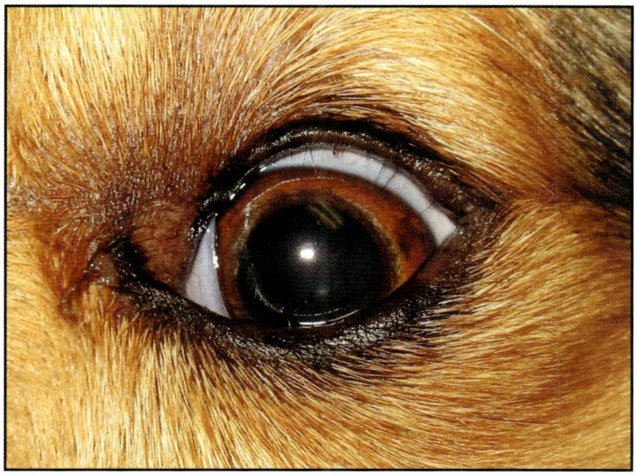

Figure 10.2 Canine distichiasis. Aberrant eyelid hairs are most readily identified against the pale conjunctival and episcleral tissues.

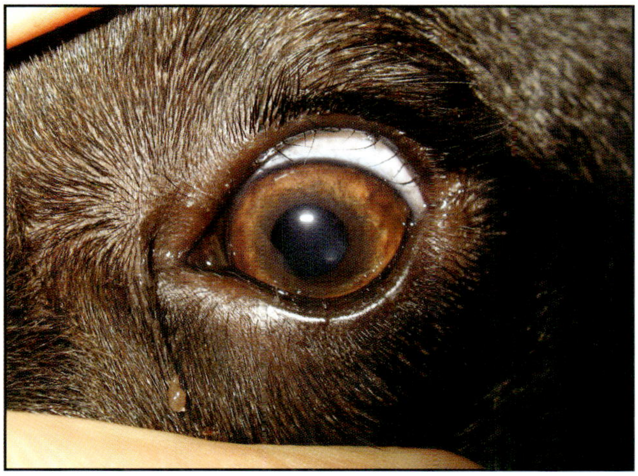

Figure 10.3 Canine distichiasis. Aberrant eyelid hairs are most readily identified against the pale conjunctival and episcleral tissues.

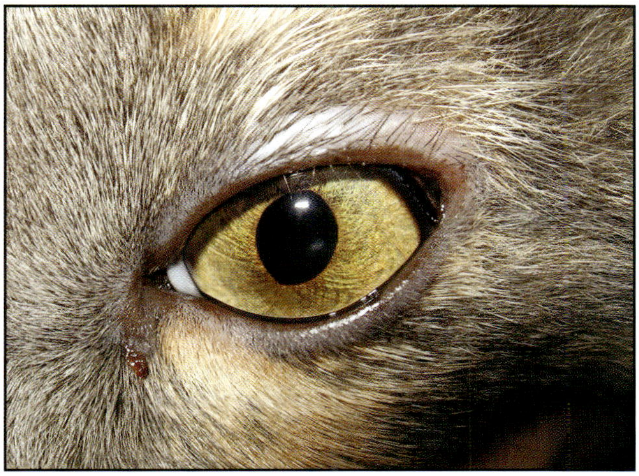

Figure 10.4 Feline distichiasis.

CHAPTER 11
ECTOPIC CILIA

PRESENTATION

Ectopic cilia are abnormal hairs arising from the inner aspect of the eyelid margin and are most commonly encountered within the upper eyelids of young dogs. Presentation is frequently unilateral. Either a single or group of ectopic hairs may be present. In most cases, ectopic cilia result in keratitis and/or corneal ulceration, with discomfort marked by blepharospasm and epiphora. Ectopic cilia may be challenging to identify, particularly in painful or uncooperative patients, those with significant conjunctival swelling, and/or light-colored hair coats. Where ectopic cilia are suspected, sedation, and/or magnification may be required in order to confirm their presence. Commonly affected breeds include the English Bulldog, French Bulldog, and Golden Retriever.

DIAGNOSIS AND TREATMENT

The appropriate treatment of ectopic cilia represents en bloc removal of both the hair(s) and associated follicle, with or without adjunctive cryotherapy in a double freeze–thaw cycle. Manual epilation alone will provide temporary relief only. Cryotherapy should only be undertaken using an appropriate nitrous-oxide cooled cryo unit. Focal swelling and eyelid depigmentation are common following cryoepilation; however, affected tissues typically repigment with time. Extreme care should be taken to preserve the eyelid margins and to avoid excessive eyelid tissue damage or necrosis and the generation of excessive fibrosis, which may lead to cicatricial entropion. Postoperative care comprises routine systemic antimicrobial (if indicated), anti-inflammatory, and analgesic care. An Elizabethan collar should be placed in order to prevent self-trauma and corneal health should be frequently monitored until eyelid healing is complete.

Keratitis and/or corneal ulceration should be managed using routine topical antimicrobial therapy as well as the judicious use of a lubricating and protective agent.

SELECTED REFERENCES

D'Anna N, Sapienza JS, Guandalini A, Guerriero A. Use of a dermal biopsy punch for removal of ectopic cilia in dogs: 19 cases. *Vet Ophthalmol.* 2007;**10**(1):65–67.

Hase K, Kase S, Noda M, Ohashi T, Shinkuma S, Ishida S. Ectopic cilia: a histopathological study. *Case Rep Dermatol.* 2012;**4**(1):37–40. doi: 10.1159/000336887. Epub 2012 Feb 10.

Lackner PA. Techniques for surgical correction of adnexal disease. *Clin Tech Small Anim Pract.* 2001;**16**(1):40–50.

Clinical Atlas of Canine and Feline Ophthalmic Disease, First Edition. Douglas Esson.

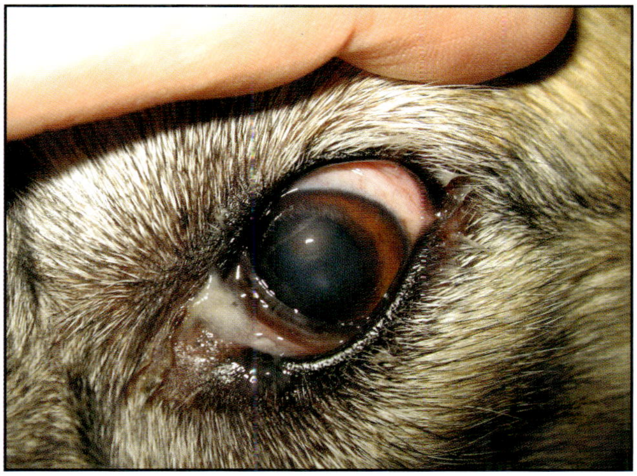

Figure 11.1 Typical, solitary, ectopic cilium, within the upper fornix at the 2 o'clock position. Keratitis as a result of chronic irritation is present.

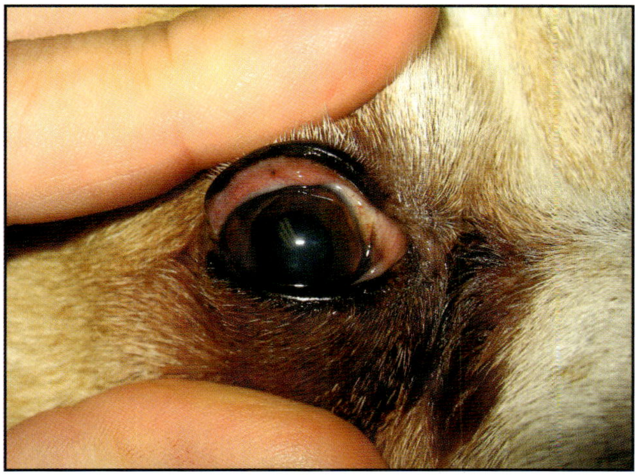

Figure 11.2 Solitary, thick, ectopic cilium within the upper fornix at the 12 o'clock position.

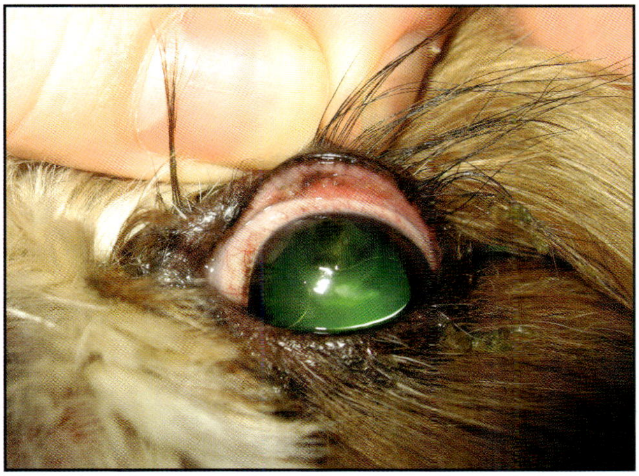

Figure 11.3 Multiple ectopic cilia within the upper fornix at the 12 o'clock position. Keratitis as a result of chronic irritation is present.

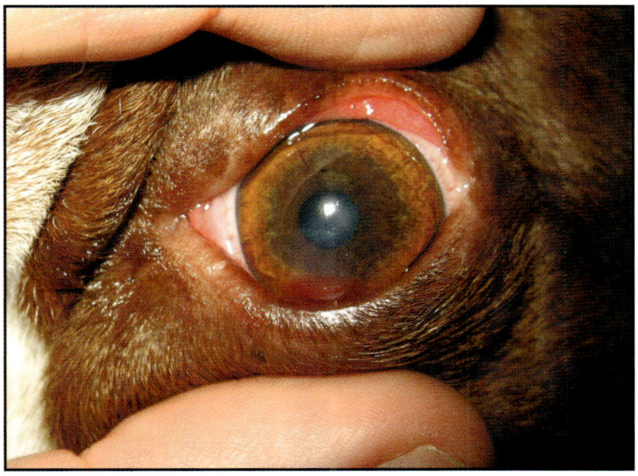

Figure 11.4 An ectopic cilium within the ventral fornix at the 6 o'clock position. Secondary ulcerative keratitis is present.

CHAPTER 12
TRICHIASIS

PRESENTATION

Trichiasis describes contact between hairs from normal hair-bearing periocular skin and the corneal surface. This may involve hairs from the upper lid, medial canthus, or nasal fold region. Corneal irritation may result in discomfort, keratitis, and/or corneal ulceration. Commonly affected breeds include the Cocker Spaniel, Shih Tzu, Pug, and Miniature Poodle.

DIAGNOSIS AND TREATMENT

Selected patients may be successfully managed by careful and regular grooming of periocular hair. More definitive treatment involves judicious cryoepilation of offending hairs and/or surgical resection of hair-bearing skin, where appropriate. Several surgical techniques have been described including that for partial upper eyelid resection by Stades and that for nasal fold resection by Severin. Cryoepilation should only be undertaken using an appropriate nitrous-oxide cryo unit. Focal depigmentation and swelling is common following cryoepilation; however, affected tissues typically repigment with time. Extreme care should be taken to preserve the eyelid margins and to avoid excessive eyelid tissue damage or necrosis and the generation of excessive fibrosis, which may lead to cicatricial entropion. Postoperative care comprises routine systemic antimicrobial (if indicated), anti-inflammatory, and analgesic care. An Elizabethan collar should be placed in order to prevent self-trauma and corneal health should be frequently monitored until eyelid healing is complete. Keratitis and/or corneal ulceration should be managed using routine topical antimicrobial therapy as well as the judicious use of a lubricating and protective agent.

SELECTED REFERENCES

Gelatt KN *et al.* 2013. *Veterinary Ophthalmology*, Vol **2**, pp. 867–871, Wiley-Blackwell, Oxford.

Severin GA. 2000. *Severin's Veterinary Ophthalmology Notes*, 3rd ed., Fort Collins, Co.

Stades FC, van de Sandt RR, Boevé MH. Clinical aspects and surgical procedures in trichiasis. *Tijdschr Diergeneeskd.* 1993;**118** Suppl 1:38S-39S.

Clinical Atlas of Canine and Feline Ophthalmic Disease, First Edition. Douglas Esson.

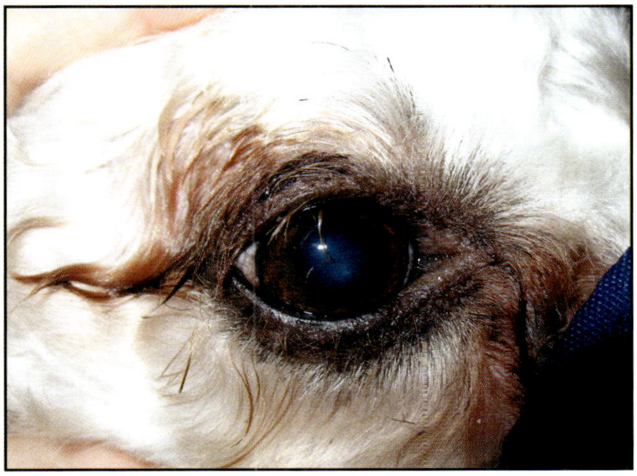

Figure 12.1 Conformational trichiasis associated with the upper eyelid.

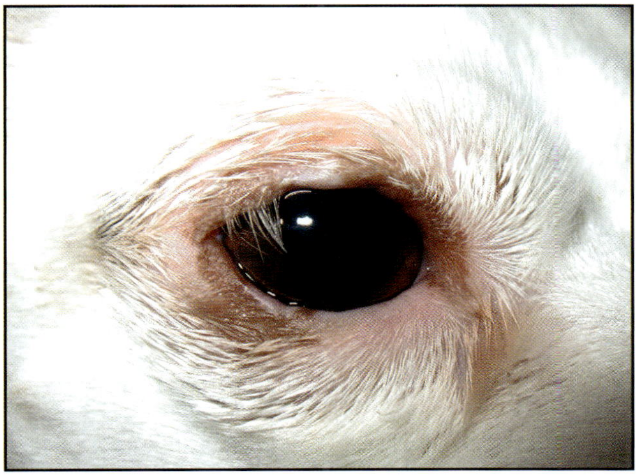

Figure 12.2 Trichiasis associated with the upper eyelid following inappropriate removal of distichia and cicatricial upper eyelid entropion.

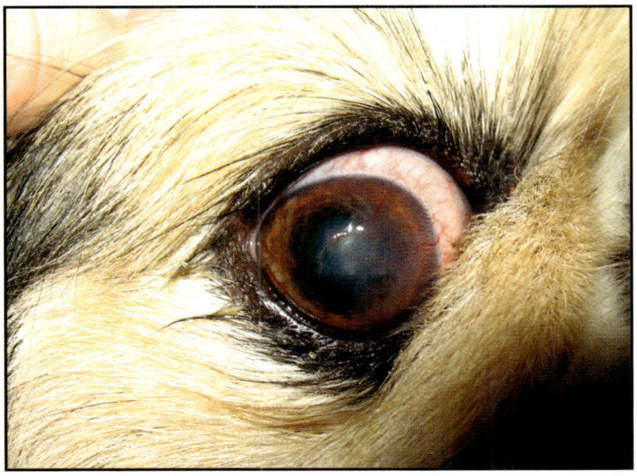

Figure 12.3 Trichiasis in association with prominent nasal folds. Significant secondary keratitis is present.

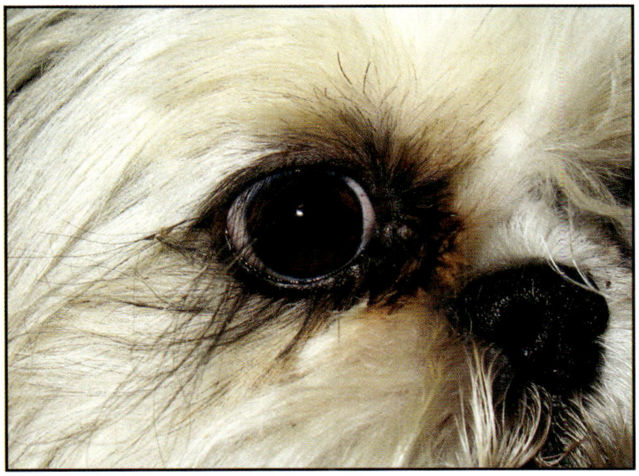

Figure 12.4 Chronic keratitis secondary to conformational hypertrichiasis.

CHAPTER 13
TEAR FILM WICKING SYNDROME

PRESENTATION

The medial canthal caruncle describes the region of haired tissue at the base of the third eyelid. In many canine breeds, particularly small breeds, this region contains an excessive amount of hair which may contact the corneal surface, acting as a "wick" and drawing the pre-corneal tear film out onto the haired skin surrounding the medial canthus. This may lead to secondary tear staining and in severe cases, recurrent moist dermatitis. Clinical signs may be exacerbated by stenotic or imperforate nasolacrimal puncta and/or ducts. The patency of the nasolacrimal drainage system may be evaluated via the "Jones test" during which a small amount of fluorescein dye is instilled into the ventral fornix. In animals with adequate nasolacrimal drainage, the dye will be noted to exit the ipsilateral nostril within 5–10 min. In patients affected by wicking syndrome, fluorescein dye will be noted to stream out onto the haired eyelid skin around the medial canthal region. Commonly affected breeds include the Shih Tzu, Lhasa Apso, Miniature Poodle, and Bichon Frise.

DIAGNOSIS AND TREATMENT

Tear film wicking may be significantly reduced by the permanent removal of hairs in the medial caruncular region. This is most effectively achieved using judicious cryoepilation in a double freeze–thaw cycle. Manual epilation alone may provide temporary relief but will result in regrowth of hairs. Cryotherapy should only be undertaken using an appropriate nitrous-oxide cooled unit. Significant swelling and eyelid depigmentation are common following cryoepilation; however, affected tissues typically repigment with time. Postoperative care comprises routine systemic antimicrobial (if indicated), anti-inflammatory, and analgesic care. An Elizabethan collar should be placed in order to prevent self-trauma and corneal health should be frequently monitored until eyelid healing is complete. Stenotic nasolacrimal systems may be cannulated and flushing attempted. In rare cases of punctual aplasia, nasolacrimal openings may be surgically reestablished. Postoperative indwelling stents using nylon or silicone may help reduce the propensity for recurrent stenosis, which nevertheless remains high. Several techniques have also been described for the creation of alternative nasolacrimal drainage into the oral and sinus spaces; however, these procedures are rarely justified.

SELECTED REFERENCES

Gelatt KN, Gelatt JP. 1995. *Handbook of Small Animal Ophthalmic Surgery: Extraocular Procedures*, Vol **1**, Pergamon Press, Gainesville, FL.

Gelatt KN *et al.* 2013. *Veterinary Ophthalmology*, Vol **2**, pp. 871–873, Wiley-Blackwell, Oxford.

Ny Y *et al.* Medial canthoplasty for epiphora in dogs: a retrospective study of 23 cases. *J Am Anim Hosp Assoc*, 2006;**42**, 435–439.

Seo KM, Nam TC. Tear formation, the patency and angle of bend of nasolacrimal duct in poodle dogs with tear staining syndrome. *Korean J Vet Res*, 1995;**35**, 383–390.

Clinical Atlas of Canine and Feline Ophthalmic Disease, First Edition. Douglas Esson.

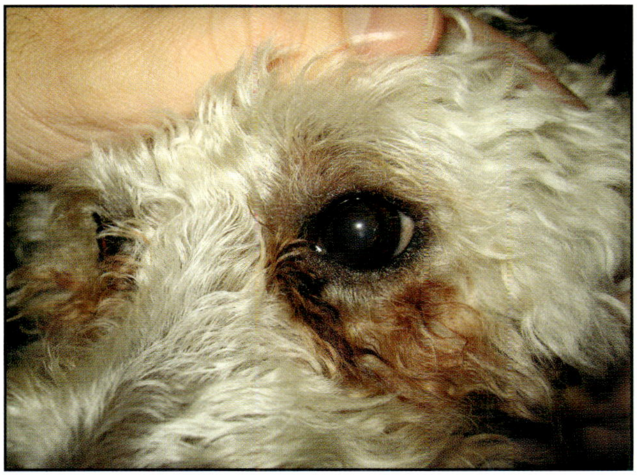

Figure 13.1 Significant tear film wicking syndrome & facial staining. Changes are most notable in animals with white hair coats.

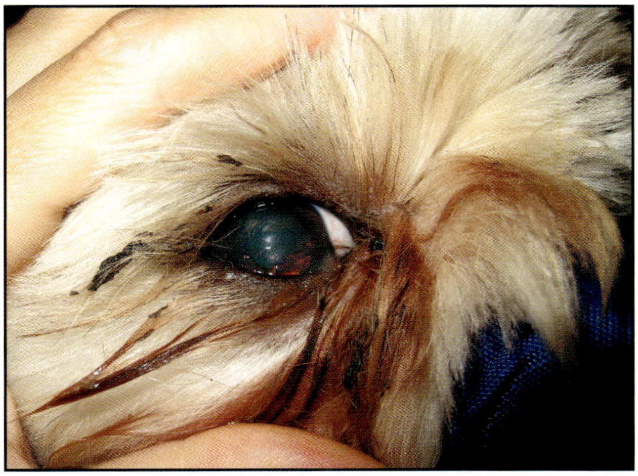

Figure 13.2 Significant tear film wicking syndrome in association with trichiasis.

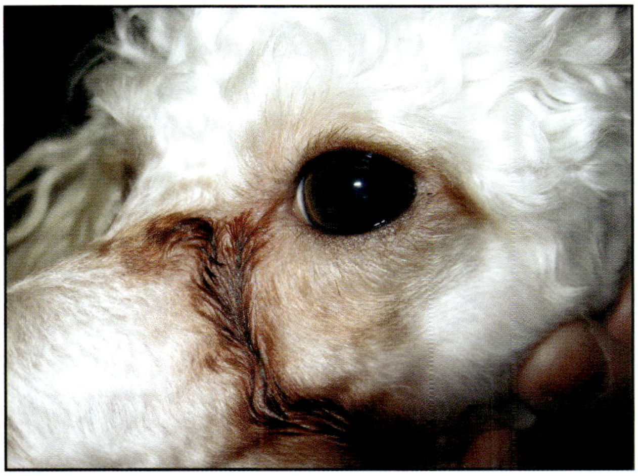

Figure 13.3 Significant tear film wicking syndrome & facial staining.

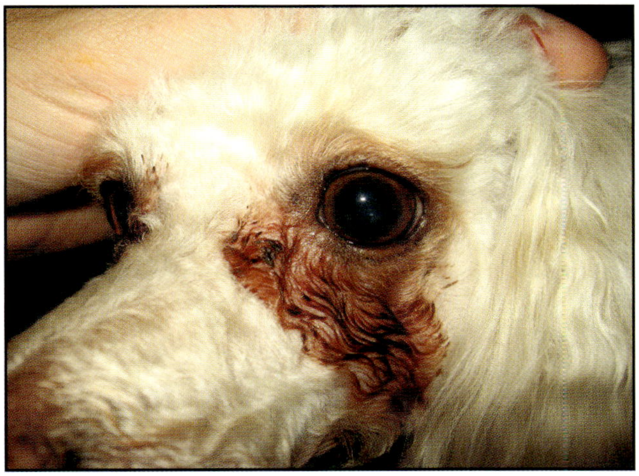

Figure 13.4 Significant tear film wicking syndrome & secondary moist dermatitis.

CHAPTER 14
ENTROPION

PRESENTATION

Entropion describes eyelid pathology such that the eyelid margin(s) are inverted toward the globe. Most typically, the lower eyelids are involved; however, upper or combined eyelid entropion may also occur. Similarly, the condition is most commonly bilateral; however, unilateral entropion may occur. Primary entropion arises because of a conformational eyelid abnormality and may additionally involve excessive eyelid length and laxity and/or brow-fold redundancy. Primary entropion is common in multiple breeds and may affect juvenile animals (particularly the English Bulldog, Chow Chow, and Shar Pei) as well as older animals (particularly the Labrador Retriever and Rottweiler). Spastic entropion arises as a result of ocular discomfort and subsequent chronic blepharospasm. Spastic entropion may be differentiated from primary entropion by the application of a topical anesthetic agent, which results in resolution of spastic symptoms. Secondary entropion may also result from abnormalities of globe positioning (most commonly enophthalmos due to orbital fat and/or muscle atrophy) or globe size (most commonly due to phthisis bulbus). Cicatricial entropion may arise secondary to postinflammatory contracture. Regardless of the etiology of entropion, corneal pathology generally arises as a result of trichiasis.

DIAGNOSIS AND TREATMENT

Pending definitive intervention, corneal tissues affected by entropion may be temporarily protected by the liberal application of petroleum-based ocular lubricants. Both juvenile primary entropion and spastic entropion may be initially treated by temporarily everting the eyelids using either nonabsorbable mattress sutures or surgical staples. Sutures or staples may be left in place (and/or replaced) for weeks to months as appropriate. Entropion in juvenile animals may resolve with increasing age and musculoskeletal conformational maturity. Multiple surgical techniques have been described for the permanent correction of primary conformational entropion, including the basic "Hotz-Celsus" procedure and its variations. These techniques are also appropriate for the management of entropion arising secondary to abnormalities of globe position or size. Postoperative care comprises routine systemic antimicrobial (if indicated), anti-inflammatory, and analgesic care. An Elizabethan collar should be placed in order to prevent self-trauma and corneal health should be frequently monitored until eyelid healing is complete. Extreme caution is advised when considering the permanent correction of entropion using techniques such as electrocautery, laser energy, and/or the injection of subcutaneous materials because the potential for surgical complication associated with these procedures is high.

SELECTED REFERENCES

Read RA, Broun HC. Entropion correction in dogs & cats using a combination Hotz-Celsus and lateral eyelid wedge resection: results in 311 eyes. *Vet Ophthalmol.* 2007;**10**(1):6–11.

Williams DL, Kim JY. Feline **entropion**: a case series of 50 affected animals (2003–2008). *Vet Ophthalmol.* 2009;**12**(4):221–226.

van der Woerdt A. Adnexal surgery in dogs and cats. *Vet Ophthalmol.* 2004;**7**(5):284–290.

Clinical Atlas of Canine and Feline Ophthalmic Disease, First Edition. Douglas Esson.

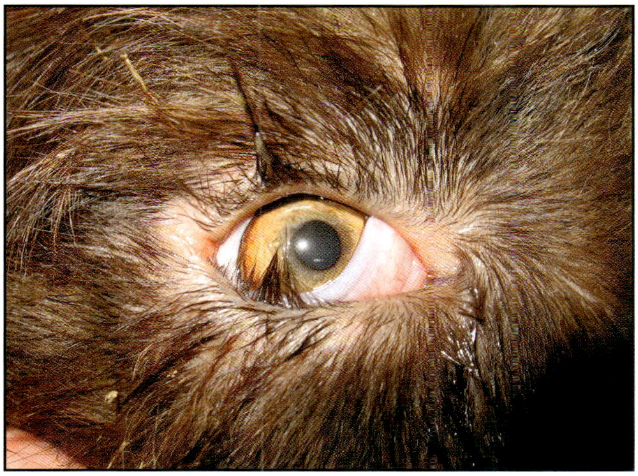

Figure 14.1 Conformational entropion, resulting in secondary trichiasis.

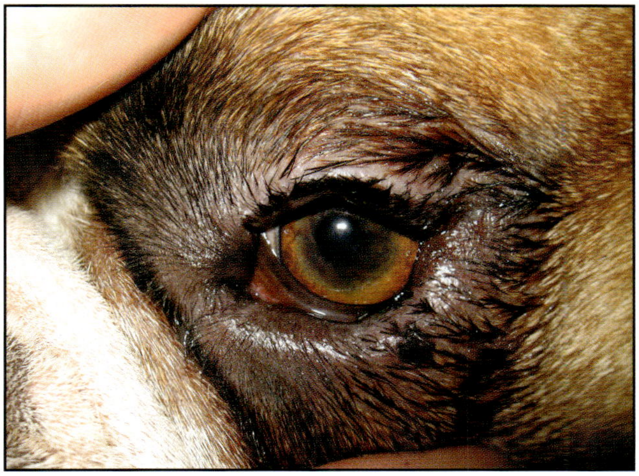

Figure 14.2 Conformational entropion, resulting from excessive lower eyelid laxity.

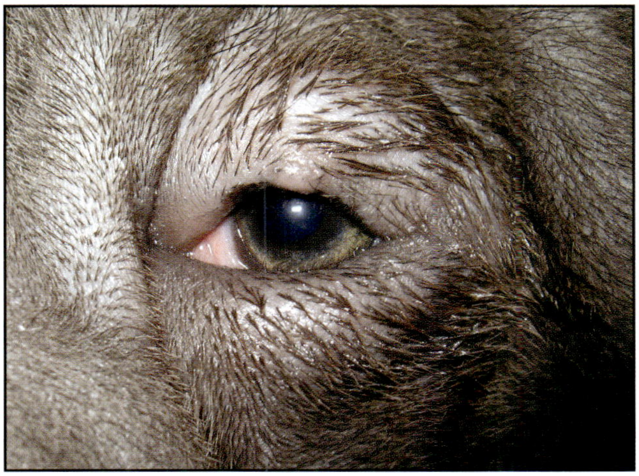

Figure 14.3 Juvenile, conformational entropion.

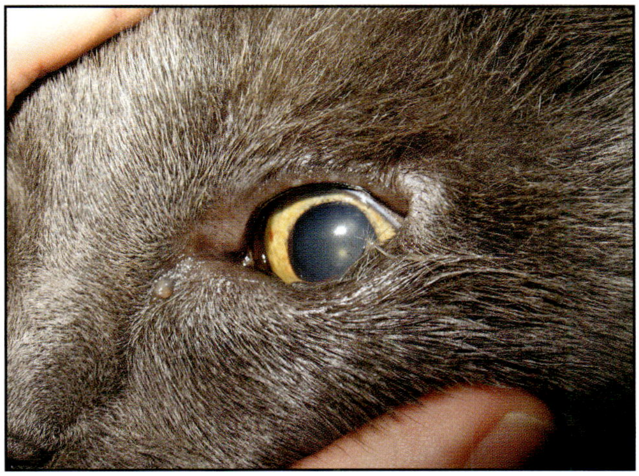

Figure 14.4 Entropion in a feline patient, resulting from enophthalmos.

CHAPTER 15
ECTROPION

PRESENTATION

Ectropion describes eversion of the eyelid(s) away from the ocular surface such that increased exposure and resultant keratoconjunctivitis may result. Ectropion is less common and less likely to result in significant corneal pathology than entropion. Ectropion may be the result of conformational abnormalities (particularly in the Bloodhound, St Bernard, Newfoundland, and Cocker Spaniel) or may occur secondary to trauma and subsequent cicatricial scarring or the inadvertent surgical overcorrection of entropion. Conformational ectropion most commonly affected the lower eyelids.

DIAGNOSIS AND TREATMENT

Ectropion may be medically managed in selected cases using a combination of anti-inflammatory as well as lubricating and protective therapy. Surgical correction of ectropion is only indicated if the condition results in significant secondary pathology. Typically, a wedge resection and/or "V to Y" procedure are employed. Surgical correction should ideally not be undertaken until patients have reached conformational maturity. Postoperative care comprises routine systemic antimicrobial (if indicated), anti-inflammatory, and analgesic care. An Elizabethan collar should be placed in order to prevent self-trauma and corneal health should be frequently monitored until eyelid healing is complete. Keratitis and/or corneal ulceration should be managed using routine topical antimicrobial therapy as well as the judicious use of a lubricating and protective agent.

SELECTED REFERENCES

Donaldson D, Smith KM, Shaw SC, Sansom J, Hartley C. Surgical management of cicatricial **ectropion** following scarring dermatopathies in two **dogs**. *Vet Ophthalmol*. 2005;**8**(5):361–366. Erratum in: Vet Ophthalmol. 2005;8(6):451.

Gelatt KN, Gelatt JN. 2001. Small animal ophthalmic surgery, pp. 101–102 Elsevier, Edinburgh.

Lackner PA. Techniques for surgical correction of adnexal disease. *Clin Tech Small Anim Pract*. 2001;**16**(1):40–50. Review

van der Woerdt A. Adnexal surgery in **dogs** and cats. *Vet Ophthalmol*. 2004;**7**(5):284–290. Review.

Clinical Atlas of Canine and Feline Ophthalmic Disease, First Edition. Douglas Esson.

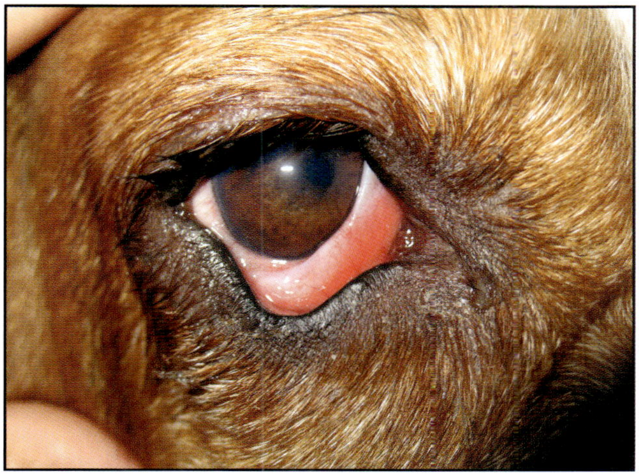

Figure 15.1 Conformational lower eyelid ectropion. Mild conjunctivitis is present.

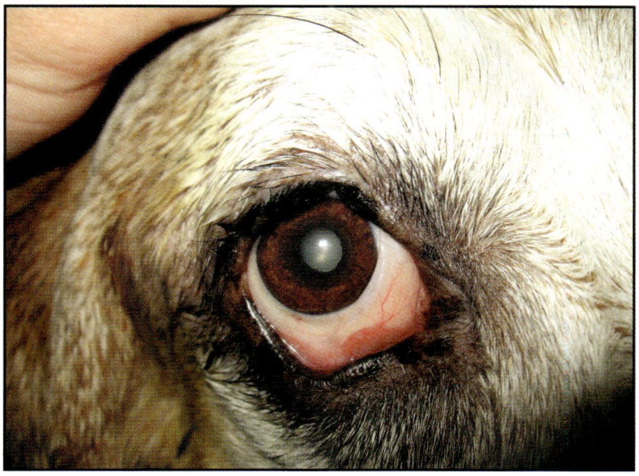

Figure 15.2 Conformational lower eyelid ectropion. Mild conjunctivitis is present.

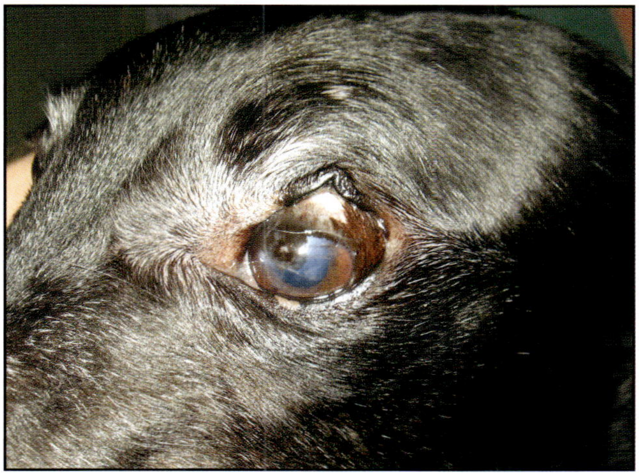

Figure 15.3 Secondary (cicatricial) ectropion affecting the upper eyelid. Moderate keratitis is present.

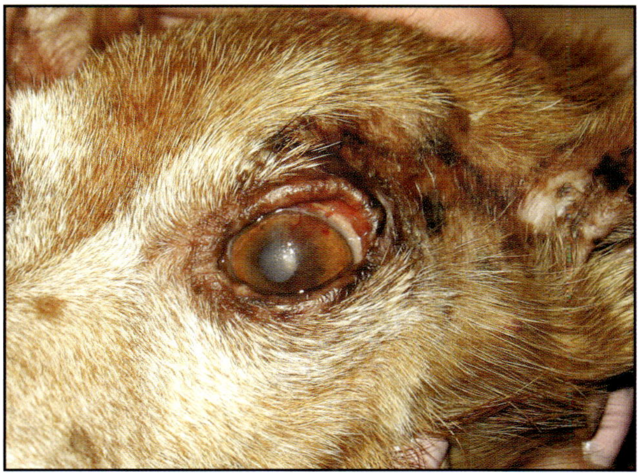

Figure 15.4 Secondary (cicatricial) ectropion affecting the upper eyelid. Moderate keratitis is present.

CHAPTER 16
COMBINED ENTROPION-ECTROPION

PRESENTATION

Combined entropion-ectropion is commonly referred to as "diamond eye." This conformation comprises lateral and/or medial entropion in combination with central ectropion of the upper and/or lower eyelids. This presentation is common in large breed dogs, particularly those with redundant facial skin (including the St Bernard, Clumber Spaniel, and English Mastiff). Secondary pathology associated with both entropic and ectropic components may result, including keratoconjunctivitis, trichiasis, and/or corneal ulceration.

DIAGNOSIS AND TREATMENT

Combined entropion-ectropion may be medically managed in selected cases using a combination of anti-inflammatory as well as lubricating and protective therapy. Surgical correction is indicated if the condition results in significant secondary pathology. A number of complex, combined blepharoplastic procedures have been described for the permanent correction of diamond eye, including the generally applicable modified Kuhnt–Szymanowski technique. Surgical correction should ideally not be undertaken until patients have reached conformational maturity. Pending this, temporary eyelid eversion, using nonabsorbable sutures or surgical staples, may be employed in young or skeletally immature animals.

SELECTED REFERENCES

Bedford PG. Technique of lateral canthoplasty for the correction of macropalpebral fissure in the dog. *J Small Anim Pract.* 1998;**39**(3):117–120.

Gelatt KN, Gelatt JN. 2001. *Small Animal Ophthalmic Surgery*, pp. 102–103, Elsevier, Edinburgh.

van der Woerdt A. Adnexal surgery in **dogs** and cats. *Vet Ophthalmol.* 2004;**7**(5):284–290. Review.

Clinical Atlas of Canine and Feline Ophthalmic Disease, First Edition. Douglas Esson.

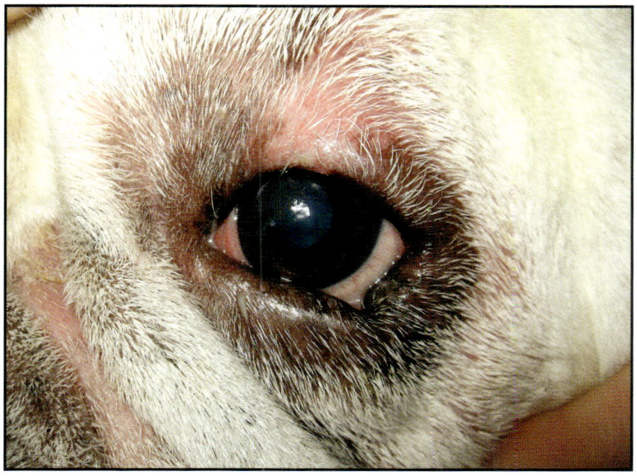

Figure 16.1 Combined entropion-ectropion (diamond eye). Moderate keratitis is present.

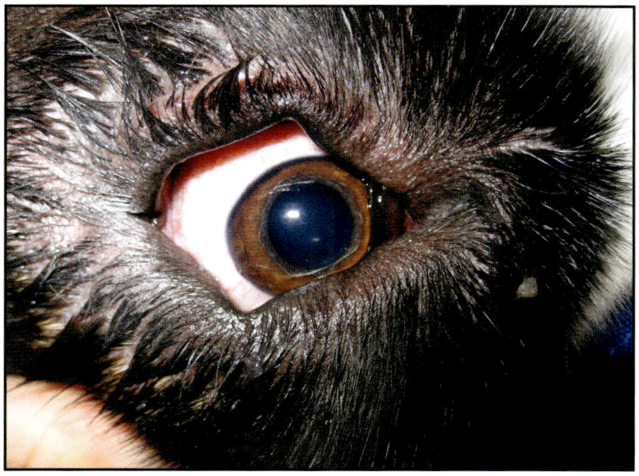

Figure 16.2 Combined entropion-ectropion (diamond eye). Moderate keratitis is present.

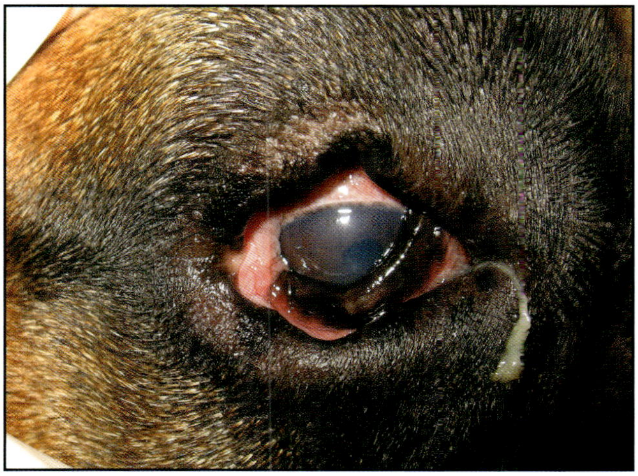

Figure 16.3 Combined entropion-ectropion (diamond eye). Moderate keratoconjunctivitis is present.

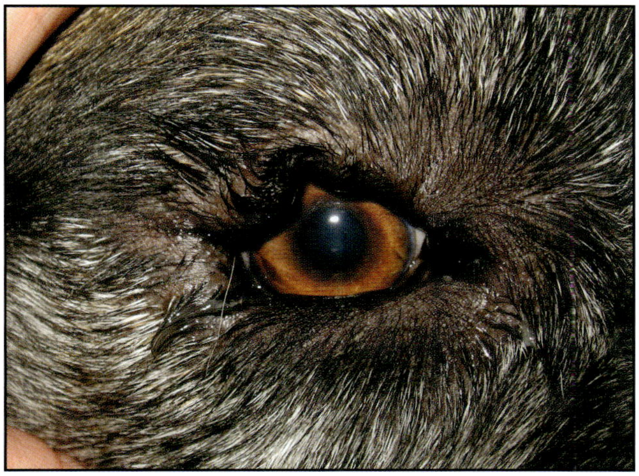

Figure 16.4 Combined entropion-ectropion (diamond eye). Mild conjunctivitis is present.

CHAPTER 17
MACROPALPEBRAL FISSURE

PRESENTATION

The term macropalpebral fissure describes a conformation comprising excessively large eyelid fissures and eyelid length. Lagophthalmos or a decreased ability to effectively close the eyelids as well as a tendency to sleep with the eyelids partially open may additionally be present. Keratoconjunctivitis, tear film abnormalities, ulcerative keratitis, and an increased risk of proptosis, result from increased exposure of the globe. Commonly affected breeds including the Pekingese, Japanese Chin, Shih Tzu, Lhasa Apso, and Pug.

DIAGNOSIS AND TREATMENT

Selected patients may be medically managed using lubricating and protective therapy (in combination with anti-inflammatory therapy if indicated). Medications to increase tear production and/or stabilize the pre-corneal tear film may also be of benefit. These include topical cyclosporine (available in various concentrations). Surgical correction is indicated if the condition results in significant pathology such as exposure keratopathy and/or ulcerative keratitis. Multiple techniques to decrease the size of the palpebral fissure have been described, including the generally appropriate Roberts/Jensen medial pocket canthoplasty.

Potential Drug-Side-Effects

Potential side effects associated with the use of cyclosporine include hypersensitivity.

SELECTED REFERENCES

Bedford PG. Technique of lateral canthoplasty for the correction of macropalpebral fissure in the dog. *J Small Anim Pract*. 1998;**39**(3):117–120.

Gelatt KN, Gelatt JN. 2001. *Small Animal Ophthalmic Surgery*, p. 109, Elsevier, Edinburgh.

van der Woerdt A. Adnexal surgery in dogs and cats. *Vet Ophthalmol*. 2004;**7**(5):284–290. Review.

Clinical Atlas of Canine and Feline Ophthalmic Disease, First Edition. Douglas Esson.

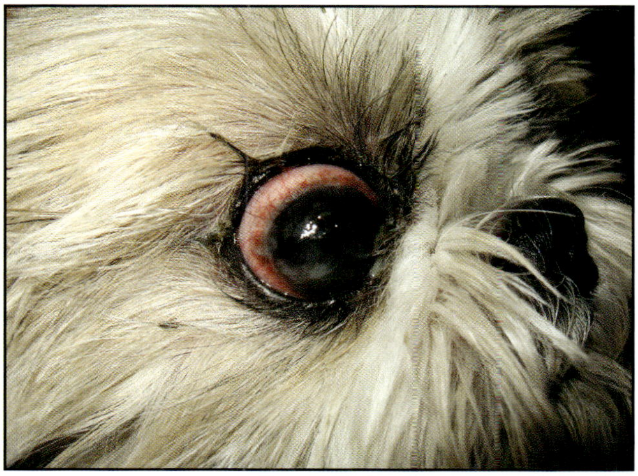

Figure 17.1 Conformational macropalpebral fissure. Severe, chronic, corneal pathology including vascular, fibrosing and pigmentary keratitis is present.

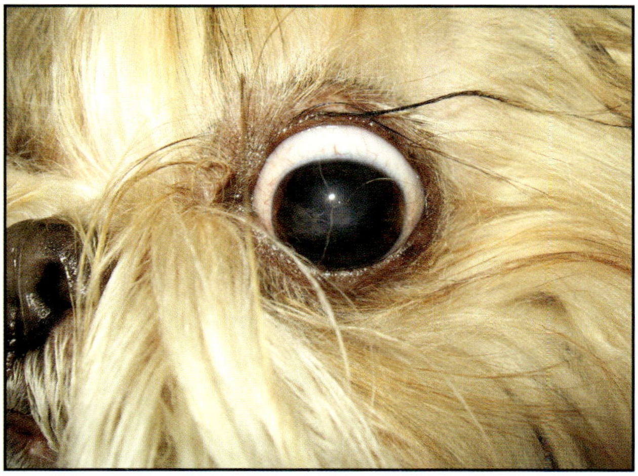

Figure 17.2 Conformational macropalpebral fissure. Mild keratitis is present.

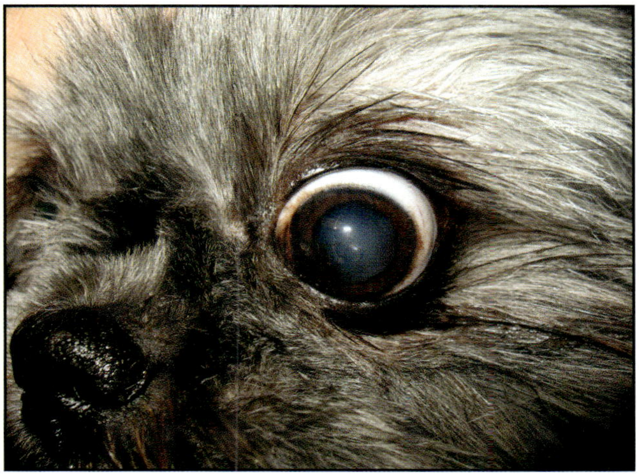

Figure 17.3 Conformational macropalpebral fissure. Mild keratitis is present.

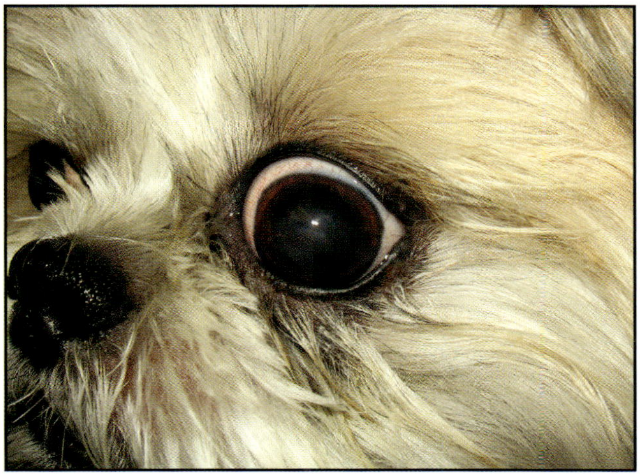

Figure 17.4 Conformational macropalpebral fissure. Mild keratitis is present.

CHAPTER 18
CHALAZION

PRESENTATION

The term chalazion describes a granulomatous reaction within the (upper or lower) eyelid, specifically affecting the meibomian gland and resulting from glandular inflammation, infection, and/or obstruction. Glandular inflammation and/or infection may be associated with more widespread blepharoconjunctivitis and/or meibomitis. Glandular obstruction is commonly the result of eyelid margin neoplasia. Clinically, these lesions comprise one or more nonpainful, firm, pale yellow swellings at or inside one or both eyelid margins. This finding is common in older dogs.

DIAGNOSIS AND TREATMENT

Topical anti-inflammatory and/or antimicrobial treatment alone is unlikely to be effective. Systemic antimicrobial therapy will address bacterial blepharitis if present; however, the granulomatous reaction which comprises a chalazion requires physical incision, drainage, and curettage in order to be effectively reduced. Any eyelid-associated neoplasia should be concurrently addressed. Appropriate antimicrobial selections include cephalosporins and tetracyclines.

Potential Drug-Side-Effects

Potential adverse effects associated with cephalosporins include hypersensitivity reactions, gastrointestinal (GI) distress and renal disease. Potential adverse effects associated with tetracyclines include GI distress, photosensitivity, and hepatic damage. Potential adverse effects associated with the use of systemic prednisone include polyphagia, polydipsia, polyuria, hair coat changes, weight gain, pancreatitis, enteritis, muscular damage, hepatic impairment, and diabetes.

Postoperatively, warm-compressing and/or systemic anti-inflammatory therapy (typically steroidal) will speed the resolution of clinical signs; however, new or recurrent lesions may occur.

SELECTED REFERENCES

Acharya N, Pineda R. 2nd, Uy HS, Foster CS. Discoid lupus erythematosus masquerading as chronic blepharoconjunctivitis. *Ophthalmology*. 2005;**112**(5):e19–e23.

Dubielzig R. *et al*. 2010. *Veterinary Ocular Pathology*, 162, Elsevier, Edinburgh.

Grahn BH, Sandmeyer LS. Diagnostic ophthalmology. *Can Vet J*. 2010;**51**(3):327.

Peiffer RL Jr. Ocular immunology and mechanisms of ocular inflammation. *Vet Clin North Am Small Anim Pract*. 1980;**10**(2):281–302.

Clinical Atlas of Canine and Feline Ophthalmic Disease, First Edition. Douglas Esson.

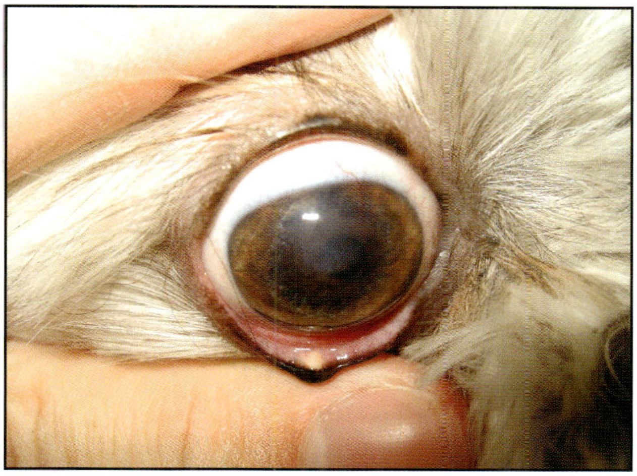

Figure 18.1 A chalazion affecting the lower eyelid.

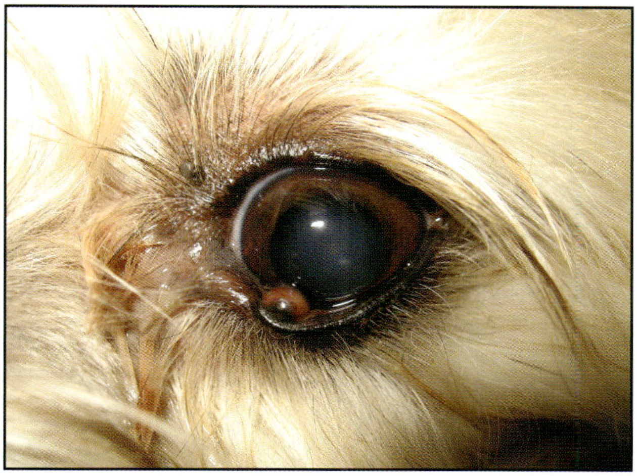

Figure 18.2 A chalazion affecting the lower eyelid.

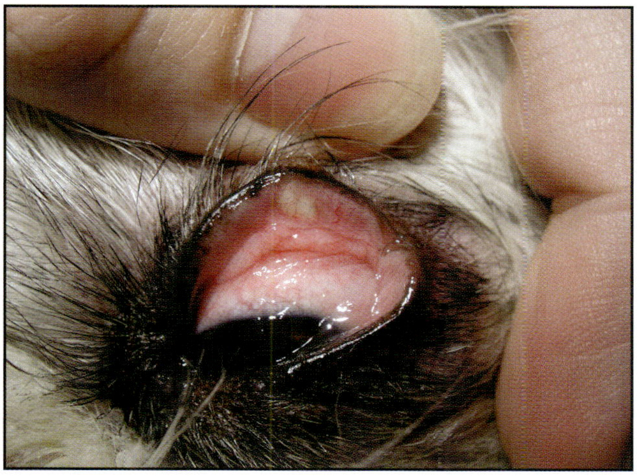

Figure 18.3 A chalazion affecting the upper eyelid.

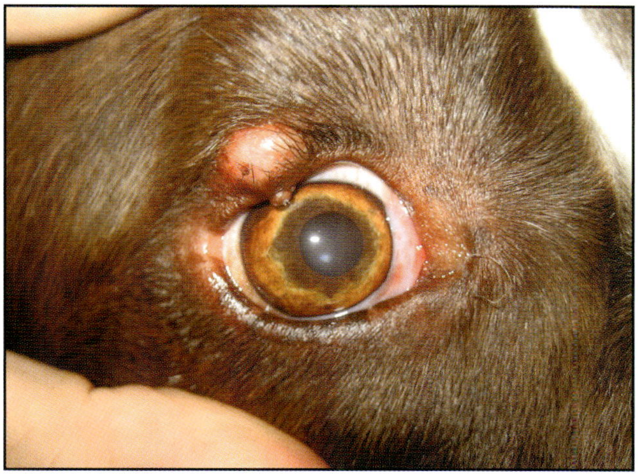

Figure 18.4 A chalazion secondary to the obstruction of a meibomian gland by a small, benign eyelid tumor.

CHAPTER 19
JUVENILE PYODERMA

PRESENTATION

Juvenile pyoderma (also referred to as "juvenile cellulitis," "juvenile dermatitis," or "puppy-strangles") describes a pyogranulomatous condition affecting young dogs, generally within the first 6 months of life. Clinical symptoms comprise variable combinations of symmetrical pustular dermatitis of the muzzle, face, periocular tissues, and/or ears as well as external ear canal inflammation and/or regional (submandibular) reactive lymphadenopathy. In some cases, more generalized dermatitis may also be present. The disease is postulated to be an immune-mediated reaction; however, secondary bacterial infection may be present. Commonly affected breeds include the Golden Retriever, Labrador Retriever, and the Dachshund.

DIAGNOSIS AND TREATMENT

The diagnosis of juvenile pyoderma is based on clinical findings, confirmed via histological assessment of skin biopsies if necessary. Bacterial culture and sensitivity testing is frequently unrewarding. Treatment comprises the administration of systemic corticosteroids, with or without adjunctive systemic antimicrobial therapy. Appropriate empirical antimicrobial selections include cephalosporins and tetracyclines (with or without adjunctive niacinamide).

Potential Drug-Side-Effects

Potential adverse effects associated with the use of systemic corticosteroids include polyphagia, polydipsia, polyuria, hair coat changes, weight gain, pancreatitis, enteritis, muscular damage, hepatic impairment, and diabetes. Potential adverse effects associated with cephalosporins include hypersensitivity reactions, gastrointestinal (GI) distress, and renal disease. Potential adverse effects associated with tetracyclines include GI distress, photosensitivity, and hepatic damage. Potential adverse effects associated with niacinamide include GI distress.

SELECTED REFERENCES

Gortel K. Recognizing pyoderma: more difficult than it may seem. *Vet Clin North Am Small Anim Pract*. 2013;**43**(1):1–18. doi: 10.1016/j.cvsm.2012.09.004.

Hutchings SM. Juvenile cellulitis in a puppy. *Can Vet J*. 2003;**44**(5):418–419.

White SD, Rosychuk RA, Stewart LJ, Cape L, Hughes BJ. Juvenile cellulitis in dogs: 15 cases (1979–1988). *J Am Vet Med Assoc*. 1989;**195**(11):1609–1611.

Clinical Atlas of Canine and Feline Ophthalmic Disease, First Edition. Douglas Esson.

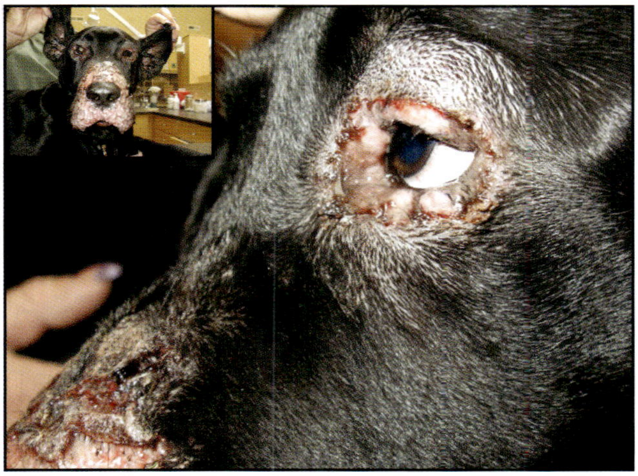

Figure 19.1 Findings associated with juvenile pyoderma, marked by symmetrical, facial, and periocular pustular dermatitis (the inset demonstrates typical bilateral presentation).

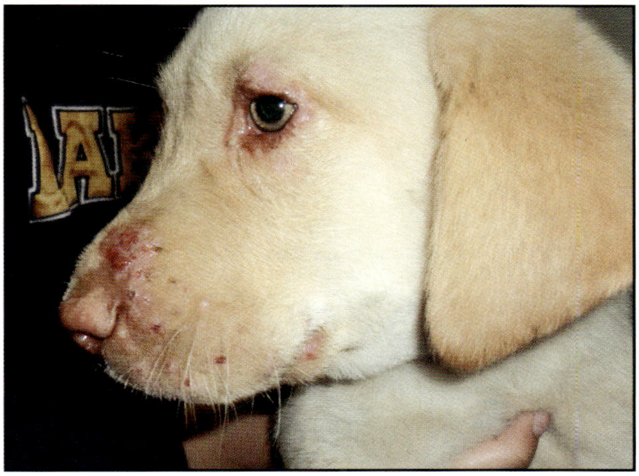

Figure 19.2 Juvenile pyoderma.

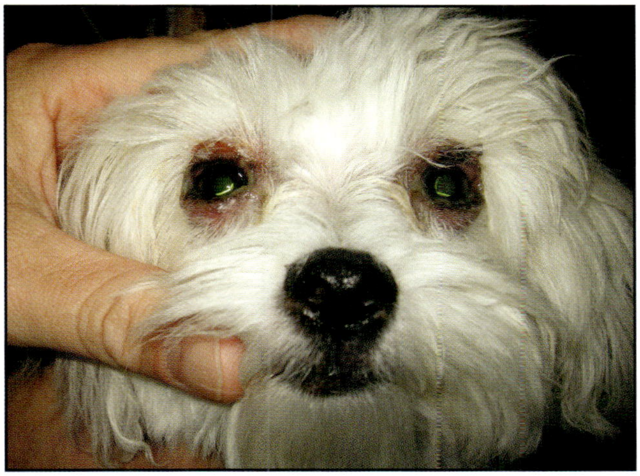

Figure 19.3 Juvenile pyoderma.

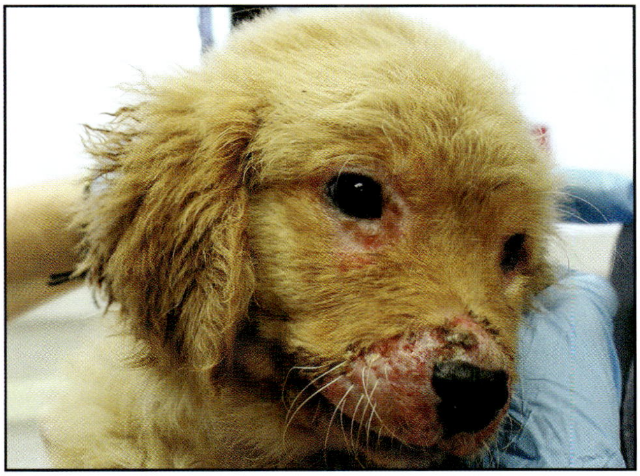

Figure 19.4 Juvenile pyoderma.

CHAPTER 20
IMMUNE-MEDIATED BLEPHAROCONJUNCTIVITIS

PRESENTATION

The term "blepharoconjunctivitis" defines a severe, acute, bilateral inflammation of the eyelid tissues that occurs relatively frequently, particularly in small breed dogs. Clinical symptoms may include irregular erythema and/or swelling of the eyelids and marked patient discomfort manifesting as blepharospasm and epiphora. An associated conjunctivitis is also typically present. This condition may or may not be associated with inflammation or infection of the meibomian glands or "meibomitis" and may additionally coincide with the incidence and severity of more generalized atopic dermatitis. Commonly affected breeds include the Chihuahua, Miniature Pinscher, Papillon, and Dachshund.

DIAGNOSIS AND TREATMENT

The diagnosis of immune-mediated blepharoconjunctivitis is made based on clinical findings. It is likely that a sterile hypersensitivity reaction to commensal bacterial eyelid flora plays a role in many cases and bacterial culture and sensitivity testing frequently fails to identify the presence of specific pathogens. The concurrent presence of parasitic mites may be ruled out by skin-scraping. Biopsy may be indicated in severe or poorly responsive cases in order to differentiate them from autoimmune and/or neoplastic processes (see also Autoimmune Blepharitis). Topical therapy alone is unlikely to result in clinical resolution and effective treatment usually comprises aggressive and lengthy systemic antimicrobial and anti-inflammatory and/or immune-modulating therapy (typically encompassing steroidal therapy). Appropriate empirical antimicrobial selections include cephalosporins and tetracyclines (with or without niacinamide).

Potential Drug-Side-Effects

Potential adverse effects associated with the use of systemic corticosteroids include polyphagia, polydipsia, polyuria, hair coat changes, weight gain, pancreatitis, enteritis, muscular damage, hepatic impairment, and diabetes. Potential adverse effects associated with cephalosporins include hypersensitivity reactions, GI distress, and renal disease. Potential adverse effects associated with tetracyclines include gastrointestinal (GI) distress, photosensitivity, and hepatic damage. Potential adverse effects associated with niacinamide include GI distress.

Warm compressing may help facilitate the opening of inflamed meibomian glands and focal lesions may also be curettaged if necessary. The use of an Elizabethan collar will prevent self-trauma until active inflammation is controlled. Blepharoconjunctivitis may be chronic, frustrating to treat, and/or recurrent.

SELECTED REFERENCES

Bistner S. Allergic- and immunologic-mediated diseases of the eye and adnexae. *Vet Clin North Am Small Anim Pract*. 1994;**24**(4):711–734. Review.

Chambers ED, Severin GA. Staphylococcal bacterin for treatment of chronic staphylococcal blepharitis in the dog. *J Am Vet Med Assoc*. 1984;**185**(4):422–425.

Furiani N, Scarampella F, Martino PA, Panzini I, Fabbri E, Ordeix L. Evaluation of the bacterial microflora of the conjunctival sac of healthy dogs and dogs with atopic dermatitis. *Vet Dermatol*. 2011;**22**(6):490–496. doi: 10.1111/j.1365-3164.2011.00979.x. Epub 2011 May 2.

Peña MA, Leiva M. Canine conjunctivitis and blepharitis. *Vet Clin North Am Small Anim Pract*. 2008;**38**(2):233–249, v. doi: 10.1016/j.cvsm.2007.12.001. Review.

Sansom J, Heinrich C, Featherstone H. Pyogranulomatous blepharitis in two dogs. *J Small Anim Pract*. 2000;**41**(2):80–83.

Clinical Atlas of Canine and Feline Ophthalmic Disease, First Edition. Douglas Esson.

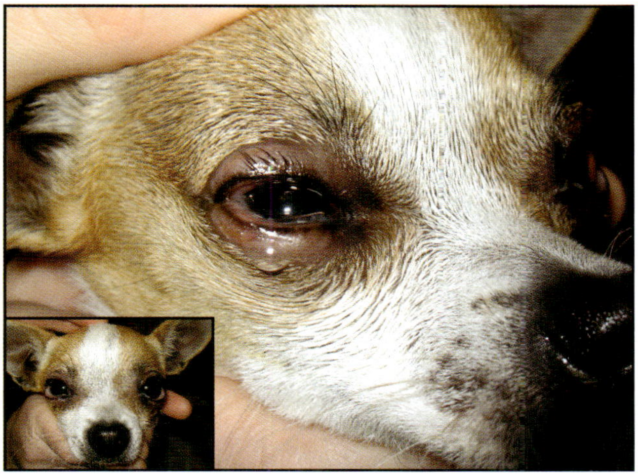

Figure 20.1 Immune-mediated blepharoconjunctivitis (the inset demonstrates typical bilateral presentation).

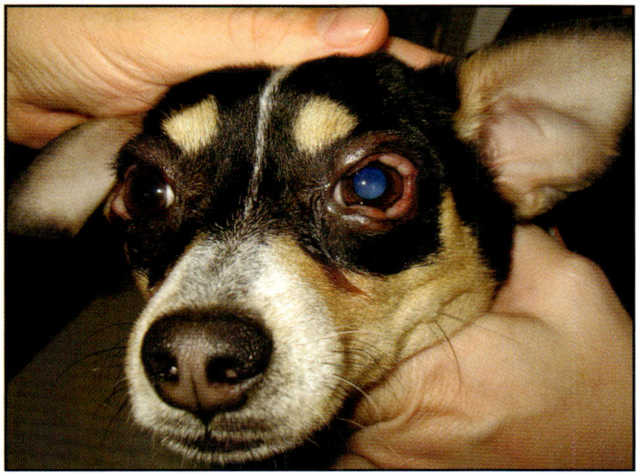

Figure 20.2 Immune-mediated blepharoconjunctivitis, demonstrating a significant conjunctival component.

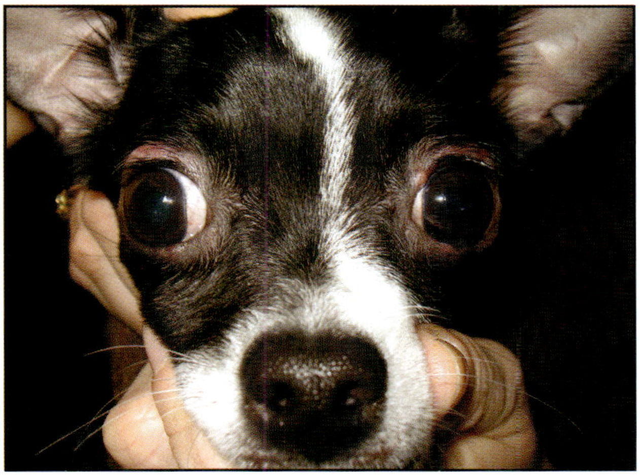

Figure 20.3 Typical clinical presentation associated with immune-mediated blepharoconjunctivitis.

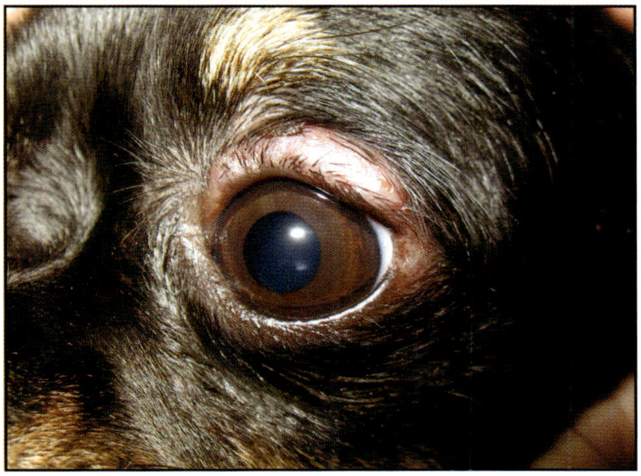

Figure 20.4 Immune-mediated blepharoconjunctivitis, broken hair-shafts are the result of self-trauma.

CHAPTER 21
AUTOIMMUNE BLEPHARITIS

PRESENTATION

Primary dermal autoimmune disease may affect multiple areas including the facial, nasal, and periocular regions, mucocutaneous junctions and/or external pinnae, manifesting as papular erosions, ulceration, dermatitis, and/or depigmentation. The classification of these diseases is complex, encompassing the pemphigus (auto-antibody-mediated acantholysis) diseases, lupus (immune-cellular dysfunction) diseases, vasculitis-related diseases, and uveodermatological syndrome (also described as "Vogt-Koyanagi-Harada-like" or "VKH-like" disease). Of the pemphigus diseases, pemphigus foliaceus (PF) is more commonly encountered, notably affecting the Akita, Chow Chow, and Labrador Retriever. Of the lupus diseases, discoid lupus erythematosus (DLE), also described as "cutaneous lupus erythematosus," is more commonly encountered, notably affecting the Akita, Chow Chow, Siberian Husky, German Shepherd, and Australian herding and Collie-breeds. Uveodermatological syndrome typically involves not only dermal tissues (manifesting as nasal, periocular, and mucocutaneous ulceration and/or depigmentation) but also the uveal tract where it may result in uveitis, retinal detachment, hyphema, and/or glaucoma. Breeds commonly affected by uveodermatological syndrome include the Akita, Chow Chow, and Siberian Husky (see also Uveodermatologic Syndrome (UDS) Associated Uveitis and Uveodermatologic Syndrome (UDS) Associated Chorioretinitis).

DIAGNOSIS AND TREATMENT

The diagnosis of autoimmune blepharitis is made on the basis of clinical findings in conjunction with the interpretation of representative dermal biopsies, ideally taken from the interface of affected/non-affected tissue. In all cases, treatment comprises long-term immune modulation, typically encompassing steroidal therapy with or without the adjunctive use of immunosuppressive agents including azathioprine, chlorambucil, mycophenolate, and/or cyclosporine.

Potential Drug-Side-Effects

Potential adverse effects associated with the use of systemic corticosteroids include polyphagia, polydipsia, polyuria, hair coat changes, weight gain, pancreatitis, gastrointestinal (GI) distress, muscle damage, hepatic impairment, and diabetes. Potential adverse effects associated with the use of systemic azathioprine, chlorambucil and mycophenolate include GI distress, pancreatitis, hepatotoxicity, and myelosuppression. Potential adverse affects associated with the use of cyclosporine include hypersensitivity and GI distress.

Secondary pyoderma, if present, is treated using appropriate systemic antimicrobials.

SELECTED REFERENCES

Griffin CE. Diagnosis and management of primary autoimmune skin diseases: a review. *Semin Vet Med Surg (Small Anim).* 1987;**2**(3):173–185. Review.

Ihrke PJ, Stannard AA, Ardans AA, Griffin CE. Pemphigus foliaceus in dogs: a review of 37 cases. *J Am Vet Med Assoc* 1985;**186**(1):59–66.

Mueller RS, Krebs I, Power HT, Fieseler KV. Pemphigus foliaceus in 91 dogs. *J Am Anim Hosp Assoc* 2006;**42**(3):189–196.

Pye CC. Uveodermatologic syndrome in an Akita. *Can Vet J* 2009;**50**(8):861–864.

White SD, Rosychuk RA, Reinke SI, Paradis M. Use of tetracycline and niacinamide for treatment of autoimmune skin disease in 31 **dogs**. *J Am Vet Med Assoc* 1992;**200**(10):1497–1500.

Clinical Atlas of Canine and Feline Ophthalmic Disease, First Edition. Douglas Esson.

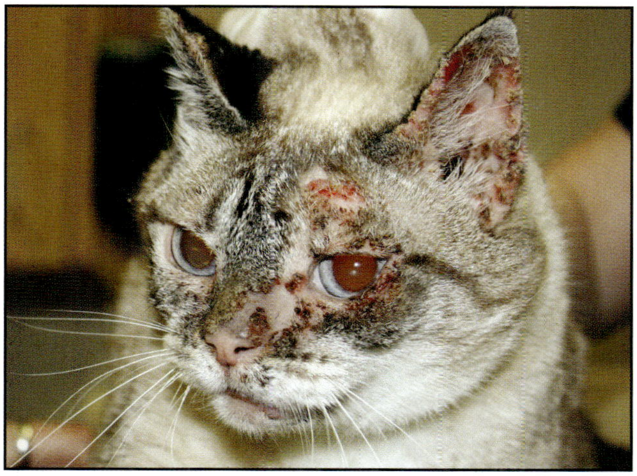

Figure 21.1 Periocular and facial findings associated with feline pemphigus foliaceus (PF).

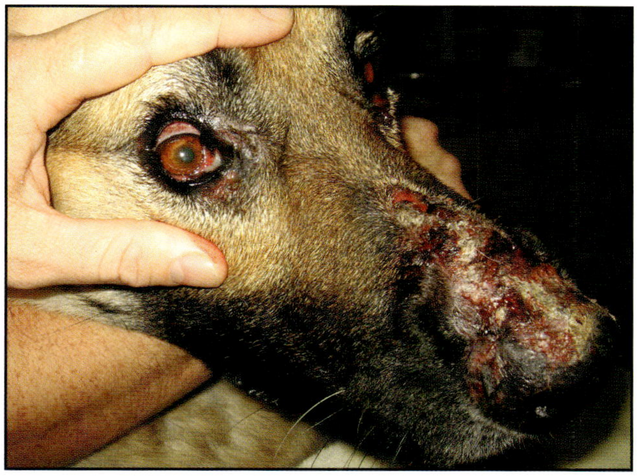

Figure 21.2 Periocular and facial findings associated with canine pemphigus foliaceus (PF).

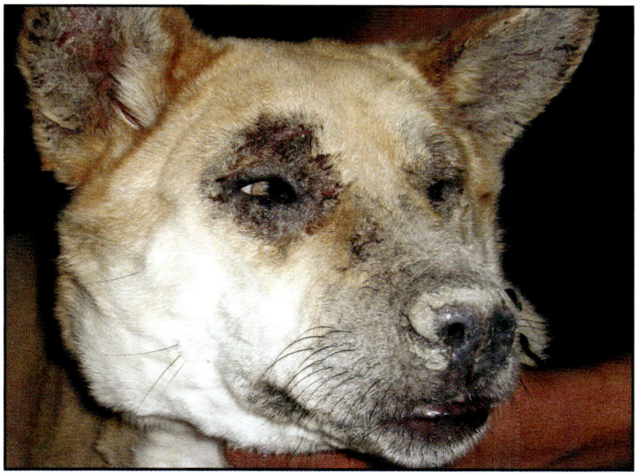

Figure 21.3 Periocular and facial findings associated with canine discoid lupus erythematosus (DLE).

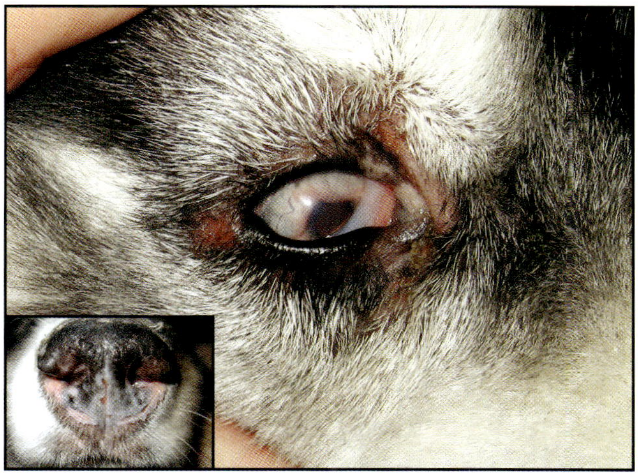

Figure 21.4 Findings associated with uveodermatological syndrome or "VKH-like disease", including blepharitis, vitiligo and active uveitis (the inset demonstrates typical nasal changes).

CHAPTER 22
EOSINOPHILIC FOLLICULITIS/FURUNCULOSIS

PRESENTATION

Folliculitis describes inflammation of the dermis and hair follicles. Furunculosis describes a deep necrotizing folliculitis. Eosinophilic folliculitis/furunculosis represents a severe, rapid-onset, nodular, and/or ulcerative dermatitis, typically affecting the muzzle, face, and periocular regions. Occasionally more generalized dermal lesions may also occur. The etiology of this condition is unclear; however, a hypersensitivity reaction has been proposed. Affected animals are typically young, large-breed dogs, with no breed predisposition noted.

DIAGNOSIS AND TREATMENT

The diagnosis of eosinophilic folliculitis/furunculosis is made on the basis of clinical findings, supported by histological interpretation of a representative incisional skin biopsy, indicating a mixed inflammatory and marked eosinophilic infiltration. Treatment comprises the systemic administration of prednisone at an anti-inflammatory to immunosuppressive dose. Secondary bacterial dermatitis, if present, should be managed using a systemic antimicrobial agent. Appropriate empirical selections include cephalosporins and tetracyclines.

Potential Drug-Side-Effects

Potential adverse effects associated with the use of systemic corticosteroids include polyphagia, polydipsia, polyuria, hair coat changes, weight gain, pancreatitis, gastrointestinal (GI) distress, muscle damage, hepatic impairment, and diabetes. Potential adverse effects associated with cephalosporins include GI distress, hypersensitivity reactions, and renal toxicity. Potential adverse effects associated with tetracyclines may include GI distress, hepatotoxicity, and photosensitivity.

SELECTED REFERENCES

Fraser M. What is your diagnosis? Eosinophilic folliculitis and furunculosis. *J Small Anim Pract*. 2002;**43**(4):150, 187.

Mauldin EA, Palmeiro BS, Goldschmidt MH, Morris DO. Comparison of clinical history and dermatologic findings in 29 dogs with severe eosinophilic dermatitis: a retrospective analysis. *Vet Dermatol* 2006;**17**(5):338–347.

Van Poucke S. What is your diagnosis? Canine eosinophilic furunculosis (folliculitis) of the face. *J Small Anim Pract*. 2000;**41**(11):485, 524–525.

Clinical Atlas of Canine and Feline Ophthalmic Disease, First Edition. Douglas Esson.

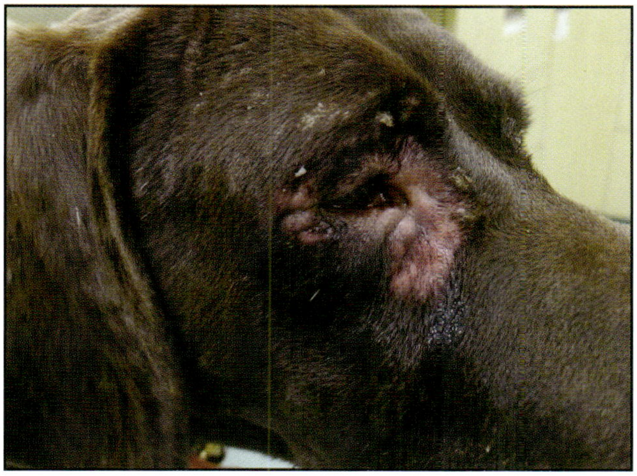

Figure 22.1 Nodular lesion characteristic of eosinophilic folliculitis/furunculosis, affecting the muzzle and periocular regions.

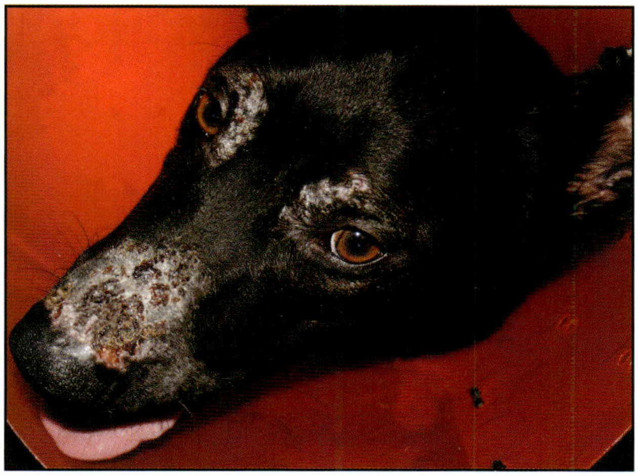

Figure 22.2 Nodular lesion characteristic of eosinophilic folliculitis/furunculosis, affecting the muzzle and periocular regions.

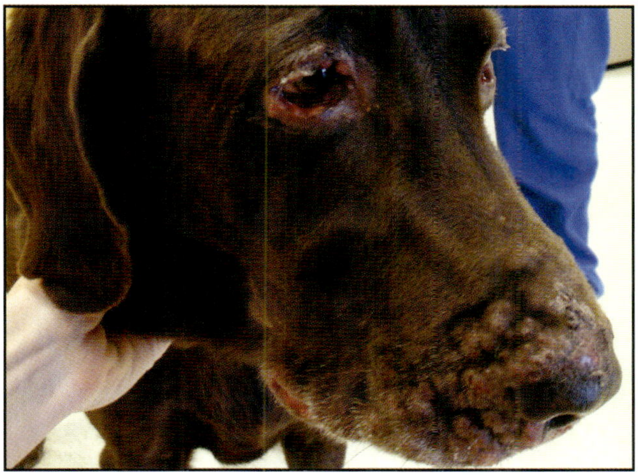

Figure 22.3 Nodular lesion characteristic of eosinophilic folliculitis/furunculosis, affecting the muzzle and periocular regions.

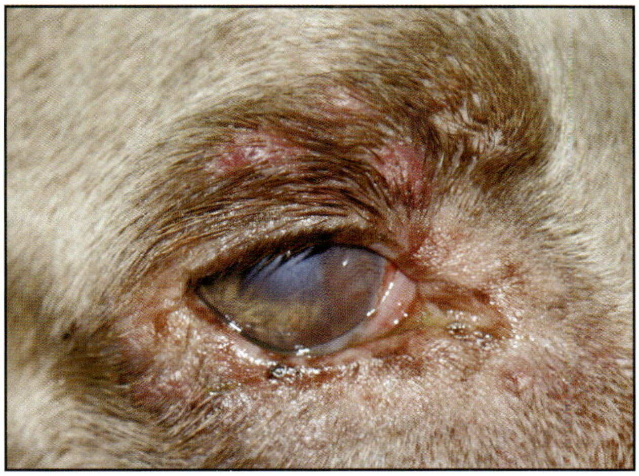

Figure 22.4 Nodular lesion characteristic of eosinophilic folliculitis/furunculosis, affecting the muzzle and periocular regions.

CHAPTER 23
ADVERSE DRUG REACTIONS (ADRs)

PRESENTATION

Adverse (cutaneous) drug reactions (ADRs) may occur as a result of pharmacologic factors as well as patients' individual immune responses. Symptoms may include severe facial and/or periocular erythema, bullous, and/or pustular eruptions, as well as more generalized lesions. Mechanisms of ADRs include immediate, delayed and antigen-antibody reactions as well as complement activation and mast cell degranulation. Medications more frequently associated with ADRs include sulfa-containing antimicrobials (particularly those potentiated with trimethoprim), penicillins, cephalosporins, neomycin, and cyclosporine. More commonly affected breeds may include the Shetland Sheepdog, Australian Shepherd, Doberman Pinscher and Yorkshire Terrier.

DIAGNOSIS AND TREATMENT

The diagnosis of an ADR is supported by medical history, histopathologic interpretation of incisional dermal biopsy, and response to drug withdrawal. Differentials include erythema multiforme, toxic epidermal necrolysis and cutaneous vasculitis as well as autoimmune disease. Treatment comprises the withdrawal of medications suspected to be resulting in ADR. Glucocorticoid therapy may additionally help speed the resolution of clinical signs. The symptomatic management of secondary bacterial pyoderma, if present, is also recommended.

Potential Drug-Side-Effects

Potential adverse effects associated with the use of systemic corticosteroids include polyphagia, polydipsia, polyuria, hair coat changes, weight gain, pancreatitis, gastrointestinal (GI) distress, muscle damage, hepatic impairment, and diabetes.

SELECTED REFERENCES

Mason KV. Cutaneous drug eruptions. *Vet Clin North Am Small Anim Pract*. 1990;**20**(6):1633–1653. Review.

Niza MM, Félix N, Vilela CL, Peleteiro MC, Ferreira AJ. Cutaneous and ocular adverse reactions in a dog following meloxicam administration. *Vet Dermatol* 2007;**18**(1):45–49.

Noli C, Koeman JP, Willemse T. A retrospective evaluation of adverse reactions to trimethoprim-sulphonamide combinations in dogs and cats. *Vet Q* 1995;**17**(4):123–128.

Scott DW, Miller WH Jr. Idiosyncratic cutaneous adverse drug reactions in the dog: literature review and report of 101 cases (1990–1996). *Canine Pract* 1999;**24**:16–22.

Clinical Atlas of Canine and Feline Ophthalmic Disease, First Edition. Douglas Esson.

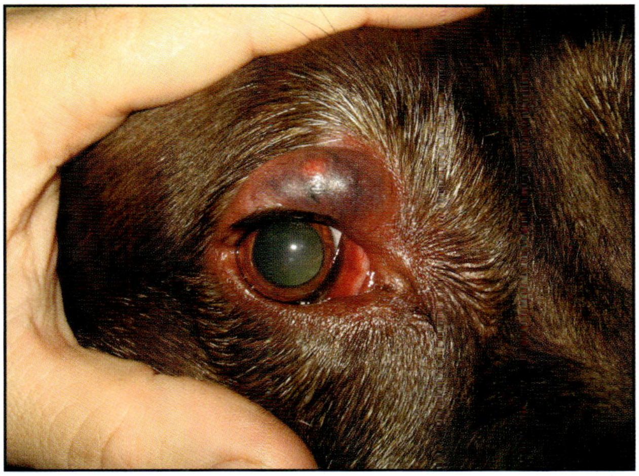

Figure 23.1 Adverse reaction associated with the topical use of sulfacetamide.

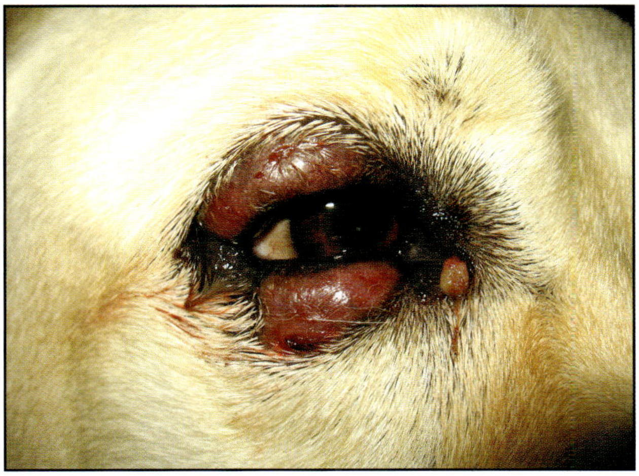

Figure 23.2 Adverse reaction associated with the topical use of sulfacetamide.

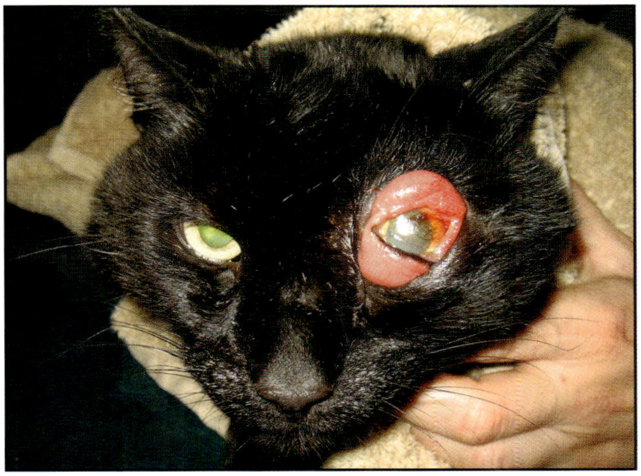

Figure 23.3 Adverse reaction associated with the topical use of neomycin.

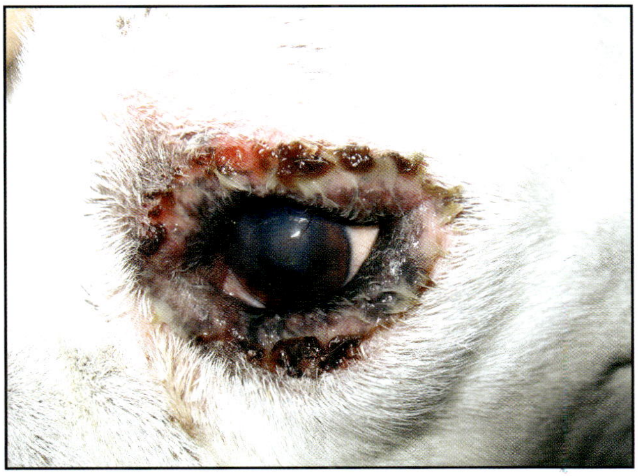

Figure 23.4 Adverse reaction associated with the topical use of cyclosporine.

CHAPTER 24
DERMATOMYOSITIS

PRESENTATION

Dermatomyositis describes an inflammatory condition affecting the dermis, connective tissues, and, to a variable degree, muscular tissues of young dogs. Dermal lesions typically comprise erythema, dermatitis, and/or alopecia of the extremities, digits, ears, and face. Affected animals are typically less than 1 year of age. Many develop subsequent myositis (notably affecting the muscles of mastication and/or locomotion). Commonly affected breeds include the Shetland Sheepdog and the Collie breeds.

DIAGNOSIS AND TREATMENT

The diagnosis of dermatomyositis is made on the basis of clinical findings, supported by histopathological interpretation of representative skin and muscle by biopsies. Affected animals may display variably elevated creatine kinase levels. Treatment comprises the systemic administration of corticosteroids, with or without adjunctive pentoxifylline and/or vitamin E.

Potential Drug-Side-Effects

Potential adverse effects associated with the use of systemic corticosteroids include polyphagia, polydipsia, polyuria, hair coat changes, weight gain, pancreatitis, gastrointestinal (GI) distress, muscle damage, hepatic impairment, and diabetes. Potential adverse effects associated with the use of pentoxifylline include GI distress, central nervous system (CNS) excitement, and/or hypersensitivity reactions.

Dermal lesions typically resolve (with the formation of scar tissue); however, myopathy may persist.

SELECTED REFERENCES

Evans J, Levesque D, Shelton GD. Canine inflammatory myopathies: a clinicopathologic review of 200 cases. *J Vet Intern Med*. 2004;**18**(5):679–691.

Ferguson EA, Cerundolo R, Lloyd DH, Rest J, Cappello R. Dermatomyositis in five Shetland sheepdogs in the United Kingdom. *Vet Rec*. 2000 Feb 19;**146**(8):214–217.

Rees CA, Boothe DM. Therapeutic response to pentoxifylline and its active metabolites in dogs with familial canine dermatomyositis. *Vet Ther*. 2003;**4**(3):234–241.

Clinical Atlas of Canine and Feline Ophthalmic Disease, First Edition. Douglas Esson.

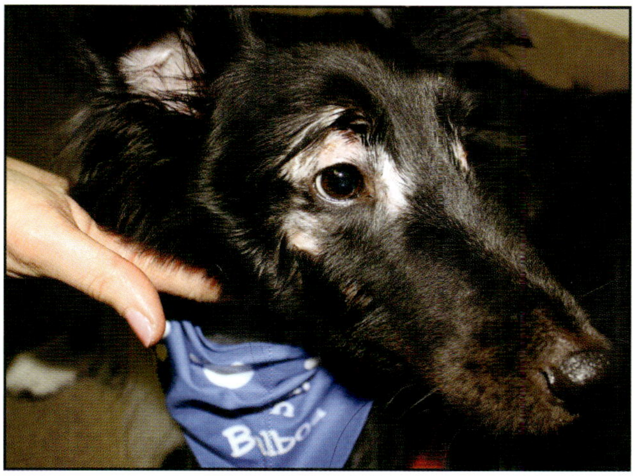

Figure 24.1 Typical presentation associated with canine dermatomyositis.

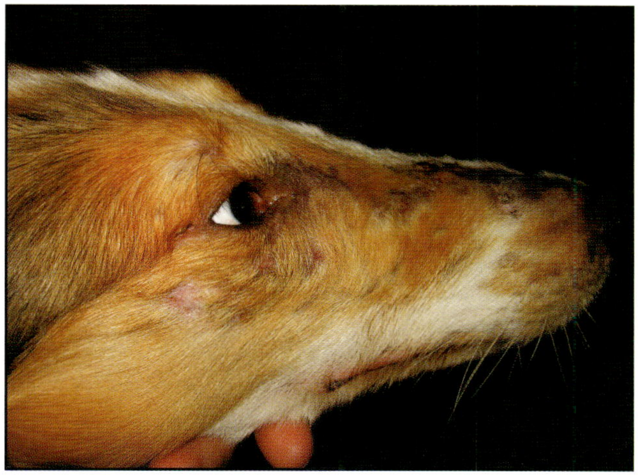

Figure 24.2 Typical presentation associated with canine dermatomyositis.

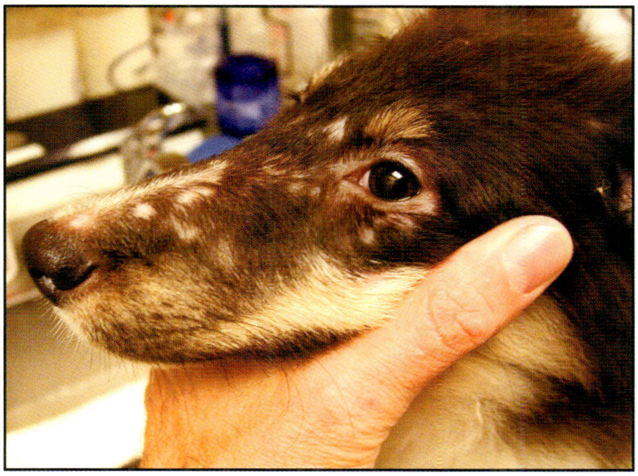

Figure 24.3 Typical presentation associated with canine dermatomyositis.

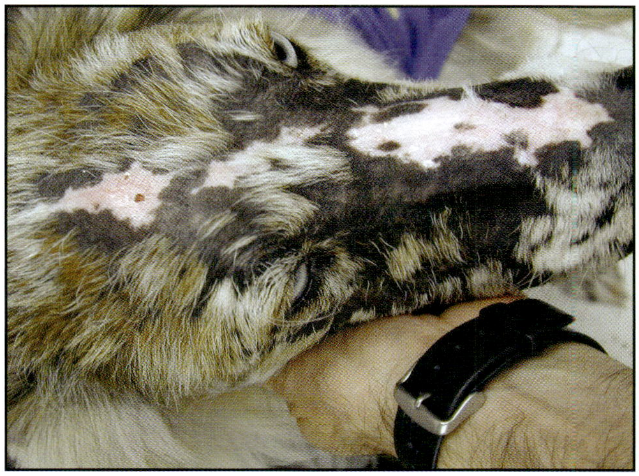

Figure 24.4 Chronic scarring associated with resolved dermatomyositis.

CHAPTER 25
DEMODEX-ASSOCIATED BLEPHARITIS

PRESENTATION

Clinical cases of canine demodicosis arise as a result of significantly increased numbers of commensal *Demodex Canis* or *Demodex Cati* mites within hair follicles. Poor body condition, debilitating disease, stress, corticosteroid-induced immunosuppression and/or hereditary factors may play a role in the development of clinical disease. Affected patients typically display erythema, moist dermatitis, alopecia, and/or lichenification and hyperpigmentation in either a localized or generalized pattern, particularly around the periocular regions. Multiple regions of the body may be affected and significant self-trauma as well as secondary bacterial pyoderma may result. Both canine and feline species of any breed or crossed breed may be affected (cats also potentially being affected by *Notoedres cati*). Commonly affected canine breeds include the Old English sheepdog, Lhasa Apso, Shih Tzu, and English Bulldog.

DIAGNOSIS AND TREATMENT

The diagnosis of demodicosis is made on the basis of cytological assessment following manual follicular expression in combination with deep skin scraping, demonstrating large numbers of adult parasites, and/or an increased ratio of immature parasite forms (ova, larvae, nymphs). The use of localized, topical treatments in the management of demodicosis is frequently unrewarding. Appropriate therapy comprises miticidal treatments, most commonly ivermectins, administered at a frequency of Q24–Q48 h over the course of three to six months, until two negative skin scrapings are achieved with an interval of 2–3 months.

Potential Drug-Side-Effects

Potential adverse reactions associated with use of ivermectins include neurotoxicity and retinal damage, particularly in the Collie breeds.

Secondary pyoderma should be treated using appropriate systemic antimicrobials (with or without the adjunctive use of medicated shampoos as indicated).

Clinical Atlas of Canine and Feline Ophthalmic Disease, First Edition. Douglas Esson.

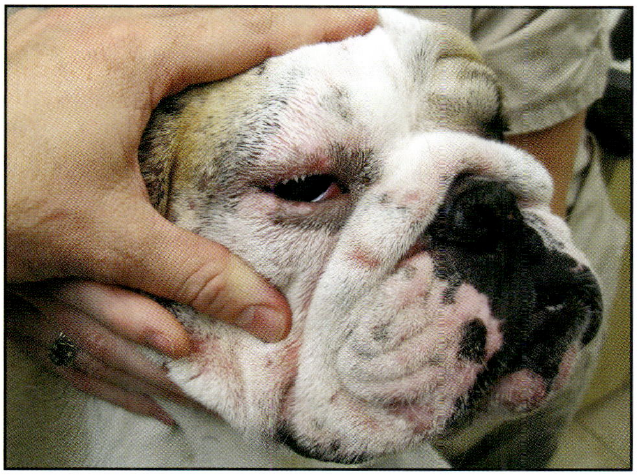

Figure 25.1 Clinical presentation associated with generalized canine demodicosis.

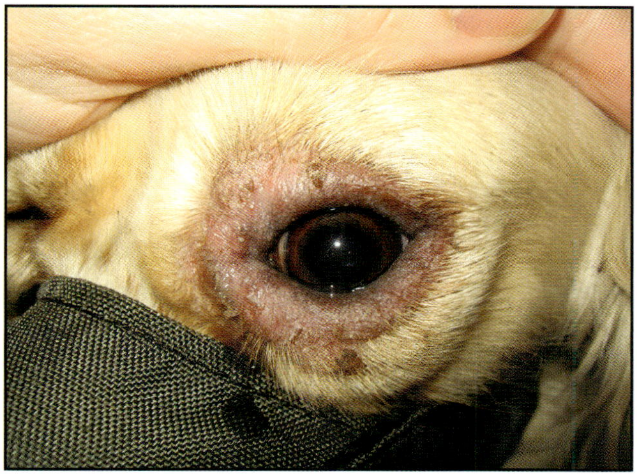

Figure 25.2 Clinical presentation associated with localized canine demodicosis.

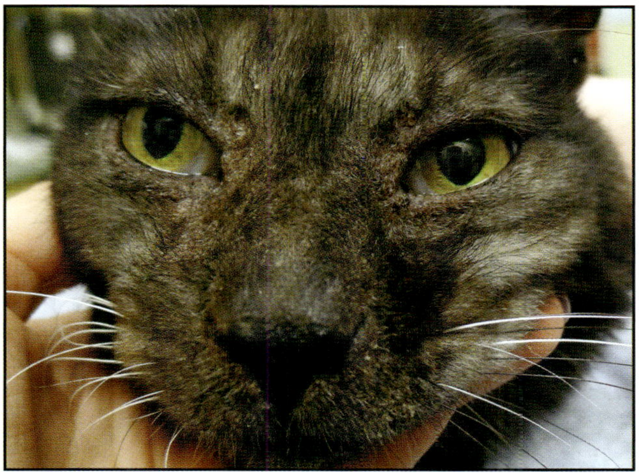

Figure 25.3 Clinical presentation associated with generalized feline demodicosis.

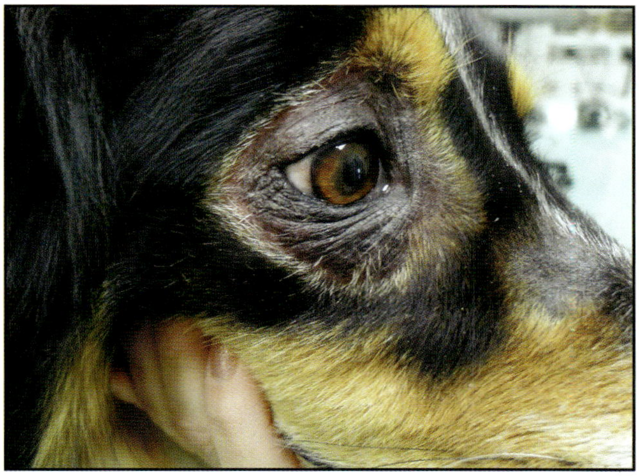

Figure 25.4 Lichenification and hyperpigmentation associated with chronic demodicosis.

CHAPTER 26
DERMATOPHYTOSIS

PRESENTATION

Dermatophytosis describes dermal infection with one of a number of fungal organisms. The confusing name "ringworm" has been used as a blanket term to describe these infections. Commonly identified organisms include *Microsporum canis*, *Microsporum gypseum*, and *Trichophyton mentagrophytes*. Clinically, affected patients display erythematous and/or crusting dermatitis, with or without secondary bacterial infection. Changes frequently affect the face, periocular tissues, pinnae, and/or forelimbs. Chronic lesions may display alopecia and/or lichenification. Both canine and feline species of any breed or crossed breed may be affected.

DIAGNOSIS AND TREATMENT

The diagnosis of dermatophytosis is made on the basis of clinical findings as well as the results of incubating samples on dermatophyte test media (DTM), with or without adjunctive cytological or histological assessment of representative samples. Infectious organisms represent potentially contagious zoonoses. Treatment typically comprises the systemic administration of fungicidal agents including fluconazole and itraconazole (with or without adjunctive antibiotic agents if secondary bacterial infection is present).

Potential Drug-Side-Effects

Potential adverse effects associated with the use of fluconazole and itraconazole include gastrointestinal (GI) distress and hepatotoxicity.

SELECTED REFERENCES

Bond R. Superficial veterinary mycoses. *Clin Dermatol.* 2010;**28**(2):226–236. doi: 10.1016/j.clindermatol.2009.12.012.
Moriello KA. Treatment of dermatophytosis in dogs and cats: review of published studies. *Vet Dermatol.* 2004;**15**(2):99–107.
Outerbridge CA. Mycologic disorders of the skin. *Clin Tech Small Anim Pract.* 2006;**21**(3):128–134.

Clinical Atlas of Canine and Feline Ophthalmic Disease, First Edition. Douglas Esson.

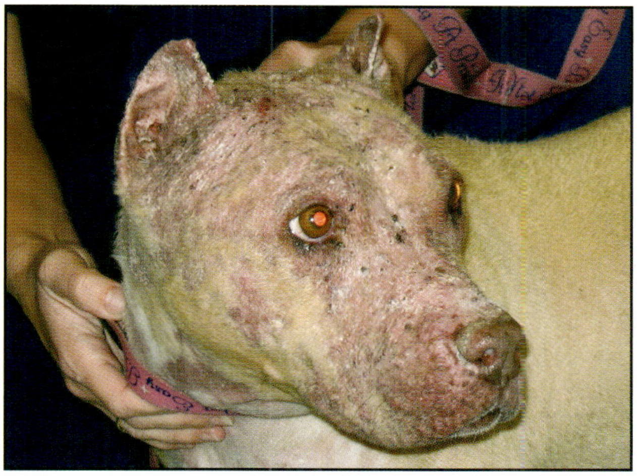

Figure 26.1 Clinical presentation associated with severe dermatophytosis, resulting in facial and periocular alopecia and crusting.

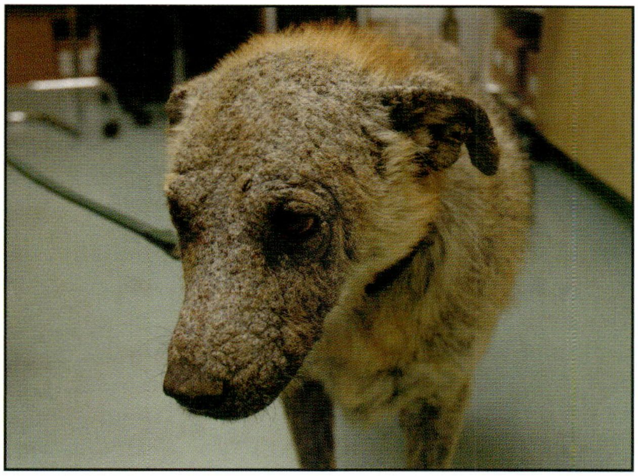

Figure 26.2 Clinical presentation associated with severe dermatophytosis, resulting in facial and periocular alopecia and crusting.

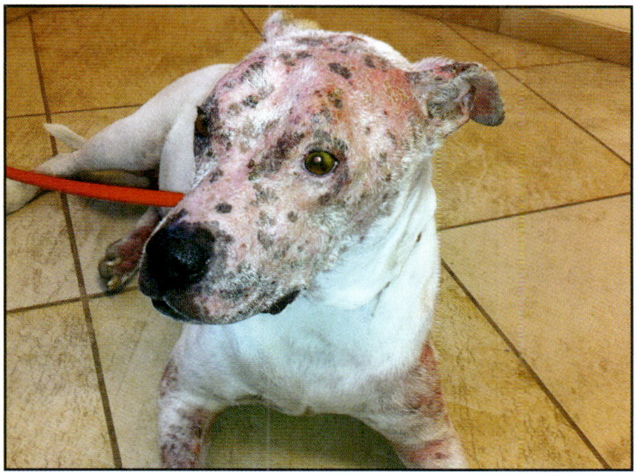

Figure 26.3 Clinical presentation associated with severe dermatophytosis, resulting in facial and periocular alopecia and crusting.

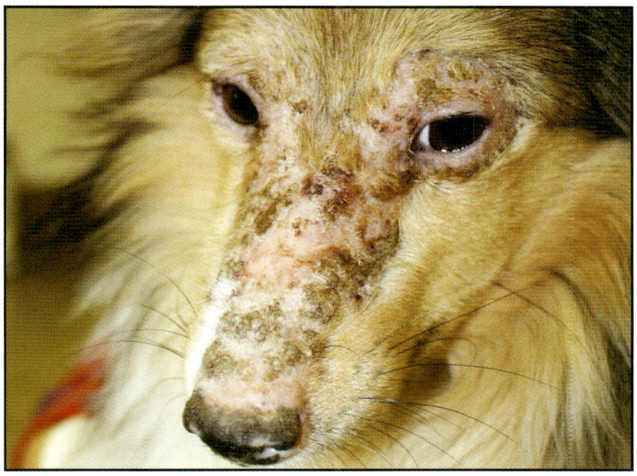

Figure 26.4 Clinical presentation associated with severe dermatophytosis, resulting in facial and periocular alopecia and crusting.

CHAPTER 27
RADIATION INDUCED BLEPHAROCONJUNCTIVITIS

PRESENTATION

Radiation therapy for the treatment of canine and feline patients affected by neoplasia of the cranial, orbital, or sinus regions, has become significantly more commonplace. The therapeutic radiation beam is generated in much the same way as an X-ray beam and similarly collimated. Where possible, an effort is made to avoid including ocular structures in the primary radiation beam. Radiation impairs the mitotic ability of exposed tissues in a manner that is both dose-dependent and cumulative. Tissues with significant metabolic turnover are most severely affected and ocular complications associated with radiation exposure include severe periocular dermatitis (tissue necrosis marked by moist dermatitis, secondary bacterial infection, and subsequent fibrosis), keratoconjunctivitis sicca (KCS), ulcerative keratitis, cataract formation and/or retinal necrosis (leading to degeneration)

DIAGNOSIS AND TREATMENT

The diagnosis of radiation-induced changes is made on the basis of clinical findings as well as history. Moist periocular dermatitis should be managed with appropriate systemic antimicrobial and anti-inflammatory therapy. KCS should be addressed using a combination of lacrimomimetic and anti-inflammatory therapy. Ulcerative keratitis should be managed by the debridement of devitalized tissue, routine antimicrobial cover, and the use of lubricating and protective agent. It should be anticipated that by definition, the healing of irradiated eyelid and corneal tissues may be slow and frustrating. Uveitis, including that associated with the presence of cataract(s), should managed using a topical anti-inflammatory agent in order to minimize the risk of secondary glaucoma. Affected patients are not usually suitable candidates for cataract surgery.

SELECTED REFERENCES

Ching SV, Gillette SM, Powers BE, Roberts SM, Gillette EL, Withrow SJ. Radiation-induced ocular injury in the dog: a histological study. *Int J Radiat Oncol Biol Phys*. 1990;**19**(2):321–328.

Lawrence JA, Forrest LJ, Turek MM, Miller PE, Mackie TR, Jaradat HA, Vail DM, Dubielzig RR, Chappell R, Mehta MP. Proof of principle of ocular sparing in dogs with sinonasal tumors treated with intensity-modulated radiation therapy. *Vet Radiol Ultrasound*. 2010;**51**(5):561–570.

Pinard CL, Mutsaers AJ, Mayer MN, Woods JP. Retrospective study and review of ocular radiation side effects following external-beam Cobalt-60 radiation therapy in 37 dogs and 12 cats. *Can Vet J*. 2012;**53**(12):1301–1307.

Roberts SM, Lavach JD, Severin GA, Withrow SJ, Gillette EL. Ophthalmic complications following megavoltage irradiation of the nasal and paranasal cavities in dogs. *J Am Vet Med Assoc*. 1987;**190**(1):43–47.

Clinical Atlas of Canine and Feline Ophthalmic Disease, First Edition. Douglas Esson.

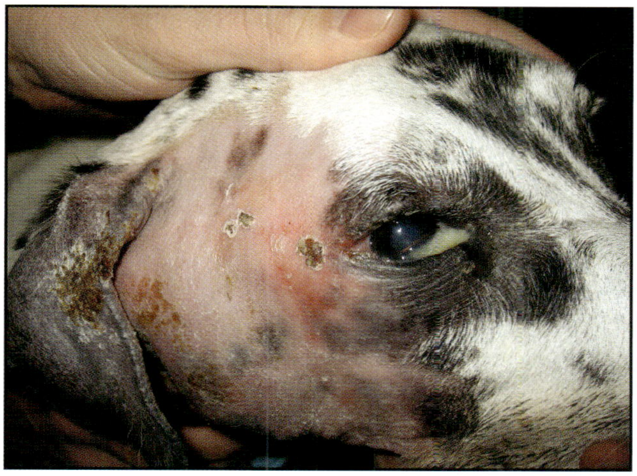

Figure 27.1 Changes associated with exposure to therapeutic radiation. The tenacious mucoid discharge visible in this figure is suggestive of associated KCS.

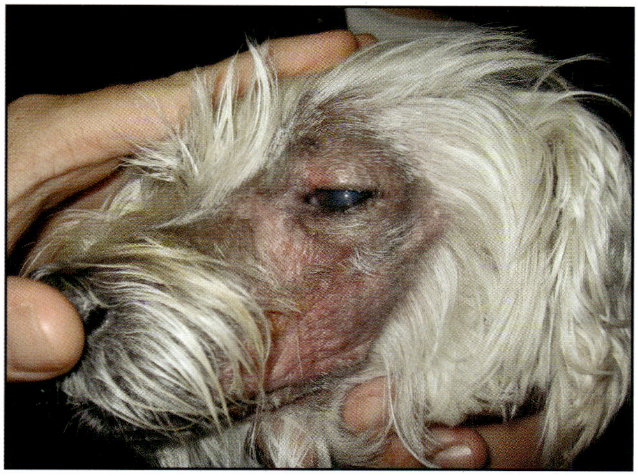

Figure 27.2 Changes associated with exposure to therapeutic radiation. Keratitis is present.

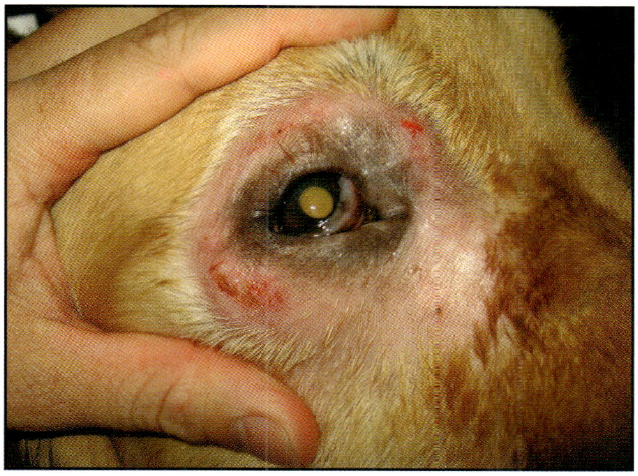

Figure 27.3 Changes associated with exposure to therapeutic radiation.

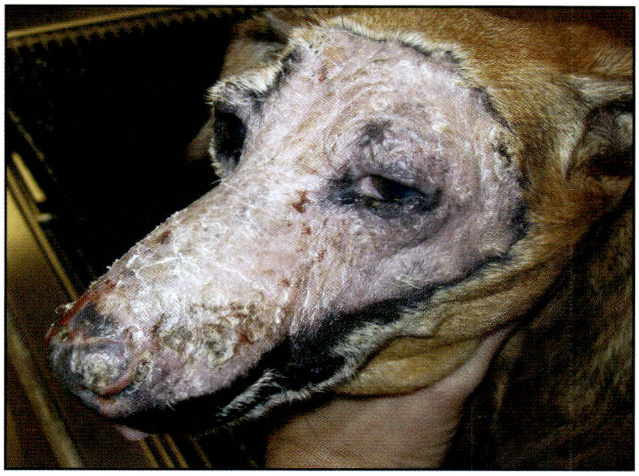

Figure 27.4 Chronic dermal alopecia and scarring following the resolution of radiation-associated, periocular inflammation.

CHAPTER 28
APOCRINE HIDROCYSTOMA

PRESENTATION

Apocrine hidrocystomas are relatively common eyelid masses affecting cats, predominantly the Persian and Himalayan breeds. These lesions appear as one or more focal to coalescing, raised, gray, cystic masses affecting one or both eyelid margins (upper and/or lower) and/or the periocular region. Histologically, these masses comprise adenomatous tissue and dilated epithelial cysts, which contain viscous tan- to brown-colored proteinaceous debris.

DIAGNOSIS AND TREATMENT

Apocrine hidrocystomas are benign and generally do not result in significant discomfort or secondary pathology. If necessary, however, these lesions may be removed by either surgical excision or more ideally by CO_2 laser ablation. In all cases, an attempt should be made to preserve eyelid margins. New or recurrent lesions may occur following removal.

SELECTED REFERENCES

Cantaloube B, Raymond-Letron I, Regnier A. Multiple eyelid apocrine hidrocystomas in two Persian cats. *Vet Ophthalmol.* 2004;**7**(2):121–125.

Chaitman J, van der Woerdt A, Bartick TE. Multiple eyelid cysts resembling apocrine hidrocystomas in three Persian cats and one Himalayan cat. *Vet Pathol.* 1999;**36**(5):474–476.

Giudice C, Muscolo MC, Rondena M, Crotti A, Grieco V. Eyelid multiple cysts of the apocrine gland of Moll in Persian cats. *J Feline Med Surg.* 2009;**11**(6):487–491. doi: 10.1016/j.jfms.2008.11.006. Epub 2008 Dec 21.

Yang SH, Liu CH, Hsu CD, Yeh LS, Lin CT. Use of chemical ablation with trichloroacetic acid to treat eyelid apocrine hidrocystomas in a cat. *J Am Vet Med Assoc.* 2007;**230**(8):1170–1173.

Clinical Atlas of Canine and Feline Ophthalmic Disease, First Edition. Douglas Esson.

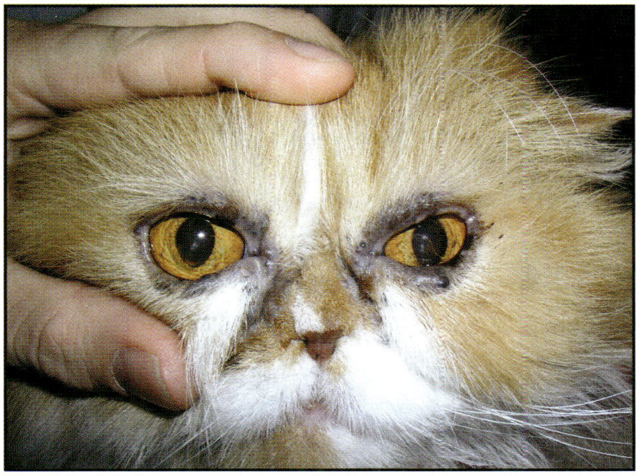

Figure 28.1 Clinical presentation associated with apocrine hidrocystomas affecting both eyelids.

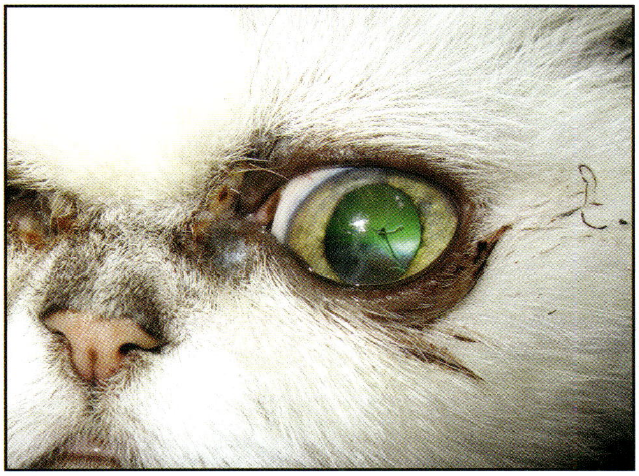

Figure 28.2 Clinical presentation associated with a large medial canthal apocrine hidrocystoma.

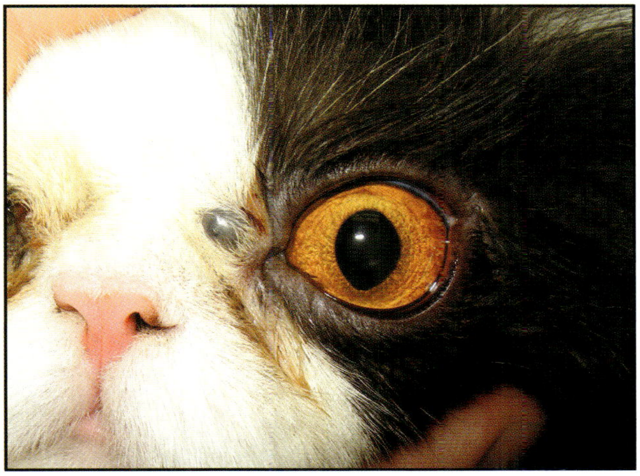

Figure 28.3 Clinical presentation associated with a large medial canthal apocrine hidrocystoma.

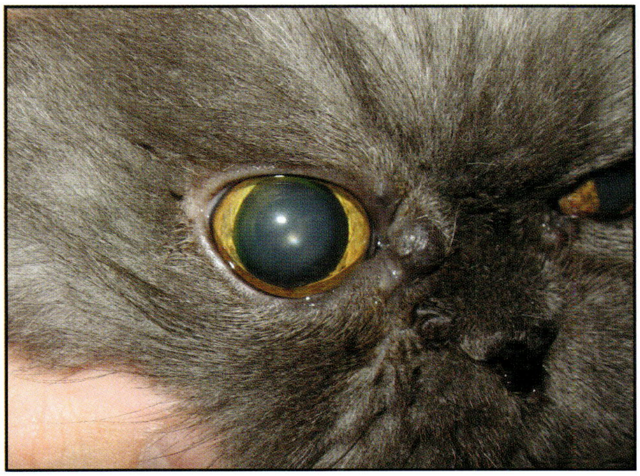

Figure 28.4 Clinical presentation associated with a large medial canthal apocrine hidrocystoma.

CHAPTER 29
SEBACEOUS ADENOMA/EPITHELIOMA

PRESENTATION

Both adenomas and epitheliomas represent relatively common benign neoplastic proliferations of sebaceous (meibomian) glandular tissue. Adenomas generally exhibit histological evidence of glandular differentiation, whereas epitheliomas generally do not; however, some degree of histological "overlap" occurs. Both lesions typically appear as pink to gray, firm irregular and proliferative eyelid masses arising from the eyelid margin (upper or lower) and display variable degrees of eyelid invasion. Secondary blepharoconjunctivitis and/or keratitis may develop as a result of abrasion and/or self-trauma. Secondary chalazia may also develop in association with these lesions as a result of glandular obstruction.

DIAGNOSIS AND TREATMENT

The diagnosis is based on clinical findings as well as histopathologic interpretation of biopsy samples where indicated. Histopathology will define the nature and extent of the neoplastic process and provide an indication as to whether complete excision has been achieved. In rare cases, malignant adenocarcinomas may be identified. Treatment comprises the surgical removal of these lesions. Small lesions (2–5 mm) may be ablated using a CO_2 laser, preserving eyelid margin function and form and frequently avoiding the need for surgical reconstruction. Larger lesions, however, require full-thickness excision and accurate subsequent eyelid repair. Ideally, the medial and lateral canthal anatomy should be preserved where possible. Resultant eyelid defects that are less than one-third of the eyelid length may be directly apposed. Larger defects typically require blepharoplastic reconstruction such as lateral canthotomy and the excellent split-lid technique described by Lewin. Postoperative care comprises routine systemic antimicrobial (if indicated), anti-inflammatory and analgesic care. An Elizabethan collar should be placed post-operatively in order to prevent self-trauma and corneal health should be frequently monitored until eyelid healing is complete.

SELECTED REFERENCES

Bussieres M, Krohne SG, Stiles J, Townsend WM. The use of carbon dioxide laser for the ablation of meibomian gland adenomas in dogs. *J Am Anim Hosp Assoc.* 2005;**41**(4):227–234.

Dubielzig R *et al.* 2010. *Veterinary Ocular Pathology*, pp. 151–152, Elsevier, Edinburgh.

Grahn BH, Sandmeyer LS. Diagnostic ophthalmology. *Tarsal gland adenoma. Can Vet J.* 2009;**50**(11):1199–1200.

Lewin G. Eyelid reconstruction in seven dogs using a split eyelid flap. *J Small Anim Pract.* 2003 Aug;**44**(8):346–351.

Roberts SM, Severin GA, Lavach JD. Prevalence and treatment of palpebral neoplasms in the dog: 200 cases (1975–1983). *J Am Vet Med Assoc.* 1986;**189**(10):1355–1359.

Clinical Atlas of Canine and Feline Ophthalmic Disease, First Edition. Douglas Esson.

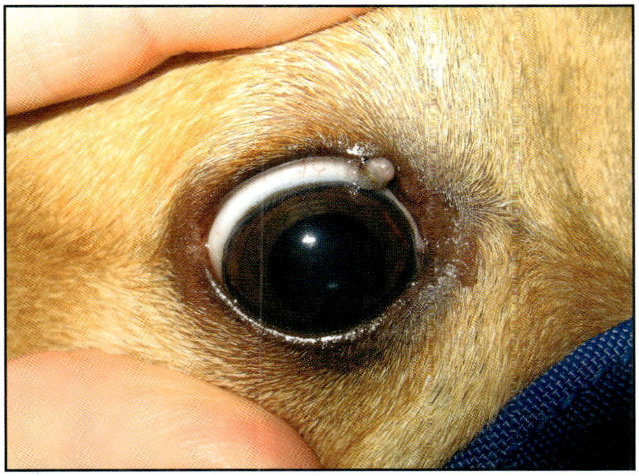

Figure 29.1 Clinical presentation associated with a sebaceous epithelioma. The small eyelid tumor is amenable to CO_2 laser ablation.

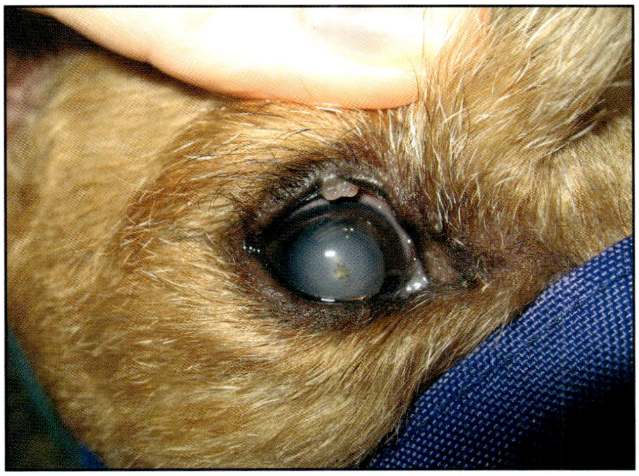

Figure 29.2 Clinical presentation associated with a sebaceous adenoma. The small eyelid tumor is amenable to CO_2 laser ablation.

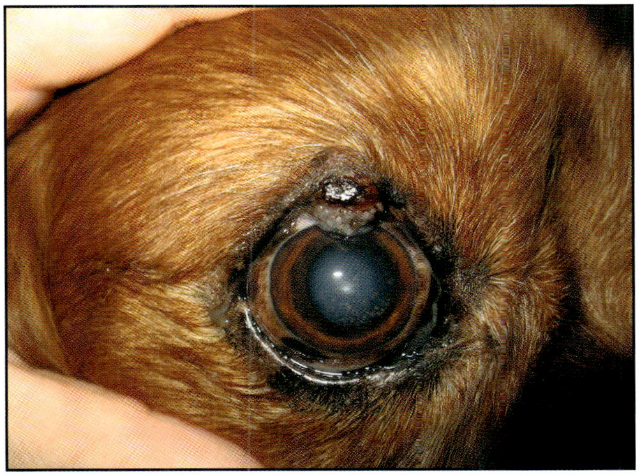

Figure 29.3 Clinical presentation associated with sebaceous adenoma. The large eyelid tumor is more appropriately surgically resected.

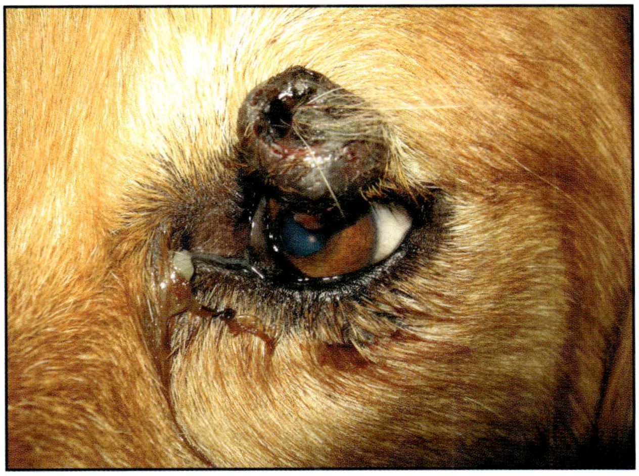

Figure 29.4 Clinical presentation associated with sebaceous adenoma. The eyelid tumor is more appropriately surgically resected.

CHAPTER 30
HISTIOCYTOMA

PRESENTATION

Histiocytomas are generally benign and frequently self-limiting dermal tumors, which may affect the eyelids or periocular regions, particularly in young dogs. Lesions present as firm, raised, pink to red, well-circumscribed masses on or close to the eyelid margin, which may or may not ulcerate. Commonly affected breeds include the Cocker Spaniel, Boxer, and Dachshund.

DIAGNOSIS AND TREATMENT

The diagnosis of histiocytoma is made on the basis of histopathologic interpretation of representative (typically excisional) biopsy. Histiocytomas in young dogs may spontaneously regress over the course of 1–3 months in association with a lymphocytic infiltrate, or may require surgical excision. In surgical cases, an attempt should be made to preserve eyelid margins. While solitary, eyelid histiocytomas are generally benign in their behavior, the spectrum of more generalized cutaneous as well as systemic histiocytosis-associated diseases (notably affecting Bernese Mountain Dogs and Labrador Retrievers) are of more concern and the behavior of much less common histiocytic sarcomas is highly malignant.

SELECTED REFERENCES

Coomer AR, Liptak JM. Canine histiocytic diseases. *Compend Contin Educ Vet*. 2008;**30**(4):202–204, 208–216; quiz 216–17.

Fulmer AK, Mauldin GE. Canine histiocytic neoplasia: an overview. *Can Vet J*. 2007;**48**(10):1041–1043, 1046–1050.

Gelatt KN. Histiocytoma of the eyelid of a dog. *Vet Med Small Anim Clin*. 1975;**70**(3):305.

Killick DR, Rowlands AM, Burrow RD, Cripps P, Miller J, Graham P, Blackwood L. Mast cell tumour and cutaneous histiocytoma excision wound healing in general practice. *J Small Anim Pract*. 2011;**52**(9):469–475. doi: 10.1111/j.1748-5827.2011.01093.x.

Schmidt JM, North SM, Freeman KP, Ramiro-Ibañez F. Canine paediatric oncology: retrospective assessment of 9522 tumours in dogs up to 12 months (1993–2008). *Vet Comp Oncol*. 2010;**8**(4):283–292. doi: 10.1111/j.1476-5829.2010.00226.x.

Clinical Atlas of Canine and Feline Ophthalmic Disease, First Edition. Douglas Esson.

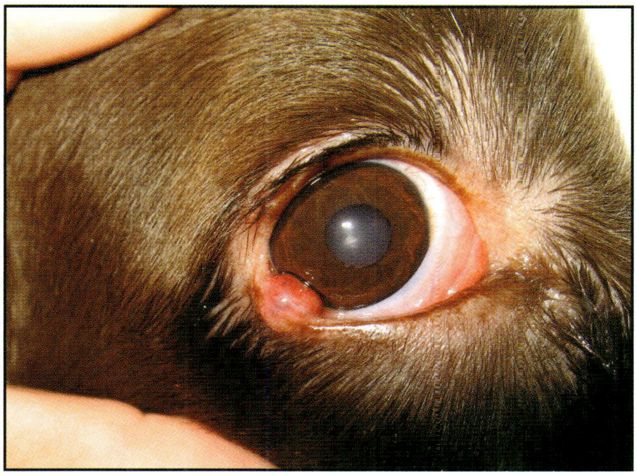

Figure 30.1 Clinical presentation associated with canine histiocytoma.

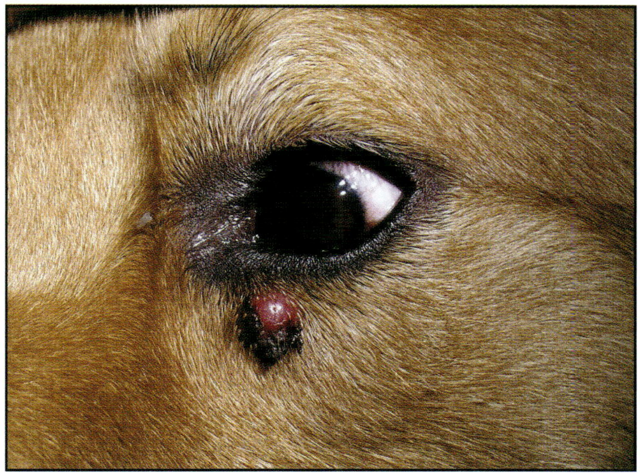

Figure 30.2 Clinical presentation associated with canine histiocytoma.

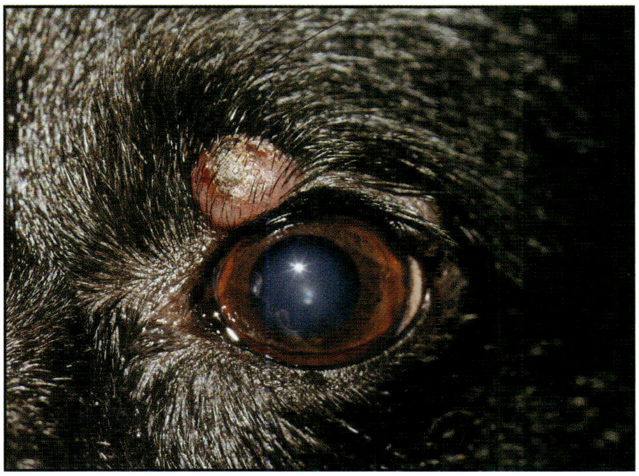

Figure 30.3 Clinical presentation associated with canine histiocytoma.

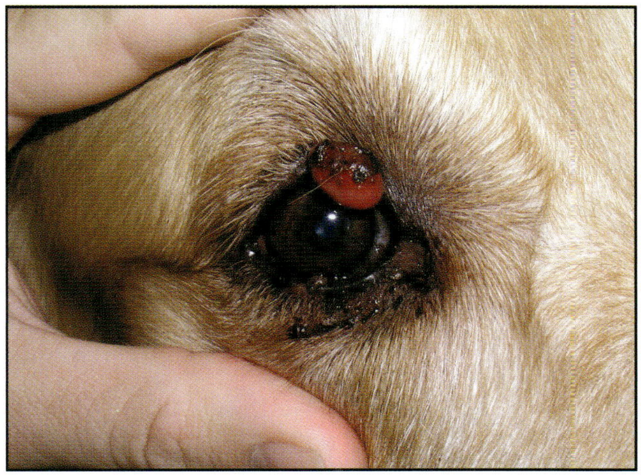

Figure 30.4 Clinical presentation associated with canine histiocytoma.

CHAPTER 31
EYELID MELANOCYTOMA

PRESENTATION

Eyelid melanocytomas represent a benign proliferation of melanocytes and present as one or frequently more, small, firm, irregular, pigmented, slowly proliferative masses along the eyelid margin(s). Commonly affected breeds include the Vizsla and Doberman Pinscher.

DIAGNOSIS AND TREATMENT

The diagnosis of melanocytoma is made on the basis of clinical findings, supported where indicated by histopathological interpretation of a representative tissue biopsy. This lesion's predication for the eyelid margin renders the surgical excision of multiple lesions challenging. Options for the management of these lesions include benign neglect, surgical resection, local treatment using cryosurgical application or more ideally CO_2-mediated laser ablation. Local recurrence as well as the development of new lesions may occur postoperatively.

SELECTED REFERENCES

Dubielzig R *et al*. 2010. *Veterinary Ocular Pathology 150*, Elsevier, Edinburgh.

Finn M, Krohne S, Stiles J. Ocular melanocytic neoplasia. *Compend Contin Educ Vet*. 2008;**30**(1):19–25; quiz 26. Review.

Roberts SM, Severin GA, Lavach JD. Prevalence and treatment of palpebral neoplasms in the dog: 200 cases (1975–1983). *J Am Vet Med Assoc*. 1986;**189**(10):1355–1359.

Clinical Atlas of Canine and Feline Ophthalmic Disease, First Edition. Douglas Esson.

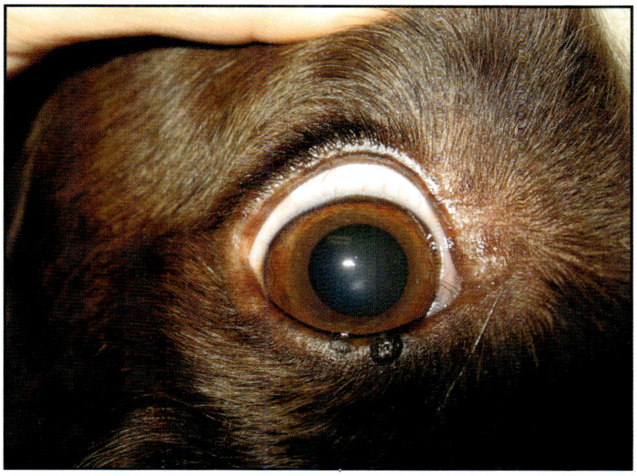

Figure 31.1 Clinical presentation associated with canine eyelid melanocytomas.

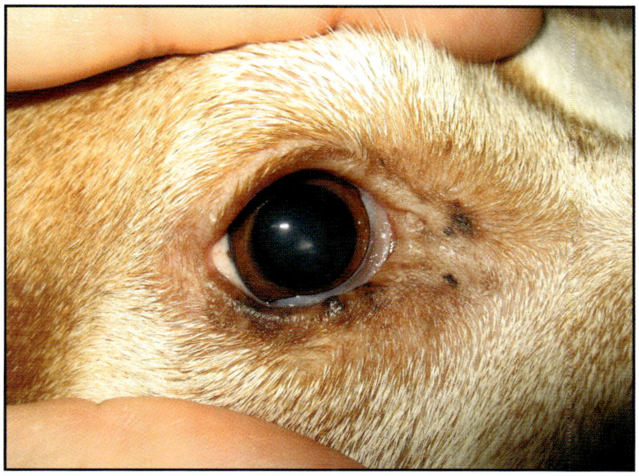

Figure 31.2 Clinical presentation associated with canine eyelid melanocytomas.

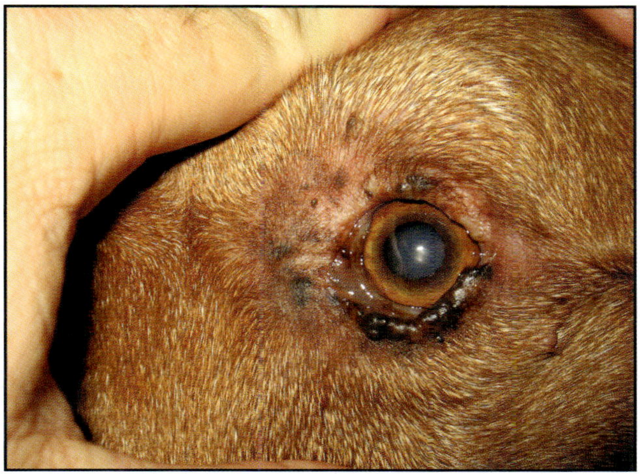

Figure 31.3 Clinical presentation associated with canine eyelid melanocytomas.

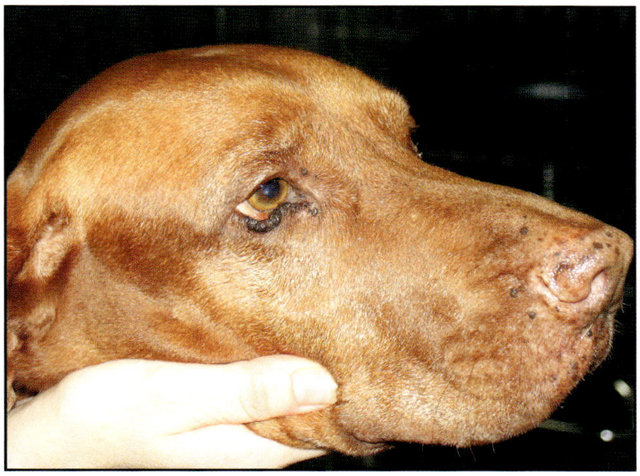

Figure 31.4 Clinical presentation associated with canine eyelid melanocytomas.

CHAPTER 32
EYELID MELANOMA

PRESENTATION

Eyelid melanomas typically present as firm, irregular, and proliferative masses. These lesions may or not be pigmented (the diagnostic spectrum encompassing amelanotic melanomas) and may occasionally be associated with hemorrhage. Eyelid melanomas typically exhibit malignant behavior, including aggressive local infiltration. Commonly affected breeds include the Doberman Pinscher and Toy Poodle.

DIAGNOSIS AND TREATMENT

Definitive diagnosis of a melanoma is made by histopathologic evaluation of representative tissue biopsy. Treatment comprises wide surgical excision where possible, as well as adjunctive chemotherapy or external beam (electron) radiation therapy and/or "metronomic therapy" (the combination of a nonsteroidal anti-inflammatory drug (NSAID) and alkylating agent to inhibit vascular growth) where indicated. The potential for metastasis exists and presurgical staging via local lymph node aspiration, three-view radiography, and complete blood count (CBC)/chemistry analysis is recommended. Cranial soft tissue imaging (magnetic resonance imaging (MRI) or computed tomography (CT)) will further facilitate accurate presurgical planning if necessary. Local blepharoplastic reconstruction may be necessary following the excision of large lesions. The potential value of vaccine-mediated immunotherapy in the treatment of eyelid melanomas has not been fully evaluated.

SELECTED REFERENCES

Aquino SM. Management of eyelid neoplasms in the dog and cat. *Clin Tech Small Anim Pract*. 2007;**22**(2):46–54. Review.

Finn M, Krohne S, Stiles J. Ocular melanocytic neoplasia. *Compend Contin Educ Vet*. 2008;**30**(1):19–25; quiz 26. Review.

Gwin RM, Alsaker RD, Gelatt KN. Melanoma of the lower eyelid of a dog. *Vet Med Small Anim Clin*. 1976;**71**(7):929–931.

Munger RJ, Gourley IM. Cross lid flap for repair of large upper eyelid defects. *J Am Vet Med Assoc*. 1981;**178**(1):45–48.

Roberts SM, Severin GA, Lavach JD. Prevalence and treatment of palpebral neoplasms in the dog: 200 cases (1975–1983). *J Am Vet Med Assoc*. 1986;**189**(10):1355–1359.

Clinical Atlas of Canine and Feline Ophthalmic Disease, First Edition. Douglas Esson.

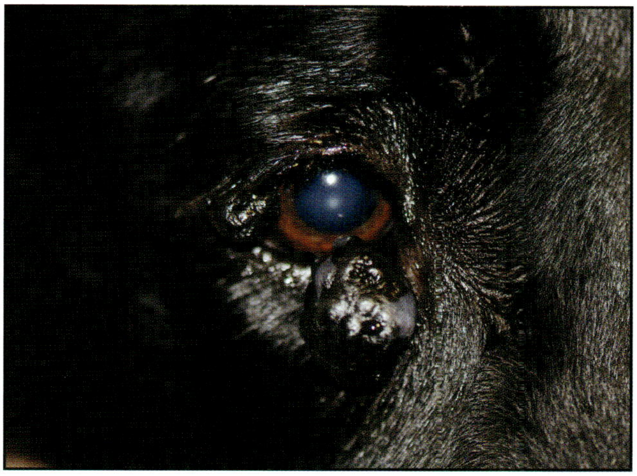

Figure 32.1 Clinical presentation associated with eyelid melanoma.

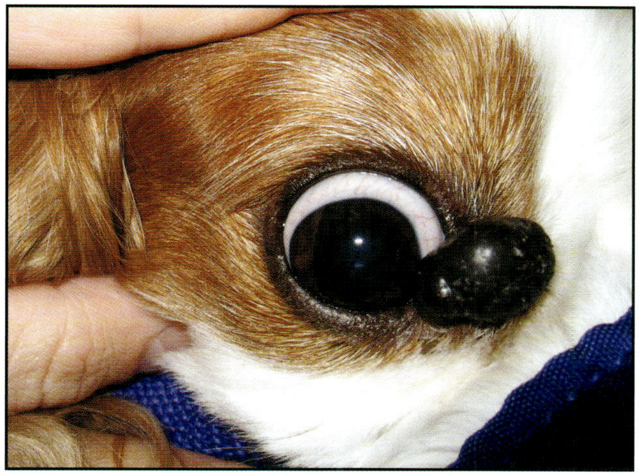

Figure 32.2 Clinical presentation associated with eyelid melanoma.

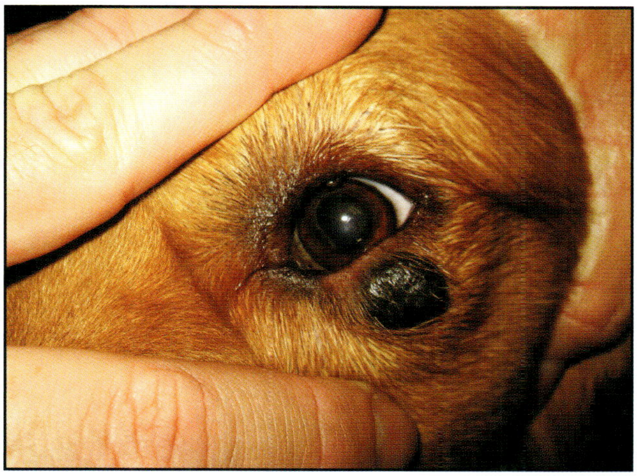

Figure 32.3 Clinical presentation associated with eyelid melanoma.

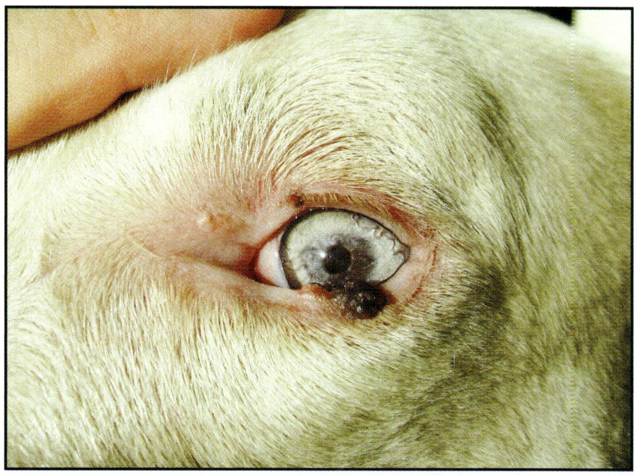

Figure 32.4 Clinical presentation associated with eyelid melanoma.

CHAPTER 33
CUTANEOUS EPITHELIOTROPIC LYMPHOMA (CEL)

PRESENTATION

Cutaneous epitheliotropic lymphoma (CEL) describes a form of lymphoma, which may specifically affect the eyelids and adnexal tissues. The somewhat confusing term "mycosis fungoides" has also been used to refer to this condition. Clinical presentation includes thickened, irregular to nodular/proliferative and/or ulcerative dermatitis/blepharitis, and/or depigmentation, which varies in severity and distribution. Mucocutaneous junctions around the eyes and mouth are commonly affected, as are nail beds and/or paw pads; however, more generalized dermal involvement may also be present. In cases affecting the periocular tissues, associated conjunctivitis and/or ocular discharge may additionally be present. Late stages of the disease may include involvement of the lymphatic, hepatic, and/or gastrointestinal systems. Commonly affected breeds include the Golden Retriever, Boxer, and American Eskimo.

DIAGNOSIS AND TREATMENT

The diagnosis of CEL is made by histologic interpretation of samples obtained by incisional biopsy. Wherever lymphoma is suspected, samples should be harvested before beginning therapy in order to facilitate the planning of an accurate treatment protocol. The potential for metastasis exists and staging via local lymph node (and/or organ/bone marrow) aspiration, three-view radiography, and complete blood count (CBC)/chemistry analysis is recommended, before the initiation of chemotherapy. Treatment comprises systemic chemotherapy as well as the management of secondary bacterial infection where present. Individual chemotherapeutic protocols are most ideally designed by a veterinary oncologist, however typically include prednisone and lomustine.

Potential Drug-Side-Effects

Potential adverse effects associated with the use of systemic corticosteroids include polyphagia, polydipsia, polyuria, hair coat changes, weight gain, pancreatitis, enteritis, muscular damage, hepatic impairment, and diabetes. Potential adverse effects associated with the use of lomustine include stomatitis, corneal epithelial toxicity, alopecia, gastrointestinal (GI) distress, renal and/or hepatotoxicity, and/or myelosuppression.

The prognosis varies based on the stage of lymphoma as well as extent of involvement representing a period, which may vary from months to years.

SELECTED REFERENCES

Fontaine J, Bovens C, Bettenay S, Mueller RS. Canine cutaneous epitheliotropic T-cell lymphoma: a review. *Vet Comp Oncol.* 2009;**7**(1):1–14. doi: 10.1111/j.1476-5829.2008.00176.x.

Fontaine J, Heimann M, Day MJ. Canine cutaneous epitheliotropic T-cell lymphoma: a review of 30 cases. *Vet Dermatol.* 2010;**21**(3):267–75. doi: 10.1111/j.1365-3164.2009.00793.x. Epub 2010 Feb 5.

Fontaine J, Heimann M, Day MJ. Cutaneous epitheliotropic T-cell lymphoma in the cat: a review of the literature and five new cases. *Vet Dermatol.* 2011;**22**(5):454–61. doi: 10.1111/j.1365-3164.2011.00972.x. Epub 2011 May 2.

Clinical Atlas of Canine and Feline Ophthalmic Disease, First Edition. Douglas Esson.

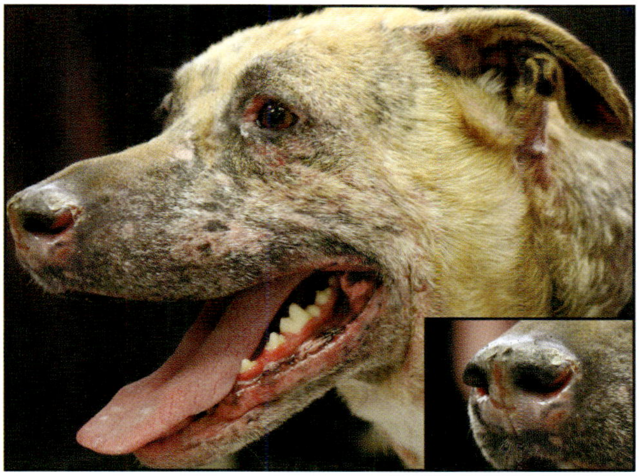

Figure 33.1 Clinical presentation associated with epitheliotropic lymphoma, displaying erosive periocular & facial lesions.

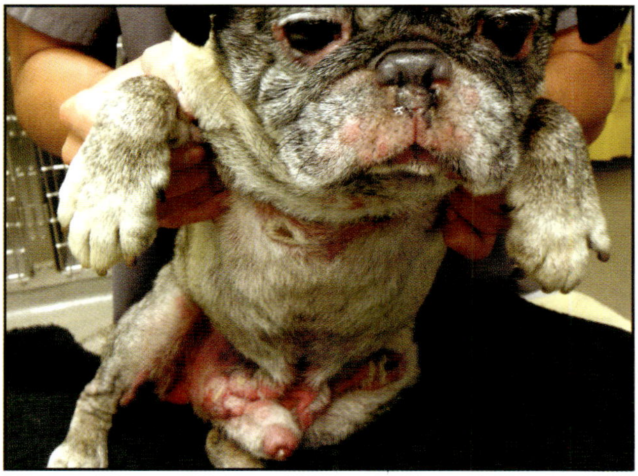

Figure 33.2 Clinical presentation associated with epitheliotropic lymphoma, displaying generalized dermal changes.

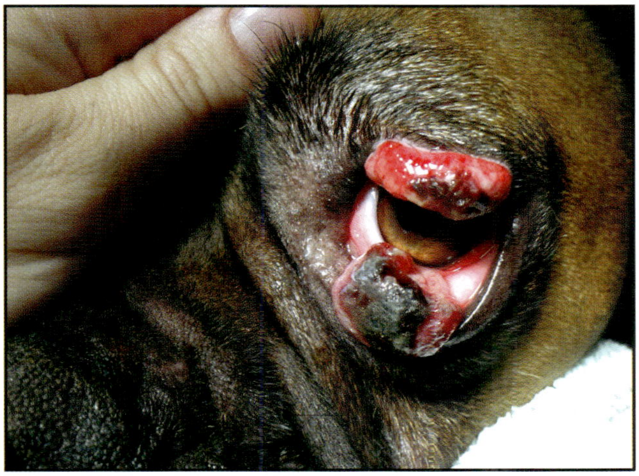

Figure 33.3 Clinical presentation associated with epitheliotropic lymphoma, displaying proliferative lesions.

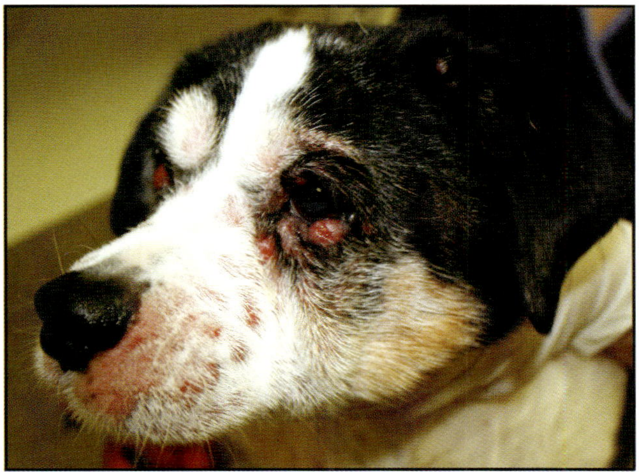

Figure 33.4 Clinical presentation associated with epitheliotropic lymphoma, displaying proliferative lesions.

CHAPTER 34
EYELID SQUAMOUS CELL CARCINOMA (SCC)

PRESENTATION

Squamous cell carcinoma (SCC) of the eyelids is a neoplastic process, which more commonly affects white or minimally pigmented animals. Hereditary factors, exposure to UV sunlight and/or chronic inflammation may contribute to the development of these lesions, which progress from focal acanthosis through carcinoma *in situ* to outright squamous cell carcinoma with time. Carcinomas affecting the eyelid are more commonly encountered in feline patients and typically present as irregular, pink to red, erosive, and/or proliferative lesions, which may be associated with local blepharoconjunctivitis, mucoid discharge, and/or hemorrhage. Carcinomas are aggressive and locally invasive tumors, which may extend into surrounding tissues, including the conjunctiva, globe, and orbit.

DIAGNOSIS AND TREATMENT

The diagnosis of SCC is based on clinical findings, supported by representative incisional tissue biopsy. Histopathology defines the degree of malignancy present. Treatment comprises wide surgical excision where possible. Local blepharoplastic reconstruction is typically necessary following excision. The potential for metastasis exists and basic staging via local lymph node aspiration, three-view radiography, and complete blood count (CBC)/chemistry analysis is recommended. Cranial soft tissue imaging (magnetic resonance imaging (MRI) or computed tomography (CT)) will facilitate accurate presurgical planning where necessary. Superficial lesions may be amenable to strontium therapy. SCC demonstrates a variable sensitivity to external beam radiation.

SELECTED REFERENCES

Murphy S. Cutaneous squamous cell carcinoma in the cat: current understanding and treatment approaches. *J Feline Med Surg*. 2013;**15**(5):401–407.

Newkirk KM, Rohrbach BW. A retrospective study of eyelid tumors from 43 cats. *Vet Pathol*. 2009;**46**(5):916–927.

Roberts SM, Severin GA, Lavach JD. Prevalence and treatment of palpebral neoplasms in the dog: 200 cases (1975–1983). *J Am Vet Med Assoc*. 1986;**189**(10):1355–1359.

Schmidt K, Bertani C, Martano M, Morello E, Buracco P. Reconstruction of the lower eyelid by third eyelid lateral advancement and local transposition cutaneous flap after "en bloc" resection of squamous cell carcinoma in 5 cats. *Vet Surg*. 2005;**34**(1):78–82.

Clinical Atlas of Canine and Feline Ophthalmic Disease, First Edition. Douglas Esson.

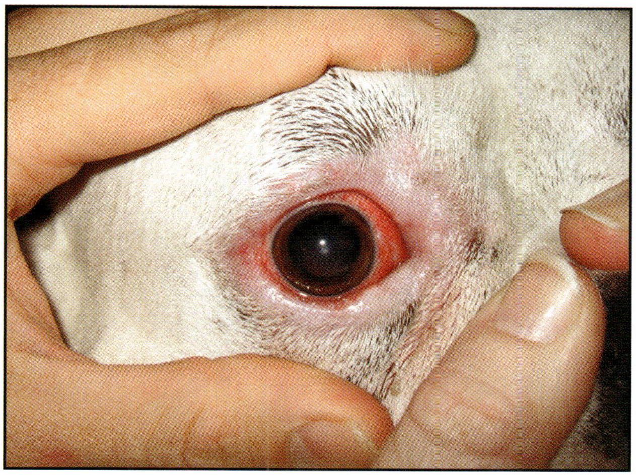

Figure 34.1 Erosive lower eyelid squamous cell carcinoma affecting a canine patient.

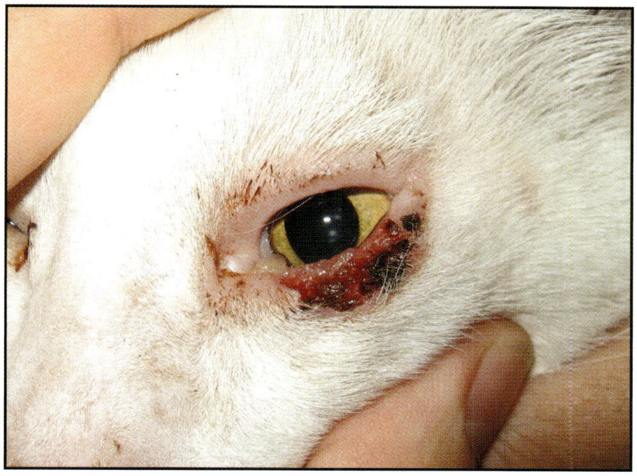

Figure 34.2 Erosive lower eyelid squamous cell carcinoma affecting a feline patient.

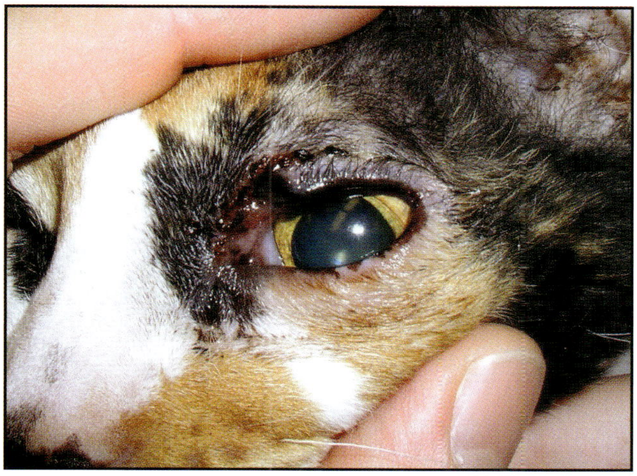

Figure 34.3 Erosive upper eyelid squamous cell carcinoma affecting a feline patient.

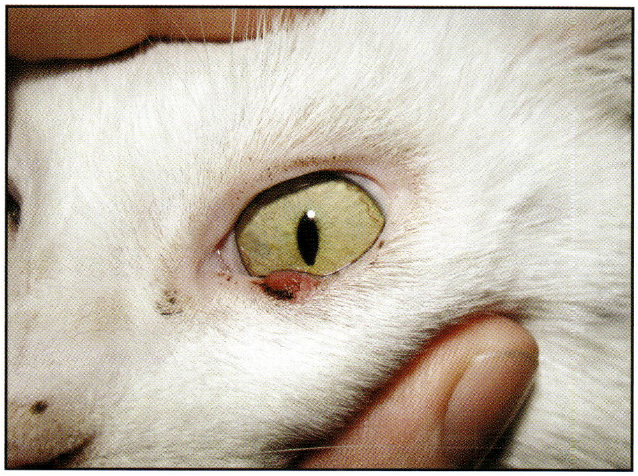

Figure 34.4 Proliferative lower eyelid squamous cell carcinoma affecting a feline patient.

CHAPTER 35
MAST CELL TUMOR (MCT)

PRESENTATION

Mast cell tumors (MCTs) are relatively common eyelid neoplasms. Lesions typically present as progressive, firm, raised masses, which may or may not ulcerate. Local extension into surrounding tissues may occur. Commonly affected breeds include the Boston Terrier, Labrador Retriever, and Boxer.

DIAGNOSIS AND TREATMENT

The diagnosis of MCT is based on representative tissue biopsy. Histopathology will confirm the diagnosis, as well as degree of malignancy of neoplasia present. Presurgical treatment using an antihistamine or corticosteroid is considered appropriate in view of the potential for neoplastic degranulation in association with manipulation. The potential for metastasis exists and staging via local lymph node aspiration, three-view radiography, and complete blood count (CBC)/chemistry analysis is recommended. Management options include wide surgical excision (where possible), local treatment with strontium, and/or external-beam (electron) radiation where appropriate.

SELECTED REFERENCES

Fife M, Blocker T, Fife T, Dubielzig RR, Dunn K. Canine conjunctival mast cell tumors: a retrospective study. *Vet Ophthalmol.* 2011;**14**(3):153–160. doi: 10.1111/j.1463-5224.2010.00857.x.

Killick DR, Rowlands AM, Burrow RD, Cripps P, Miller J, Graham P, Blackwood L. Mast cell tumour and cutaneous histiocytoma excision wound healing in general practice. *J Small Anim Pract*. 2011;**52**(9):469–475. doi: 10.1111/j.1748-5827.2011.01093.x.

Lewin G. Eyelid reconstruction in seven dogs using a split eyelid flap. *J Small Anim Pract*. 2003;**44**(8):346–351.

Roberts SM, Severin GA, Lavach JD. Prevalence and treatment of palpebral neoplasms in the dog: 200 cases (1975–1983). *J Am Vet Med Assoc*. 1986;**189**(10):1355–1359.

Clinical Atlas of Canine and Feline Ophthalmic Disease, First Edition. Douglas Esson.

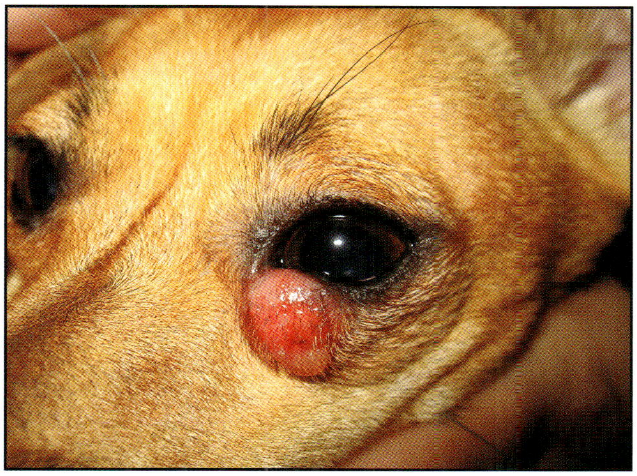

Figure 35.1 Clinical presentation associated with an eyelid mast cell tumor.

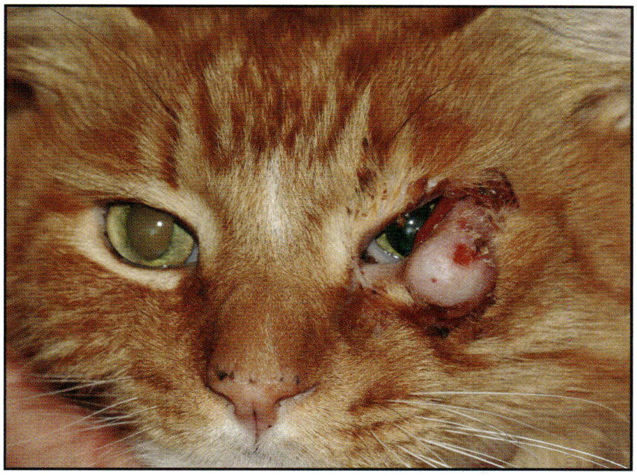

Figure 35.2 Clinical presentation associated with an eyelid mast cell tumor.

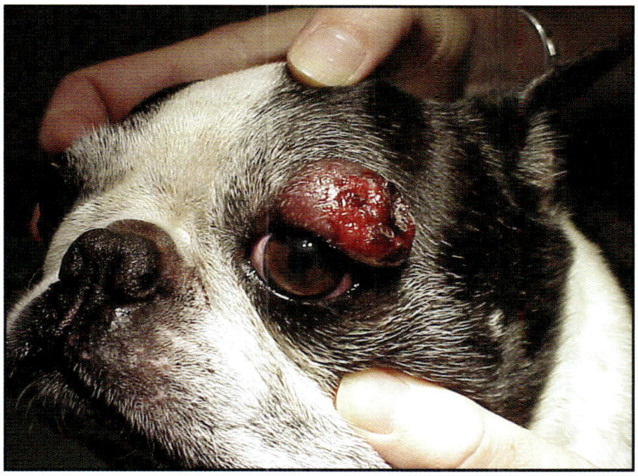

Figure 35.3 Clinical presentation associated with a significantly ulcerated eyelid mast cell tumor.

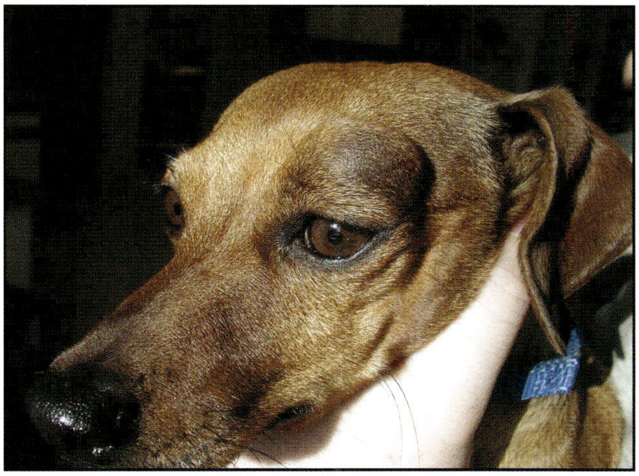

Figure 35.4 Clinical presentation associated with an eyelid mast cell tumor, displaying significant subcutaneous extension.

CHAPTER 36
FIBROSARCOMA

PRESENTATION

Fibrosarcomas represent an uncontrolled, neoplastic proliferation of fibroblasts. Large/chronic tumors affecting the eyelids frequently also involve adjacent ocular/orbital tissues. Lesions generally present as progressively enlarging, firm, poorly mobile subcutaneous swellings, which may additionally display surface ulceration. Sarcomas display varying morphological features; however, they typically behave in an aggressive and locally invasive manner. Commonly affected breeds include the Golden Retriever, Doberman Pinscher, and Rottweiler.

DIAGNOSIS AND TREATMENT

The diagnosis of fibrosarcoma is made by histologic interpretation of a representative incisional tissue biopsy. Histopathology will additionally define the degree of malignancy present. The potential for metastasis exists and staging via local lymph node aspiration, three-view radiography, and complete blood count (CBC)/chemistry analysis is recommended. Treatment comprises wide surgical excision where possible, with or without adjunctive chemotherapy. These neoplasms are generally poorly responsive to external beam radiation therapy. Cranial soft tissue imaging (magnetic resonance imaging (MRI) or computed tomography (CT)) will facilitate accurate presurgical planning where indicated. Local blepharoplastic reconstruction may be necessary following excision.

SELECTED REFERENCES

Al-Dissi AN, Haines DM, Singh B, Kidney BA. Immunohistochemical expression of vascular endothelial growth factor and vascular endothelial growth factor receptor in canine cutaneous fibrosarcomas. *J Comp Pathol.* 2009 Nov;**141**(4):229–36.

Dubielzig R *et al.* 2010. *Veterinary Ocular Pathology*, pp. 127–128, Elsevier, Edinburgh.

Frazier SA, Johns SM, Ortega J, Zwingenberger AL, Kent MS, Hammond GM, Rodriguez CO Jr, Steffey MA, Skorupski KA. Outcome in dogs with surgically resected oral fibrosarcoma (1997–2008). *Vet Comp Oncol.* 2012;**10**(1):33–43.

Clinical Atlas of Canine and Feline Ophthalmic Disease, First Edition. Douglas Esson.

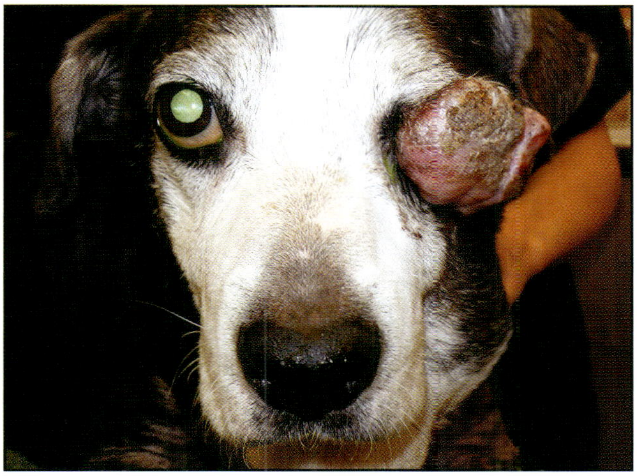

Figure 36.1 Clinical presentation associated with an eyelid fibrosarcoma.

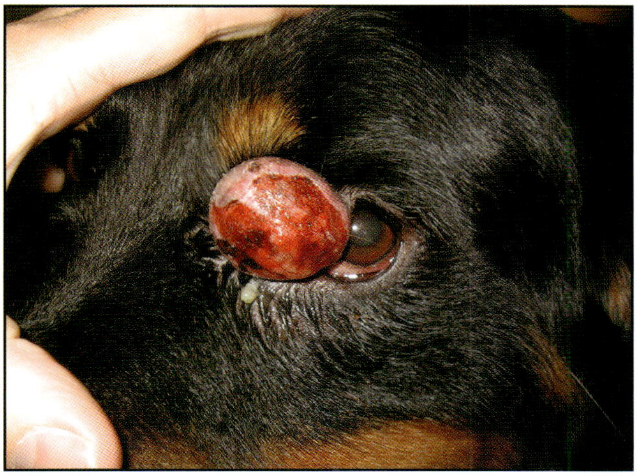

Figure 36.2 Clinical presentation associated with an eyelid fibrosarcoma.

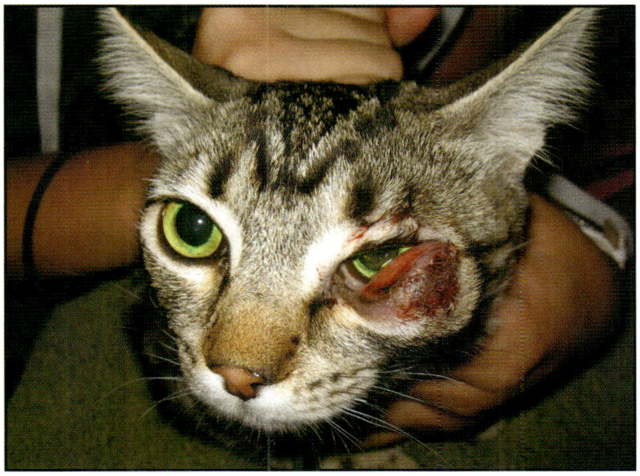

Figure 36.3 Clinical presentation associated with an eyelid fibrosarcoma.

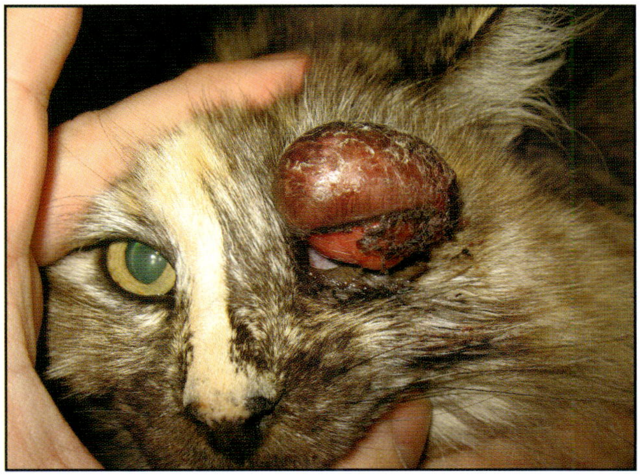

Figure 36.4 Clinical presentation associated with an eyelid fibrosarcoma.

Section 3

Diseases of the Conjunctiva, Nasolacrimal System, and Third Eyelid

CHAPTER 37
ALLERGIC CONJUNCTIVITIS

PRESENTATION

The conjunctival surfaces are richly supplied with cellular components of the immune system and represent a first line of antigenic response. As a consequence, allergic conjunctivitis is not uncommon, particularly in those patients affected by generalized dermal allergic or atopic disease. Symptoms are generally mild to moderate in severity and may include conjunctival hyperemia, chemosis, follicular proliferation, epiphora, and/or mucoid discharge. In addition, symptoms may fluctuate with generalized allergic symptoms and or seasonal allergen exposure. Commonly affected breeds include the English Bulldog and West Highland White Terrier.

DIAGNOSIS AND TREATMENT

The diagnosis of allergic conjunctivitis is typically made on the basis of a combination of clinical findings as well as the absence of significant underlying ocular abnormalities. If necessary, a conjunctival biopsy will support the diagnosis, frequently containing significantly increased numbers of mast cells. Treatment comprises the avoidance of inciting allergens where possible, the systemic management of generalized atopy where appropriate, and the application of topical anti-inflammatory therapy, the frequency, and duration of application being determined by the clinical picture. Topical steroidal therapy is frequently required, although topical nonsteroidal and/or antihistamines may also be employed in the management of this condition.

Potential Drug-Side-Effects

Potential adverse effects associated with the use of topical corticosteroids include impaired wound healing and corneal degeneration.

SELECTED REFERENCES

Bistner S. Allergic- and immunologic-mediated diseases of the eye and adnexae. *Vet Clin North Am Small Anim Pract*. 1994;**24**(4):711–734.

Glaze MB. Ocular allergy. *Semin Vet Med Surg (Small Anim)*. 1991;**6**(4):296–302.

Lourenço-Martins AM, Delgado E, Neto I, Peleteiro MC, Morais-Almeida M, Correia JH. Allergic conjunctivitis and conjunctival provocation tests in atopic dogs. *Vet Ophthalmol*. 2011;**14**(4):248–256. doi: 10.1111/j.1463-5224.2011.00874.x. Epub 2011 Apr 18.

Clinical Atlas of Canine and Feline Ophthalmic Disease, First Edition. Douglas Esson.

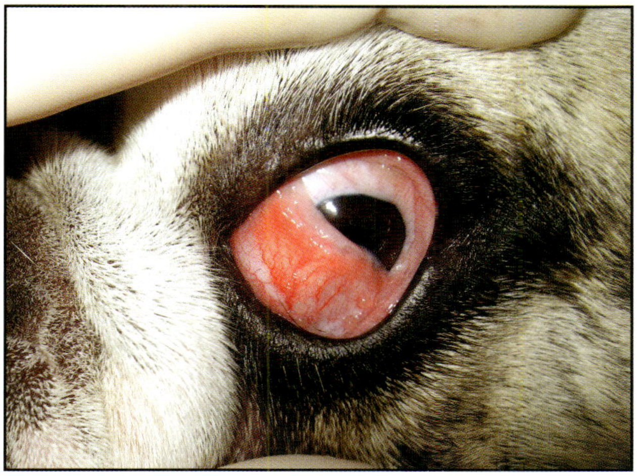

Figure 37.1 Clinical presentation associated with allergic conjunctivitis. Follicular proliferation is evident.

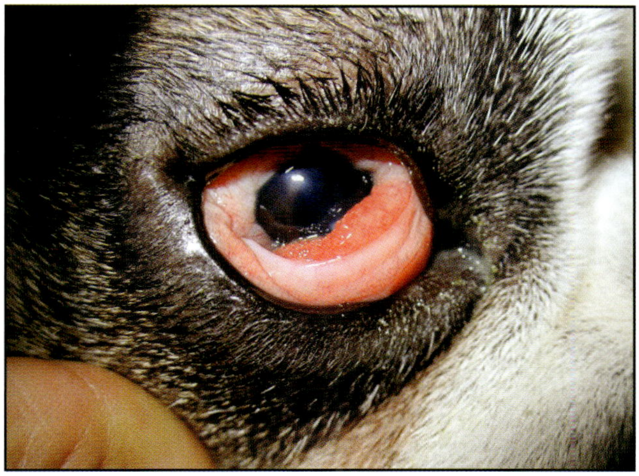

Figure 37.2 Clinical presentation associated with allergic conjunctivitis. Thickening of the third eyelid is present.

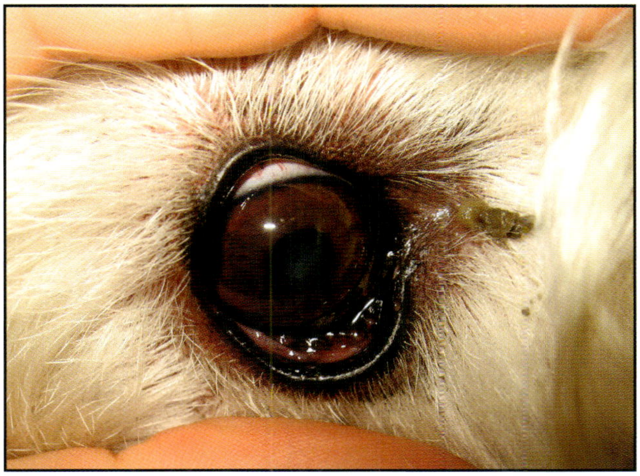

Figure 37.3 Clinical presentation associated with allergic conjunctivitis. Follicular proliferation is evident.

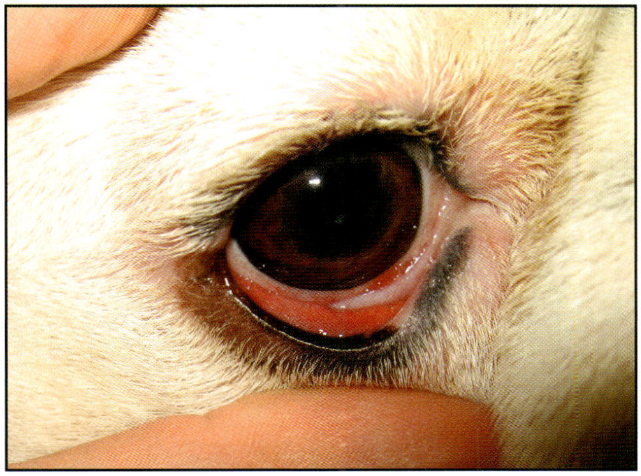

Figure 37.4 Clinical presentation associated with allergic conjunctivitis.

CHAPTER 38
DACRYOCYSTITIS

PRESENTATION

Dacryocystitis describes inflammation of the nasolacrimal drainage structures, which comprise the eyelid puncta, lacrimal canaliculi, lacrimal cavern and the sinonasal ducts that exit to the external nares. Inflammation of the nasolacrimal system may be the result of bacterial infection, extension of inflammation from adjacent structures, neoplasia, or entrapment of foreign material. Primary aplasia or hypoplasia of any part of this system may also occur, typically manifesting in young animals. Postinflammatory scarring and fibrosis is a common cause of nasolacrimal non-patency, particularly in cats previously affected by herpesviral-associated inflammation. Chronic inflammation or obstruction of the nasolacrimal ducts may also result in cystic dilation. Clinical symptoms of dacryocystitis may include conjunctivitis, fornix-based mucoid to purulent discharge, and localized swelling and/or discomfort over any part of the nasolacrimal duct system, particularly around the medial canthal region. Symptoms are typically unilateral. Both canine and feline species of any breed or mixed breed may be affected.

DIAGNOSIS AND TREATMENT

The diagnosis of dacryocystitis is made on the basis of clinical symptoms, and/or the presence of mucopurulent material noted to be arising from the nasolacrimal puncta. Nasolacrimal drainage may be impaired or absent on the affected side, marked by a negative "Jones test" such that fluorescein dye instilled into the fornix fails to exit at the ipsilateral external nares within 10–15 min. Further investigation of dacryocystitis may include sampling for cytology as well as culture and sensitivity testing, contrast radiography, and/or soft tissue imaging via magnetic resonance imaging (MRI) or computed tomography (CT). Medical therapy using topical and/or systemic antimicrobial and/or anti-inflammatory agents as well as cannulation, irrigation, stenting, and/or surgical exploration may be indicated on the basis of the severity of disease, diagnostic findings, and response to therapy. In extreme cases, the creation of alternate drainage via surgical conjunctivorhinostomy or conjunctivobuccostomy is possible; however, this is rarely indicated.

SELECTED REFERENCES

Giuliano EA, Pope ER, Champagne ES, Moore CP. Dacryocystomaxillorhinostomy for chronic dacryocystitis in a dog. *Vet Ophthalmol.* 2006;**9**(2):89–94.

Murphy JM, Severin GA, Lavach JD. Nasolacrimal catheterization for treating chronic dacryocystitis. *Vet Med Small Anim Clin.* 1977 May;**72**(5):883–887.

Singh A, Cullen CL, Gelens H, Grahn BH. Diagnostic Ophthalmology. *Left dacryocystitis with naso-lacrimal duct obstruction. Can Vet J.* 2004;**45**(11):953–955.

van der Woerdt A, Wilkie DA, Gilger BC, Smeak DD, Kerpsack SJ. Surgical treatment of dacryocystitis caused by cystic dilatation of the nasolacrimal system in three dogs. *J Am Vet Med Assoc.* 1997;**211**(4):445–447.

Clinical Atlas of Canine and Feline Ophthalmic Disease, First Edition. Douglas Esson.

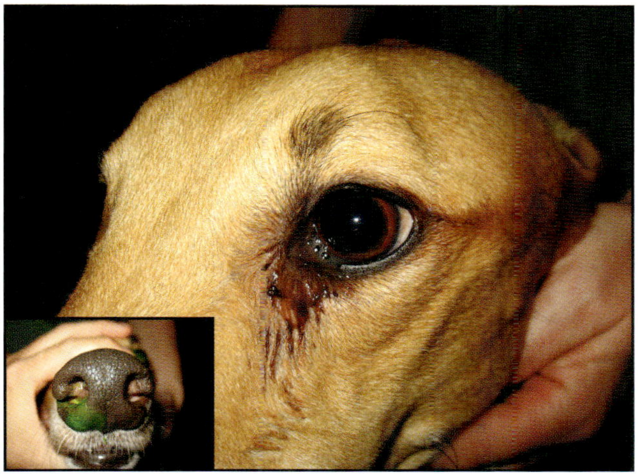

Figure 38.1 Clinical presentation associated with dacryocystitis. Inset indicates a negative "Jones test" with fluorescein dye failing to exit the external nares on the affected side as a result of nasolacrimal obstruction.

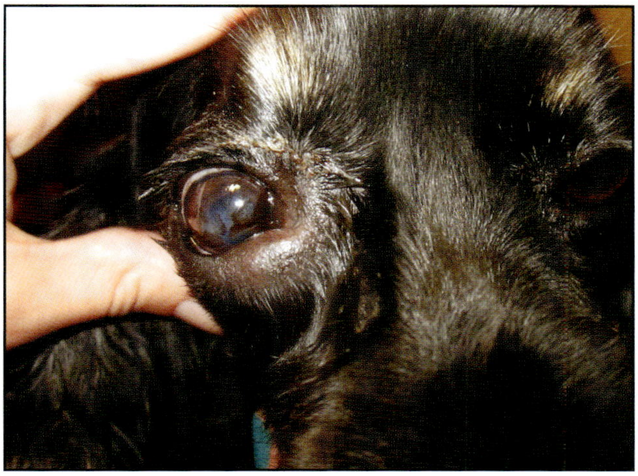

Figure 38.2 Clinical presentation associated with dacryocystitis. A fluctuant swelling of the medial canthus in association with inflammation of the lacrimal cavern is present.

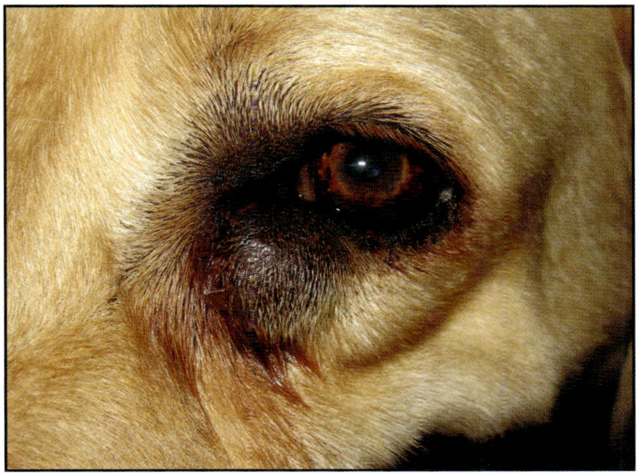

Figure 38.3 Clinical presentations associated with dacryocystitis. A fluctuant swelling of the medial canthus in association with inflammation of the lacrimal cavern is present.

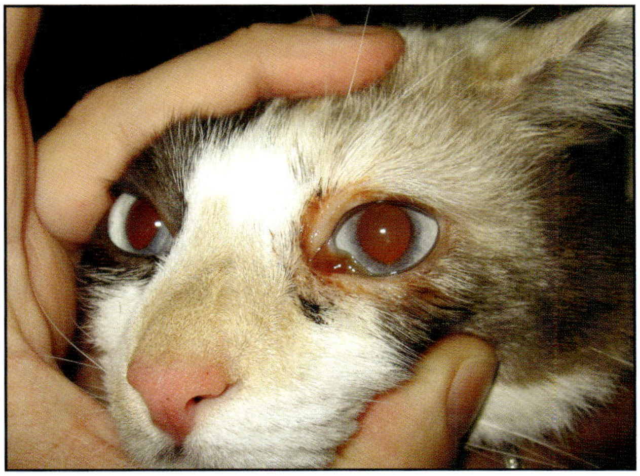

Figure 38.4 Clinical presentations associated with dacryocystitis. Discharge is arising from the nasolacrimal puncta.

CHAPTER 39
SYMBLEPHARON

PRESENTATION

Symblepharon describes varying degrees of adhesion between adjacent conjunctival surfaces (including palpebral and/or third eyelid surfaces) and/or the cornea. Clinically, varying degrees of fibrosing and/or pigmentary tissue are noted to extend across palpebral and/or corneal surfaces. Conjunctivitis, chemosis, and/or ocular discharge may additionally be present. Significant narrowing of the palpebral fissure and/or occlusion of the corneal surface may also result. Symblepharon results from loss of epithelial continuity, most commonly arising secondary to feline herpesviral disease but potentially arising secondary to any severe feline or canine conjunctival inflammation (see also Herpesviral-Associated Conjunctivitis).

DIAGNOSIS AND TREATMENT

The diagnosis of symblepharon is made based on clinical findings. Treatment comprises addressing conjunctival inflammation as well as underlying viral and/or bacterial disease. Surgical resection of conjunctival adhesions is relatively straightforward; however, the tendency for the aggressive (potentially aggravated) reformation of these adhesions is extremely high. The potential benefits of surgical intervention should consequently be carefully considered before proceeding. Surgery should not be undertaken in actively inflamed or infected eyes. The use of silicone surgical barriers to prevent re-adhesion before re-epithelialization as well as the judicious use of antimicrobial and/or anti-inflammatory agents (generally nonsteroidal in nature) may help maximize long-term success.

SELECTED REFERENCES

Jacobi S, Dubielzig RR. Feline early life ocular disease. *Vet Ophthalmol.* 2008;**11**(3):166–169.

Andrew SE. Ocular manifestations of feline herpesvirus. *J Feline Med Surg*. 2001;**3**(1):9–16. Review.

Nasisse MP. Feline herpesvirus ocular disease. *Vet Clin North Am Small Anim Pract*. 1990;**20**(3):667–680.

Clinical Atlas of Canine and Feline Ophthalmic Disease, First Edition. Douglas Esson.

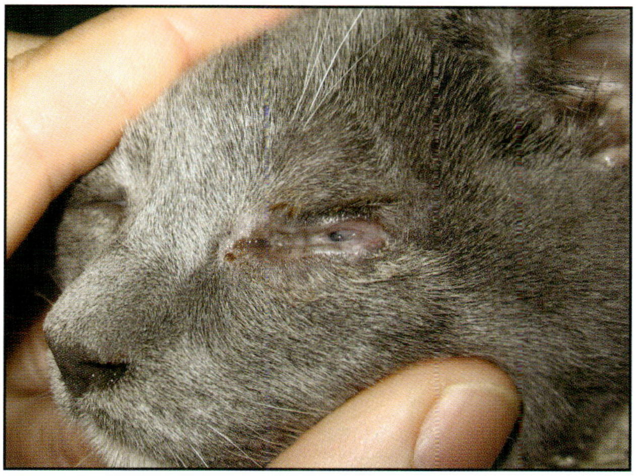

Figure 39.1 Clinical presentation associated with feline symblepharon.

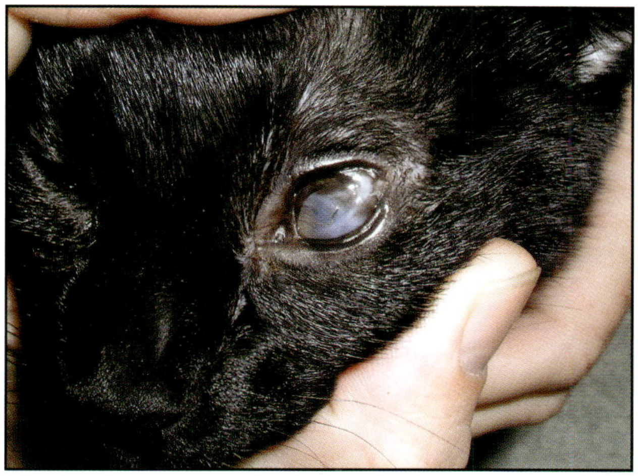

Figure 39.2 Clinical presentation associated with feline symblepharon.

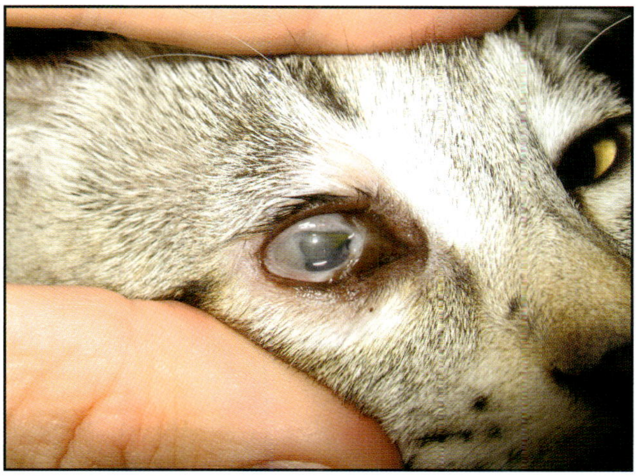

Figure 39.3 Clinical presentation associated with feline symblepharon.

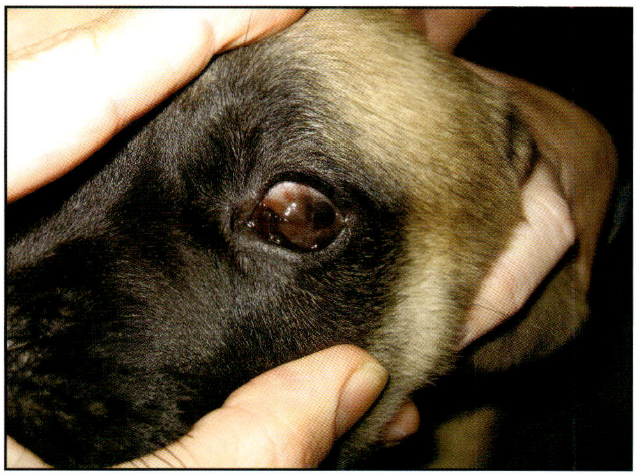

Figure 39.4 Clinical presentation associated with canine symblepharon.

CHAPTER 40
HERPESVIRAL-ASSOCIATED CONJUNCTIVITIS

PRESENTATION

Herpesviral ocular disease is highly prevalent, resulting predominantly from animal-to-animal contact, frequently via aerosolization of sneezed particles. Affected animals may display a range of symptoms including sneezing, coughing, nasal discharge, pyrexia, inappetance, lethargy, conjunctivitis, chemosis, keratitis, and/or secondary corneal ulceration (see also Herpesviral-Associated Keratitis). Young kittens are generally most severely affected, immune-competent adult cats generally exhibiting less severe symptoms. Feline patients may additionally be infected with secondary pathogens including *calicivirus*, *Chlamydophila felis*, *mycoplasma sp*., and/or bacterial pathogens. Herpes viral disease (CHV-1) should additionally be considered when investigating similar symptoms in canine patients. Other canine pathogens including *Canine adenovirus 2* (CAV-2), *Bordatella bronchiseptica*, *Canine influenza virus* (H3N8), canine parainfluenza virus, and *mycoplasma sp* should also be considered when investigating the potential role of canine herpes virus in ocular surface disease. Once a patient becomes infected, alphaherpes viral particles remain latent, with the ability to recrudesce under conditions of physiologic or pharmacologic stress (including the inappropriate administration of immunosuppressive agents). As a consequence, particular caution should be employed when considering the administration of long-acting or "depot" formulations of corticosteroids to patients who may be affected by herpesviral disease.

DIAGNOSIS AND TREATMENT

Accurate testing for the presence of FHV-1 and its correlation with ophthalmic disease is challenging; however, polymerase-chain-reaction assays, based on tissue samples, are currently considered most reliable. Ultimately, healthy cats recover spontaneously from outbreaks over the course of several weeks; however, treatment is frequently indicated. Topical and/or systemic antiviral agents may be administered, including trifluorothymidine, idoxuridine, cidofovir, and ganciclovir and/or famciclovir (metabolized to penciclovir).

Potential Drug-Side-Effects

Potential complications associated with the use of topical antiviral agents include local irritation. Potential complications associated with the use of systemic antiviral medications include gastrointestinal (GI) distress, myelosuppression, and/or hepatopathy. Potential adverse effects associated with tetracyclines and azithromycin include GI distress, photosensitivity, and hepatic damage. Potential adverse effects associated with fluoroquinolones include GI distress, hepatic disease, neurologic disease, and/or retinal toxicity.

The concurrent administration of systemic L-lysine may decrease the severity of symptoms in cats, potentially via the inhibition of herpesviral metabolism. Extreme caution is indicated when considering the use of anti-inflammatory therapy to treat herpesviral-associated disease. Nonsteroidal agents are generally considered less likely to result in complication and the use of corticosteroids are considered contraindicated in most cases. Tetracyclines, azithromycin, and fluoroquinolones represent appropriate antimicrobial choices when treating potentially complicated cases.

SELECTED REFERENCES

Ledbetter EC, Hornbuckle WE, Dubovi EJ. Virologic survey of dogs with naturally acquired idiopathic conjunctivitis. *J Am Vet Med Assoc*. 2009;**235**(8):954–959.

Maggs DJ. Update on pathogenesis, diagnosis, and treatment of feline herpesvirus type 1. *Clin Tech Small Anim Pract*. 2005;**20**(2):94–101.

Maggs DJ. Antiviral therapy for feline herpesvirus infections. *Vet Clin North Am Small Anim Pract*. 2010 Nov;**40**(6):1055–1062. DOI: 10.1016/j.cvsm.2010.07.010.

Thomasy SM, Lim CC, Reilly CM, Kass PH, Lappin MR, Maggs DJ. Evaluation of orally administered famciclovir in cats experimentally infected with feline herpesvirus type-1. *Am J Vet Res*. 2011;**72**(1):85–95. DOI: 10.2460/ajvr.72.1.85.

Clinical Atlas of Canine and Feline Ophthalmic Disease, First Edition. Douglas Esson.

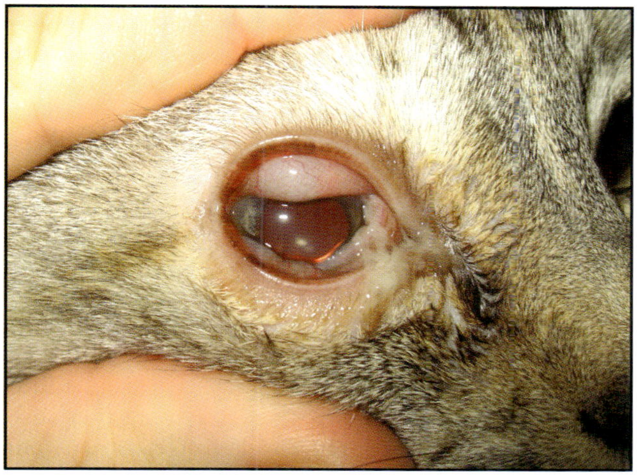

Figure 40.1 Clinical presentation associated with herpesviral disease in a feline patient. Significant chemosis and ocular discharge are present.

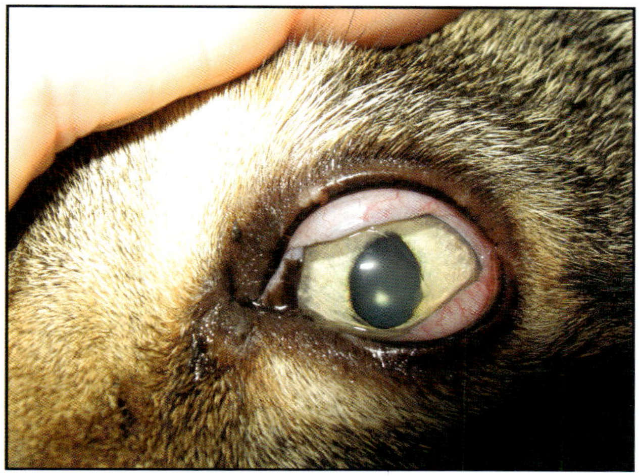

Figure 40.2 Clinical presentation associated with herpesviral disease in a feline patient. Significant chemosis is present.

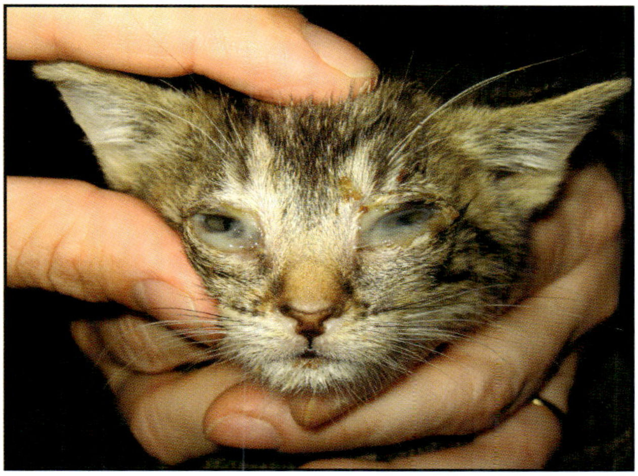

Figure 40.3 Clinical presentation associated with herpesviral disease in a young feline patient. Significant ocular discharge is present.

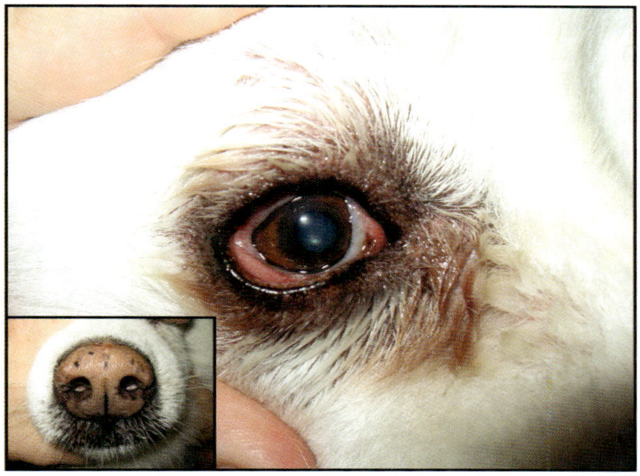

Figure 40.4 Clinical presentation associated with herpesviral disease in a canine patient. Moderate chemosis is present. Inset shows serous nasal discharge.

CHAPTER 41
THIRD EYELID GLAND PROLAPSE (CHERRY EYE)

PRESENTATION

Prolapse of the lacrimal gland of the third eyelid ("cherry eye") is relatively commonly encountered. Glandular prolapse arises as a result of defective connective tissue development and consequent glandular laxity in predisposed breeds. Partial or complete prolapse of the lacrimal gland of the third eyelid, presents as a smooth pink to red tissue mass, which protrudes from the posterior surface of one or both third eyelids. Third eyelid gland prolapse typically affects young animals. Associated symptoms may include conjunctivitis, ocular discharge, and/or decreased lacrimal function as well as secondary ulcerative keratitis. Severe secondary inflammation and or bacterial infection may develop, particularly in cases of chronic glandular prolapse. Commonly affected canine breeds include the English Bulldog, Cocker Spaniel, and Shih Tzu. This condition may also affect feline patients, with the Burmese breed being most frequently noted.

DIAGNOSIS AND TREATMENT

The ideal treatment represents surgical repositioning of prolapsed tissue. The excision of prolapsed glandular tissue should be avoided where possible, in order to avoid subsequent complications. Several techniques for repair have been described, with the "Morgan pocket" technique being most generally appropriate. Sufficient blunt dissection and the creation of a pocket into which glandular tissue can be replaced as well as the use of absorbable suture material and avoidance of knots on the bulbar surface of the third eyelid will maximize the likelihood of surgical success. More challenging cases such as those associated with chronic or severe prolapse, severe inflammation, and/or previously failed surgical intervention may be repaired via a variety of techniques that anchor prolapsed tissue to scleral or orbital tissues. Postoperative care comprises routine systemic antimicrobial (if indicated), anti-inflammatory, and analgesic care. An Elizabethan collar should be placed in order to prevent self-trauma and corneal health should be frequently monitored until third eyelid healing is complete.

SELECTED REFERENCES

Chahory S, Crasta M, Trio S, Clerc B. Three cases of prolapse of the nictitans gland in cats. *Vet Ophthalmol.* 2004;**7**(6):417–419.

Dugan SJ, Severin GA, Hungerford LL, Whiteley HE, Roberts SM. Clinical and histologic evaluation of the prolapsed third eyelid gland in dogs. *J Am Vet Med Assoc.* 1992;**201**(12):1861–1867.

Mazzucchelli S, Vaillant MD, Wéverberg F, Arnold-Tavernier H, Honegger N, Payen G, Vanore M, Liscoet L, Thomas O, Clerc B, Chahory S. Retrospective study of 155 cases of prolapse of the nictitating membrane gland in dogs. *Vet Rec.* 2012;**170**(17):443.

Clinical Atlas of Canine and Feline Ophthalmic Disease, First Edition. Douglas Esson.

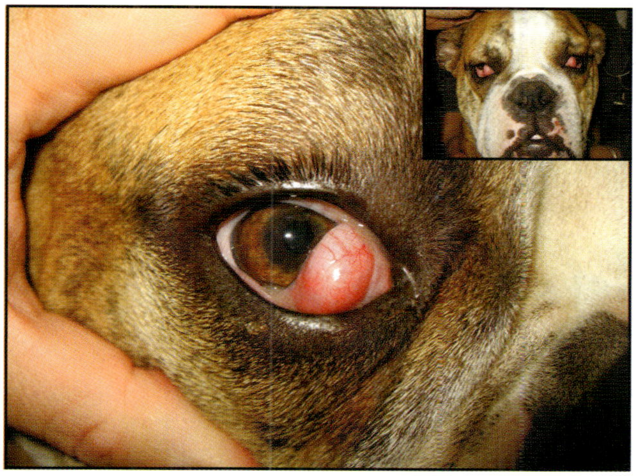

Figure 41.1 Clinical presentation associated with prolapse of the gland of the third eyelid ("cherry eye"). Inset demonstrates the frequently bilateral presentation of this condition.

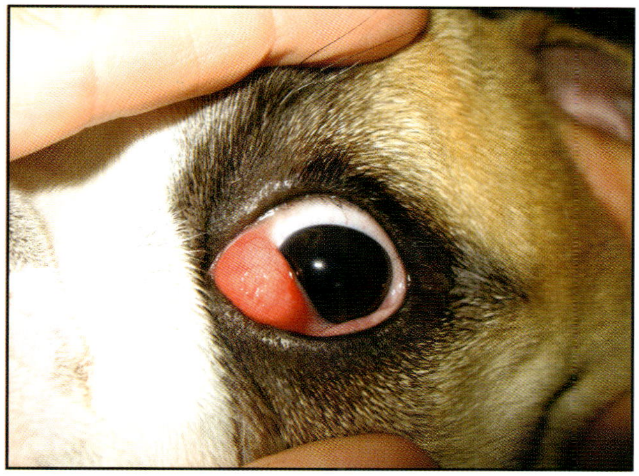

Figure 41.2 Clinical presentation associated with prolapse of the gland of the third eyelid ("cherry eye").

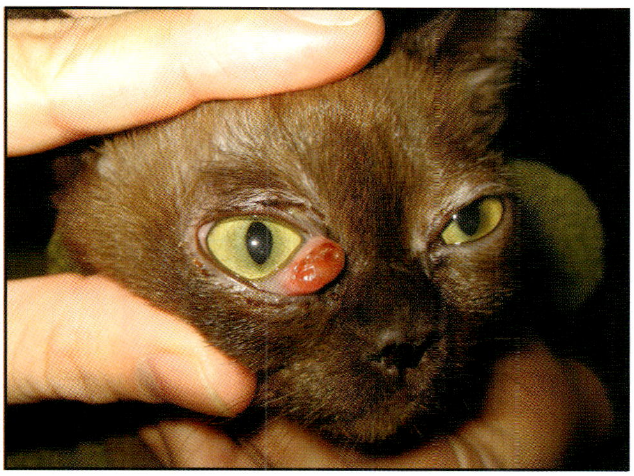

Figure 41.3 Clinical presentation associated with prolapse of the gland of the third eyelid ("cherry eye").

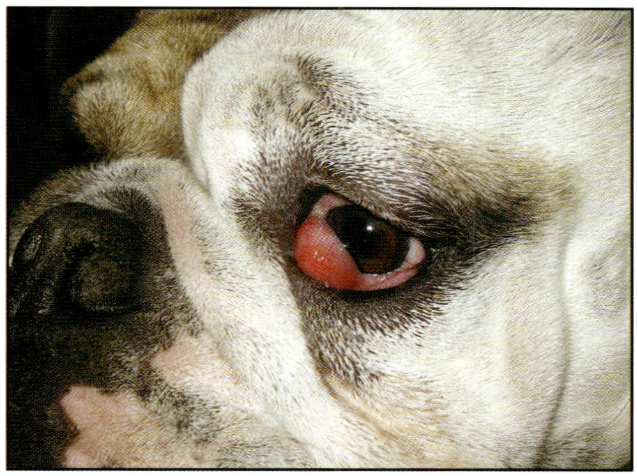

Figure 41.4 Clinical presentation associated with prolapse of the gland of the third eyelid ("cherry eye").

CHAPTER 42
KERATOCONJUNCTIVITIS SICCA (DRY EYE)

PRESENTATION

The pre-corneal tear film (PCTF) comprises an outer lipid, central aqueous, and inner mucoid component. Lipid and mucoid components are secreted by the eyelid and conjunctival glands, respectively. The aqueous portion of the PCTF is secreted by the lacrimal glands of the orbit and third eyelid. Keratoconjunctivitis sicca (KCS) may represent a qualitative deficiency resulting from insufficient lipid and/or mucous secretion and/or quantitative deficiency arising secondary to insufficient lacrimal gland secretion. Glandular dysfunction may arise secondary to immune-mediated, traumatic, inflammatory, toxic, or neurological etiologies. Pharmacological agents with the potential to cause or exacerbate KCS include etodolac and sulpha-containing antimicrobial compounds. Symptoms of KCS typically include conjunctivitis, vascular/pigmentary keratitis, secondary meibomian gland inflammation/infection, and the accumulation of green-/yellow-colored mucous in and around the fornices. Symptoms may be unilateral or bilateral, their severity correlating with the degree of tear film dysfunction. Commonly affected breeds include the English Bulldog, West Highland White Terrier and Cavalier King Charles Spaniel.

DIAGNOSIS AND TREATMENT

Qualitative KCS is diagnosed on the basis of abnormal tear films break-up times (BUTs). This represents the time taken for surface tension to break down across the corneal surface following the application of fluorescein dye and the manual opening of the eyelids. A BUT of less than 20 s is generally considered to be abnormally shortened. Quantitative KCS is diagnosed on the basis of decreased Schirmer tear test (STT) values, measured by placing graded strips into the ventral fornix for 1 min. Values of less than 15 mm/wetting per minute are generally considered suspect and those less than 10 mm, generally considered diagnostic of KCS. Values of 0 mm/wetting define “absolute” KCS and represent particularly challenging clinical cases (see also Neurogenic KCS & Xeromycteria). Treatment comprises a combination of lacrimo-stimulant and/or anti-inflammatory agents and long-term therapy is typically necessary. Lacrimo-stimulant agents include the immunosuppressive fungal cell wall extracts cyclosporine and tacrolimus. The administration of oral pilocarpine may help reestablish lacrimal function in cases of neurologic dysfunction. Anti-inflammatory agents typically encompass topical steroid agents. Secondary eyelid and/or meibomian gland inflammation/infection should be addressed where present. The ruling out of underlying endocrinopathies has been advocated. In unusually severe cases or those which fail to respond to appropriate therapy, surgical intervention in the form of parotid duct transposition may be considered; however. this procedure may be associated with a range of postoperative complications.

Potential Drug-Side-Effects

Potential adverse effects associated with the use of topical cyclosporine and tacrolimus include periocular dermatitis and alopecia. Potential adverse effects associated with the use of topical corticosteroids include impaired wound healing and corneal degeneration. Potential side effects associated with the use of oral pilocaripine include gastrointestinal (GI) distress.

SELECTED REFERENCES

Hendrix DV, Adkins EA, Ward DA, Stuffle J, Skorobohach B. An investigation comparing the efficacy of topical ocular application of tacrolimus and cyclosporine in dogs. *Vet Med Int.* 2011;**2011**:487592. DOI: 10.4061/2011/487592. Epub 2011 May 23.

Klauss G, Giuliano EA, Moore CP, Stuhr CM, Martin SL, Tyler JW, Fitzgerald KE, Crawford DA. Keratoconjunctivitis sicca associated with administration of etodolac in dogs: 211 cases (1992–2002). *J Am Vet Med Assoc.* 2007;**230**(4):541–547.

Matheis FL, Walser-Reinhardt L, Spiess BM. Canine neurogenic Keratoconjunctivitis sicca: 11 cases (2006–2010). *Vet Ophthalmol.* 2012;**15**(4):288–290. DOI: 10.1111/j.1463-5224.2011.00968.x. Epub 2011 Oct 31.

Williams DL. Immunopathogenesis of keratoconjunctivitis sicca in the dog. *Vet Clin North Am Small Anim Pract.* 2008;**38**(2):251–268, vi. DOI: 10.1016/j.cvsm.2007.12.002.

Clinical Atlas of Canine and Feline Ophthalmic Disease, First Edition. Douglas Esson.

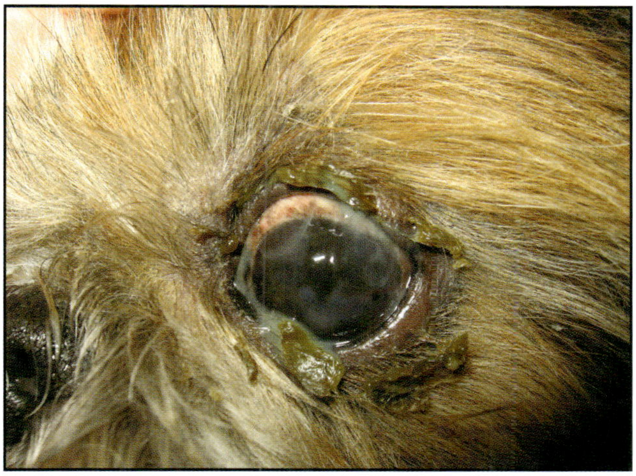

Figure 42.1 Typical clinical presentation associated with keratoconjunctivitis sicca ("dry eye"), including accumulated mucoid discharge, conjunctivitis and vascular pigmentary keratitis.

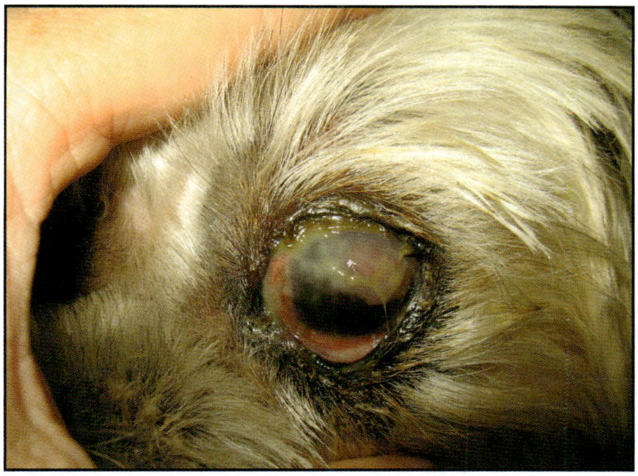

Figure 42.2 Typical clinical presentation associated with keratoconjunctivitis sicca ("dry eye"), including accumulated mucoid discharge, conjunctivitis and vascular pigmentary keratitis.

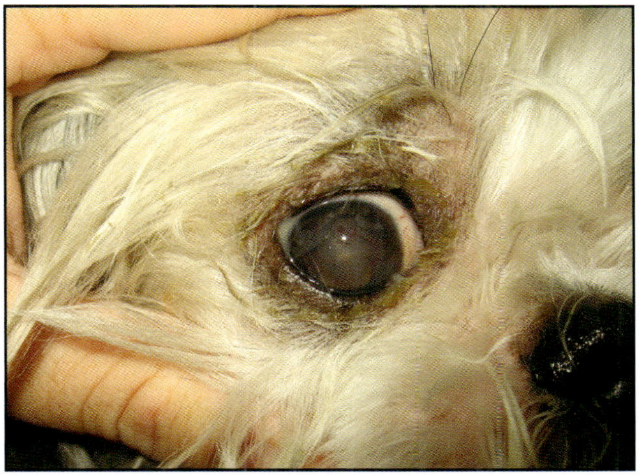

Figure 42.3 Typical clinical presentation associated with keratoconjunctivitis sicca ("dry eye"), including accumulated mucoid discharge, conjunctivitis and vascular pigmentary keratitis.

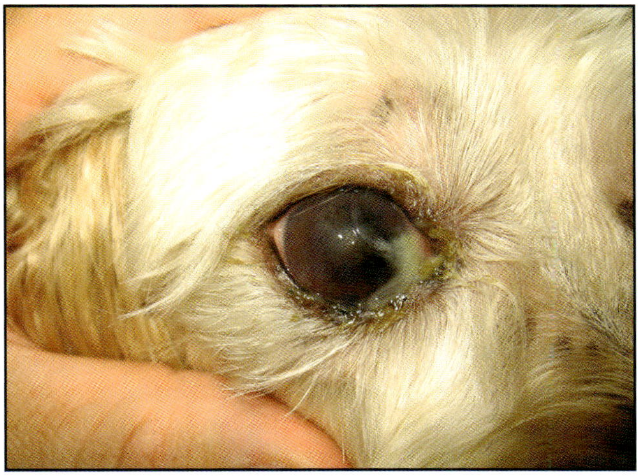

Figure 42.4 Typical clinical presentation associated with keratoconjunctivitis sicca ("dry eye"), including accumulated mucoid discharge, conjunctivitis and vascular pigmentary keratitis.

CHAPTER 43
SCROLLED THIRD EYELID CARTILAGE

PRESENTATION

The third eyelid is supported by a "T-shaped" cartilaginous structure. Occasionally, this cartilage may be malformed, typically resulting in bending or "scrolling" of the leading edge of the third eyelid and consequent eversion of these tissues away from the ocular surface. This condition is generally congenital and may be unilateral or bilateral. Secondary conjunctivitis and/or partial prolapse of the third eyelid lacrimal gland ("cherry eye") may be associated with scrolling of the third eyelid cartilage. The Great Dane is commonly affected.

DIAGNOSIS AND TREATMENT

The diagnosis is made on the basis of careful inspection of the third eyelid structures. When indicated, treatment comprises the surgical resection of malformed cartilage. In skilled hands, the prognosis for repair is excellent; however, significant potential exists for postoperative complications associated with inappropriate cartilage resection or apposition as well as the subsequent abrasion of incorrectly placed suture material against the corneal surface. Postoperative care comprises routine systemic antimicrobial (if indicated), anti-inflammatory, and analgesic care. An Elizabethan collar should be placed in order to prevent self-trauma and corneal health should be frequently monitored until eyelid healing is complete.

SELECTED REFERENCES

Allbaugh RA, Stuhr CM. Thermal cautery of the canine third eyelid for treatment of cartilage eversion. *Vet Ophthalmol.* 2013;**16**(5):392–395.

Mañé MC, Vives MA, Barrera R, Bascuas JA. Results and histological development of various surgical techniques for correcting eversion of the third eyelid in dogs. *Histol Histopathol.* 1990;**5**(4):415–425.

Williams D, Middleton S, Caldwell A. Everted third eyelid cartilage in a cat: a case report and literature review. *Vet Ophthalmol.* 2012;**15**(2):123–127. doi: 10.1111/j.1463-5224.2011.00945.x. Epub 2011 Oct 7.

Clinical Atlas of Canine and Feline Ophthalmic Disease, First Edition. Douglas Esson.

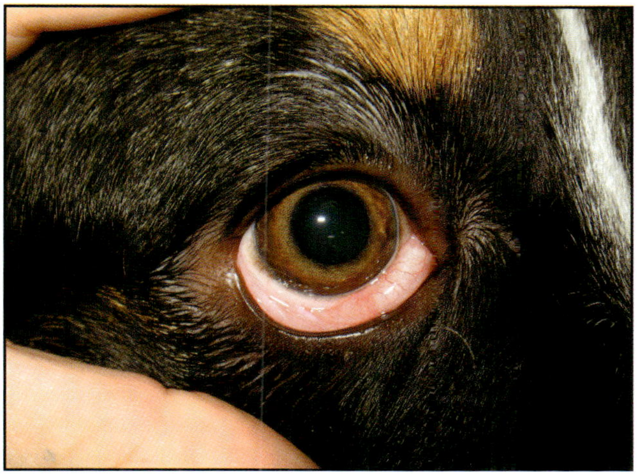

Figure 43.1 Scrolled third eyelid cartilage (canine).

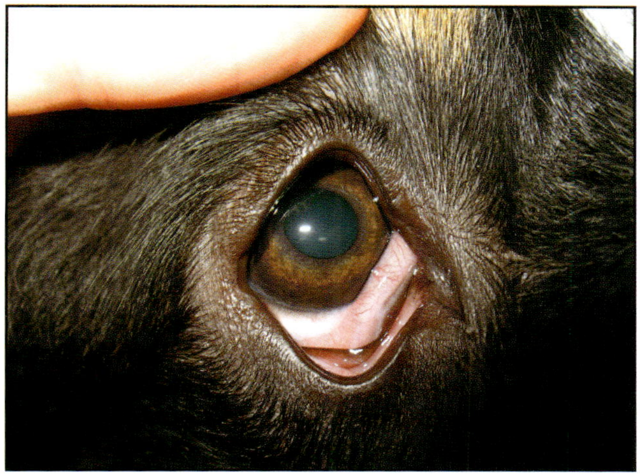

Figure 43.2 Scrolled third eyelid cartilage (canine).

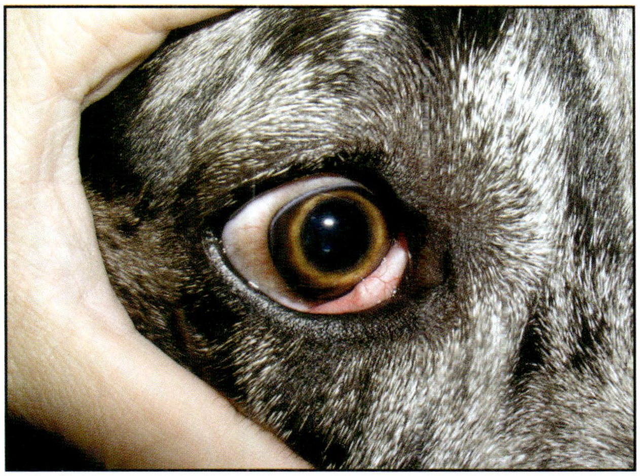

Figure 43.3 Scrolled third eyelid cartilage (canine).

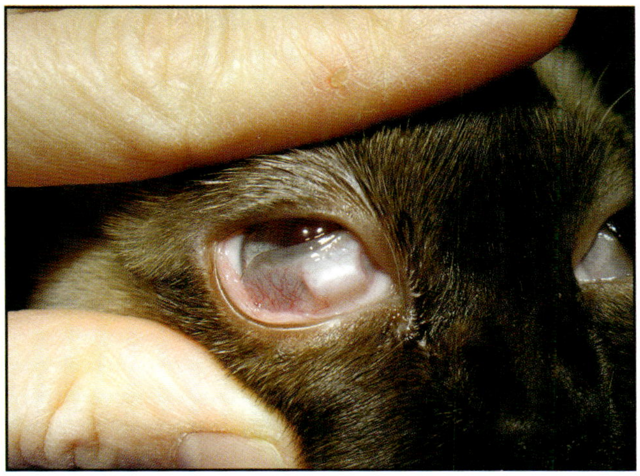

Figure 43.4 Scrolled third eyelid cartilage (feline).

CHAPTER 44
MEDIAL CANTHAL POCKET SYNDROME

PRESENTATION

Medial canthal pocket syndrome describes a relatively common presentation, particularly associated with breeds displaying deep orbits and narrow skulls such that microdebris collects in the ventral conjunctival fold or "pocket." Clinically, this condition presents as low-grade, chronic, follicular conjunctivitis affecting both the ventral palpebral fornix and tissues of the third eyelid. Mild-to-moderate associated mucoid ocular discharge is typically present and dried discharge may additionally accumulate around the medial canthus. Symptoms may be exacerbated by seasonal/atopic dermatitis. Commonly affected breeds include the Standard Poodle and Afghan Hound.

DIAGNOSIS AND TREATMENT

Treatment of this condition typically involves management rather than cure. Frequent flushing of debris and discharge from the conjunctival fornix using an ophthalmic irrigating solution as well as the application of topical anti-inflammatory agents (such as cyclosporine and/or corticosteroids) is indicated.

Potential Drug-Side-Effects

Potential adverse affects associated with the use of cyclosporine include hypersensitivity and gastrointestinal (GI) distress. Potential adverse effects associated with the use of topical corticosteroids include impaired wound healing and corneal degeneration.

Treatment may need to be continued for a significant period of time or indefinitely in select cases.

SELECTED REFERENCES

Hendrix DVH 1991. Diseases and surgery of the canine conjunctiva. In: *Veterinary Ophthalmology*, 3rd ed., Gelatt KN (Ed.), Lippincott Williams & Wilkins.

Rubin LF. 1989. *Inherited Eye Diseases in Purebred Dogs*, Williams & Wilkins, Baltimore.

Turner SM. 2008. Medial canthal pocket syndrome. In: *Small Animal Ophthalmology*.

Clinical Atlas of Canine and Feline Ophthalmic Disease, First Edition. Douglas Esson.

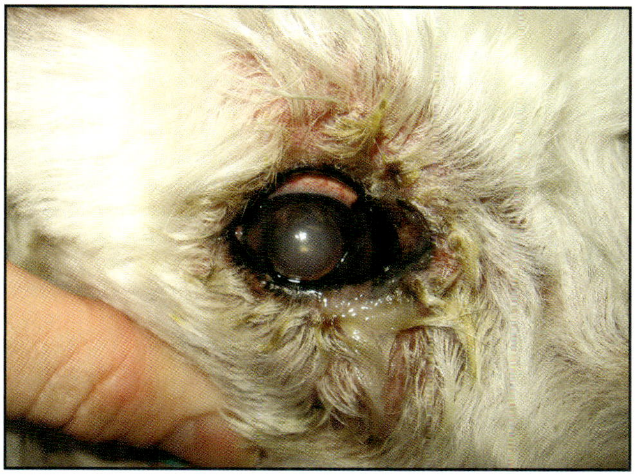

Figure 44.1 Clinical presentation associated with medial canthal pocket syndrome.

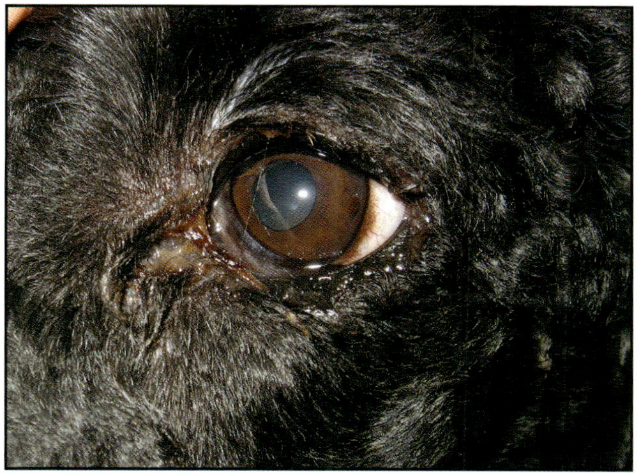

Figure 44.2 Clinical presentation associated with medial canthal pocket syndrome.

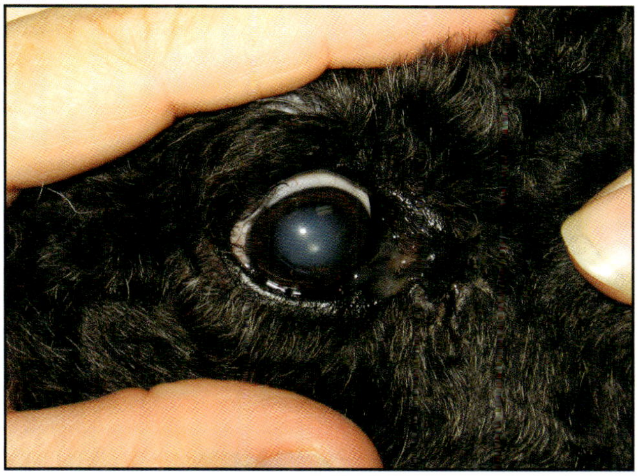

Figure 44.3 Clinical presentation associated with medial canthal pocket syndrome.

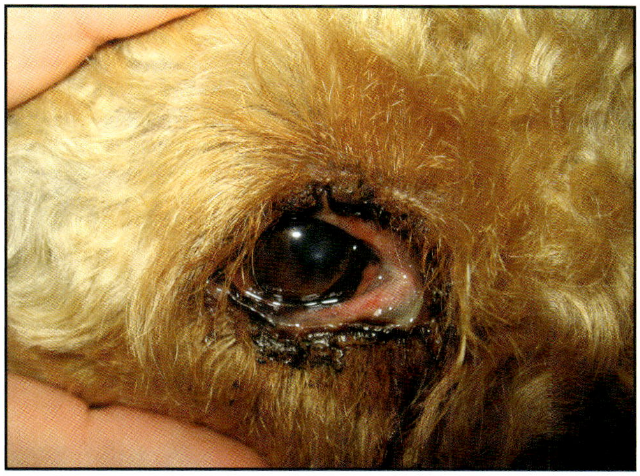

Figure 44.4 Clinical presentation associated with medial canthal pocket syndrome. This chronic and severe case has developed secondary erosive blepharitis.

CHAPTER 45
ONCHOCERCIASIS

PRESENTATION

Onchocerciasis represents a filarial nematode parasitic infection of the ocular and periocular tissues, which may affect dogs. Infection with *Onchocerca lupi* and *Onchocerca lienalis* has been described. This parasite cycles through a definitive wild host, adults mating to produce microfilariae, which may be vectored by either *Simulium* sp or *Culicoides* sp flies. Clinically, onchocerciasis may present as any combination of ocular discharge, blepharospasm, conjunctivitis, chemosis, episclerokeratitis, uveitis, and/or parasite-containing granulomas affecting the episcleral or periocular tissues.

DIAGNOSIS AND TREATMENT

The diagnosis of onchocerciasis is made on the basis of the identification of parasites and/or biopsy specimens. Treatment comprises

- surgical removal of granulomas (with or without adult parasites)
- systemic anti-inflammatory therapy (typically using corticosteroids)
- systemic antimicrobial therapy to destroy endosymbiotic *Wolbachia* sp (typically using tetracyclines)
- adulticide therapy (typically using melarsomine daily for 2 days immediately postoperatively)
- microfilaricide therapy (typically using a single dose of ivermectin 1 month following surgery, representing off-label use of this product).

Potential Drug-Side-Effects

Potential adverse effects associated with tetracyclines include gastrointestinal (GI) distress, photosensitivity, and hepatic damage. Potential side effects associated with the use of melarsomine include injection-site reactions. Potential adverse reactions associated with use of ivermectins include neurotoxicity and retinal damage, particularly in the Collie breeds.

SELECTED REFERENCES

Labelle AL, Daniels JB, Dix M, Labelle P. *Onchocerca lupi* causing ocular disease in two cats. *Vet Ophthalmol.* 2011;**14** Suppl 1:105–110.

Labelle AL, Maddox CW, Daniels JB, Lanka S, Eggett TE, Dubielzig RR, Labelle P. Canine ocular onchocerciasis in the United States is associated with *Onchocerca lupi*. *Vet Parasitol*. 2013;**193**(1–3):297–301.

Sréter T, Széll Z. onchocerciasis: a newly recognized disease in dogs. *Vet Parasitol*. 2008;**151**(1):1–13.

Zarfoss MK, Dubielzig RR, Eberhard ML, Schmidt KS. Canine ocular onchocerciasis in the United States: two new cases and a review of the literature. *Vet Ophthalmol*. 2005;**8**(1):51–57. Review.

Clinical Atlas of Canine and Feline Ophthalmic Disease, First Edition. Douglas Esson.

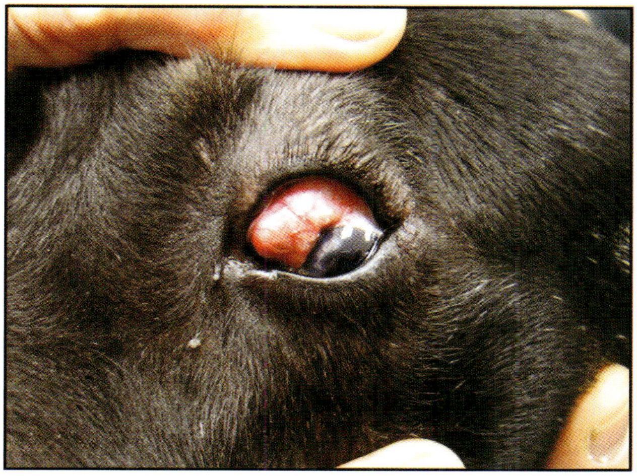

Figure 45.1 Typical episcleral granuloma and associated conjunctivitis associated with canine onchocerciasis.

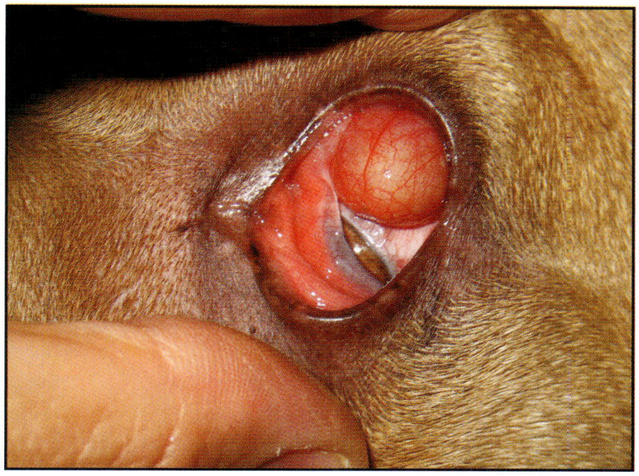

Figure 45.2 Typical episcleral granuloma and associated conjunctivitis associated with canine onchocerciasis.

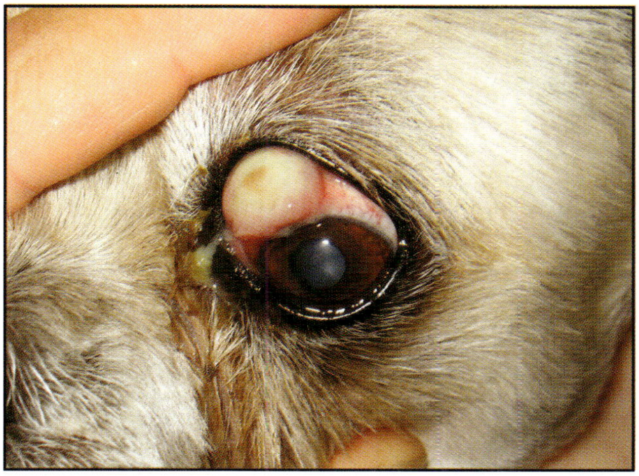

Figure 45.3 Typical episcleral granuloma and associated conjunctivitis associated with canine onchocerciasis.

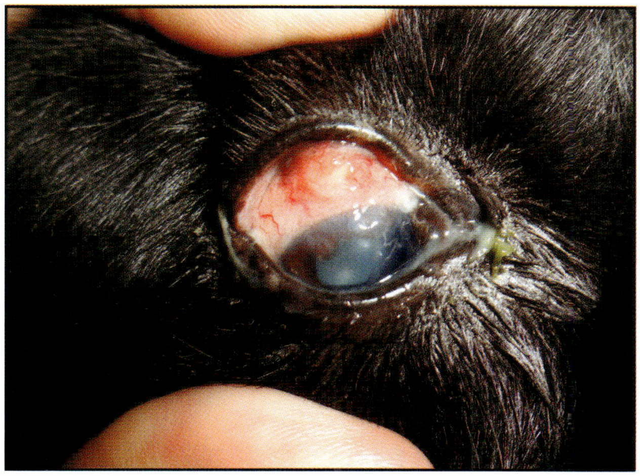

Figure 45.4 Typical episcleral granuloma and associated conjunctivitis associated with canine onchocerciasis.

CHAPTER 46
THELAZIA

PRESENTATION

Thelazia represent a genus of nematode parasites (sometimes referred to as "eye worms"), which may affect the ocular and adnexal tissues of dogs and cats. Infection with *Thelazia callipaeda* and *Thelazia californiensis* has been described. The life cycle of these parasites comprises a definitive host (including horses, ruminants, and numerous wild carnivores) and an intermediate host (notably dipteran flies). After mating, adult female parasites produce immature (first stage) larvae, which are released into the pre-corneal tear film of the definitive host. Immature larvae are subsequently ingested by flies, where they develop to third stage larvae before again being released into the tear film. Adult parasites may be found in the conjunctival fornix, nasolacrimal system, under the third eyelid or in rare cases, inside the globe. Associated symptoms may include blepharospasm, conjunctivitis, chemosis, ocular discharge, third eyelid elevation and/or uveitis, all of which may be aggravated by self-trauma.

DIAGNOSIS AND TREATMENT

The diagnosis of this condition is made on the basis of clinical findings and the identification of parasites in association with ocular and/or adnexal tissues. Adult worms are thin, linear, white to translucent in color, and approximately 1–2 cm in length. Treatment includes the removal of adult parasites, the topical administration of demecarium bromide and/or systemic anthelmintic agents including the avermectins, praziquantel, and/or mebendazole.

Potential Drug-Side-Effects

Potential complications associated with the use of demecarium bromide include ocular discomfort and gastrointestinal (GI) distress. Potential complications associated with the use of avermectins include neurologic abnormalities and retinal toxicity. Potential complications associated with the use praziquantel and mebendazole include GI distress.

SELECTED REFERENCES

Burnett HS, Lee RD, Parmelee WE, Wagner ED. A survey of Thelazia californiensis, a mammalian eye worm, with new locality records. *J Am Vet Med Assoc.* 1956;**129**(7):325–327.

Calero-Bernal R, Sánchez-Murillo JM, Alarcón-Elbal PM, Sánchez-Moro J, Latrofa MS, Dantas-Torres F, Otranto D. Resolution of canine ocular thelaziosis in avermectin-sensitive Border Collies from Spain. *Vet Parasitol.* 2014;**200**(1–2):203–206. DOI: 10.1016/j.vetpar.2013.12.014. Epub 2013 Dec 22.

Dubay SA, Williams ES, Mills K, Boerger-Fields AM. Bacteria and nematodes in the conjunctiva of mule deer from Wyoming and Utah. *J Wildl Dis.* 2000;**36**(4):783–787.

Motta B, Schnyder M, Basano FS, Nägeli F, Nägeli C, Schiessl B, Mallia E, Lia RP, Dantas-Torres F, Otranto D. Therapeutic efficacy of milbemycin oxime/praziquantel oral formulation (Milbemax‸) against Thelazia callipaeda in naturally infested dogs and cats. *Parasit Vectors.* 2012;**5**:85. DOI: 10.1186/1756-3305-5-85.

Otranto D, Traversa D. Thelazia eyeworm: an original endo- and ecto-parasitic nematode. *Trends Parasitol.* 2005;**21**(1):1–4.

Clinical Atlas of Canine and Feline Ophthalmic Disease, First Edition. Douglas Esson.

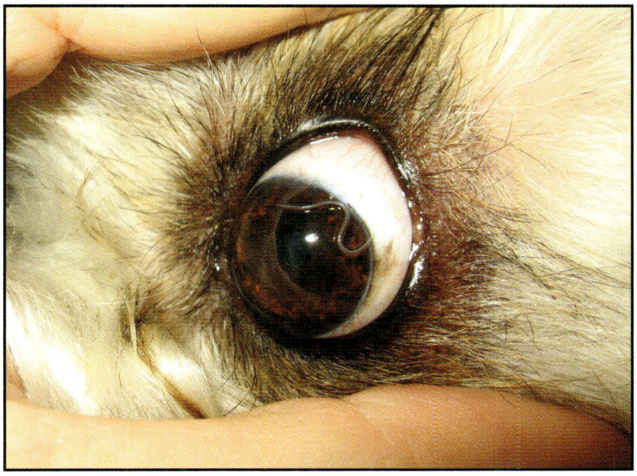

Figure 46.1 The presence of adult Thelazia parasites in the conjunctival fornix.

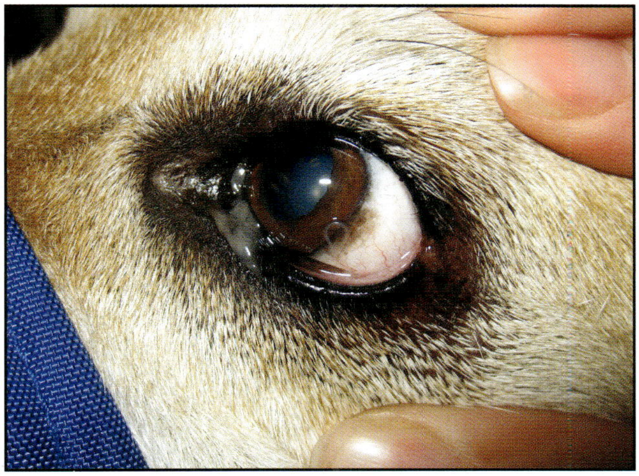

Figure 46.2 The presence of adult Thelazia parasites in the conjunctival fornix.

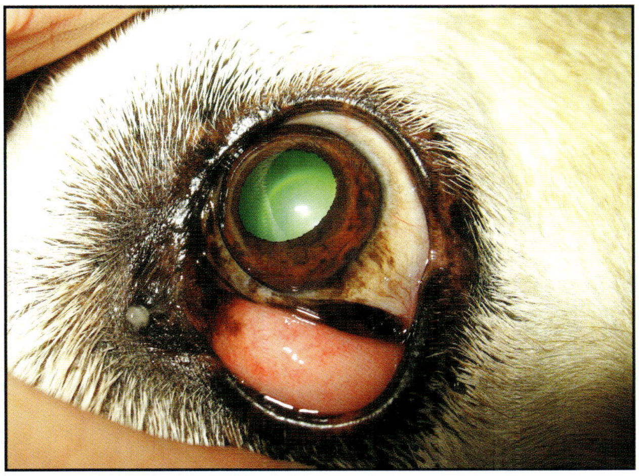

Figure 46.3 The presence of adult Thelazia parasites in the conjunctival fornix. Parasites can be difficult to identify (as indicated in this case) however, may be stimulated into vigorous movement by the instillation of topical demecarium bromide.

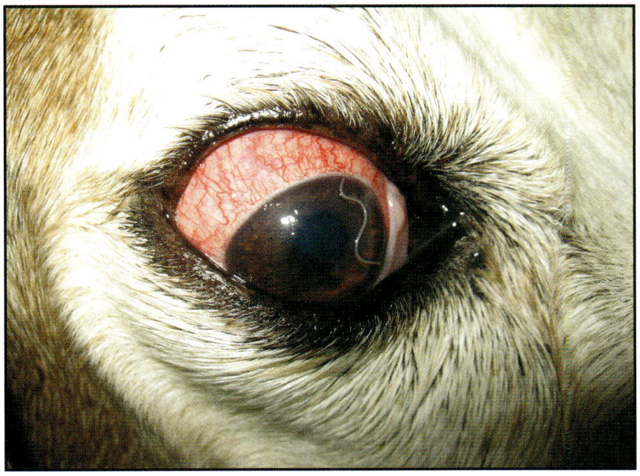

Figure 46.4 The presence of adult Thelazia parasites in the conjunctival fornix.

CHAPTER 47
PAPILLOMA

PRESENTATION

Squamous papillomas are benign neoplasms that may affect the conjunctival and mucosal surfaces. Young dogs may be affected by significant numbers of viral papillomas, typically developing on the conjunctival and eyelid surfaces as well as the mucous membranes of the oral cavity. Adult animals more frequently display single discrete papillary eyelid lesions, which are pink to tan in color and often sessile with a "stalk-like" base.

DIAGNOSIS AND TREATMENT

A tentative diagnosis of papilloma may be made on the basis of clinical presentation; however, confirmation requires incisional or excisional biopsy and adjunctive histopathology. Papillomas may be managed via benign neglect or surgical excision where indicated, the condition frequently resolving spontaneously in young animals over the course of 6–24 months. If present in large numbers, lesions may be ablated effectively using a CO_2 laser. The administration of patient-specific autoantigenic vaccines has also been advocated. Although often a frustrating, condition to manage initially, viral papillomas typically regress as the animal achieves maturity.

SELECTED REFERENCES

Bonney CH, Koch SA, Confer AW, Dice PF. A case report: a conjunctivocorneal papilloma with evidence of a viral etiology. *J Small Anim Pract*. 1980a;**21**(3):183–188.

Bonney CH, Koch SA, Dice PF, Confer AW. Papillomatosis of conjunctiva and adnexa in **dogs**. *J Am Vet Med Assoc*. 1980b;**176**(1):48–51.

Wiggans KT, Hoover CE, Ehrhart EJ, Wobeser BK, Cohen LB, Gionfriddo JR. Malignant transformation of a putative eyelid papilloma to squamous cell carcinoma in a dog. *Vet Ophthalmol*. 2013;**16** Suppl 1:105–112. DOI: 10.1111/j.1463-5224.2012.01062.x. Epub 2012 Aug 9.

Clinical Atlas of Canine and Feline Ophthalmic Disease, First Edition. Douglas Esson.

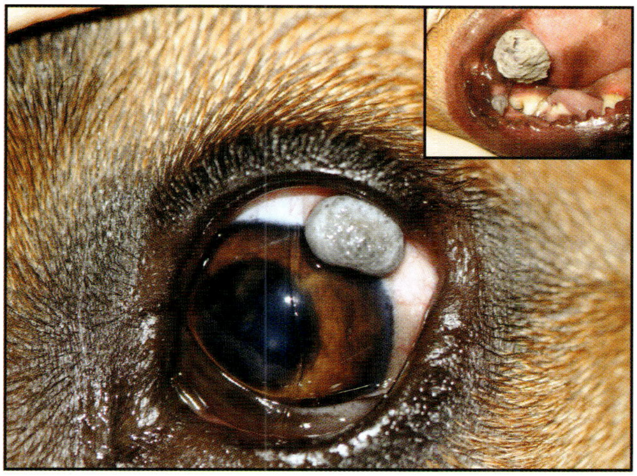

Figure 47.1 Typical presentation of a viral papilloma in a young dog. Inset shows oral lesions.

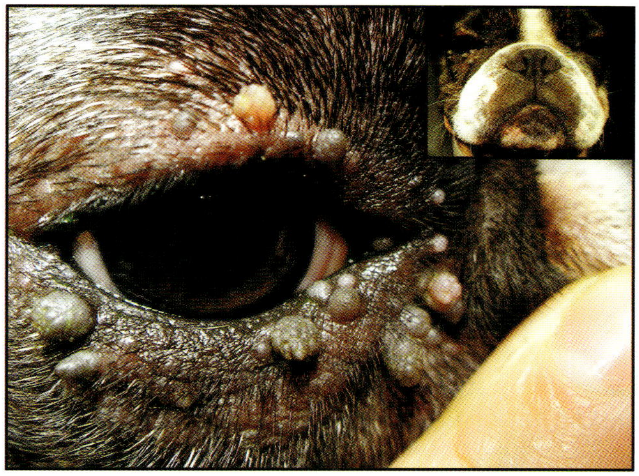

Figure 47.2 Typical presentation of viral papillomas in a young dog. Inset shows oral lesions.

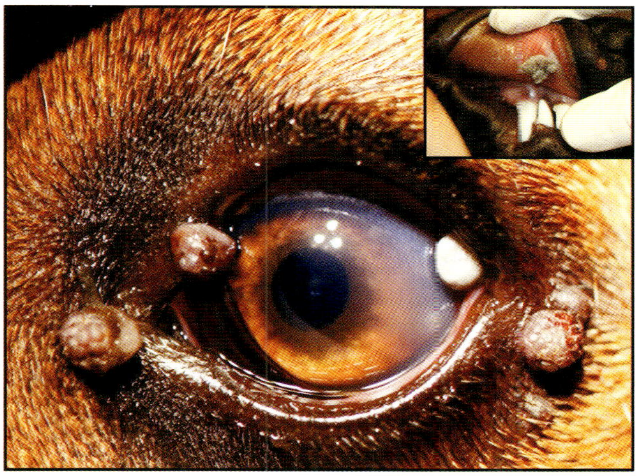

Figure 47.3 Typical presentation of viral papillomas in a young dog. Inset shows oral lesions.

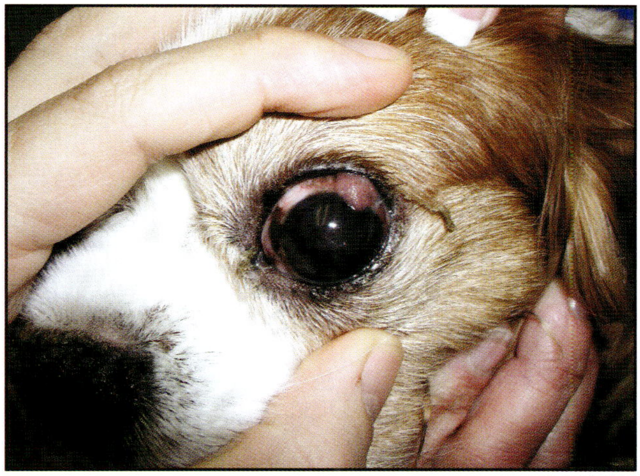

Figure 47.4 A sessile papilloma in an adult dog.

CHAPTER 48
CONJUNCTIVAL MELANOMA

PRESENTATION

Melanomas may be associated with the ocular mucocutaneous junctions, typically presenting as firm irregular and proliferative masses. Lesions may or not be pigmented (the diagnostic spectrum encompassing amelanotic melanomas) and may occasionally be associated with hemorrhage. Conjunctival melanomas typically exhibit malignant behavior including aggressive local infiltration. Canine and feline species of any breed or crossbreed may be affected.

DIAGNOSIS AND TREATMENT

The diagnosis of melanoma is made by histopathological interpretation of a representative biopsy sample. The potential for metastasis exists and basic staging via local lymph node aspiration, three-view radiography, and complete blood count (CBC)/chemistry analysis is recommended. Treatment comprises surgical excision where possible (sometimes extending to exenteration), with or without adjunctive chemotherapy, external beam radiation, and/or "metronomic therapy" (the combination of a nonsteroidal anti-inflammatory drug (NSAID) and alkylating agent to inhibit vascular growth) where indicated. Cranial soft tissue imaging (magnetic resonance imaging (MRI) or computed tomography (CT)) will facilitate accurate presurgical planning if necessary. The value of vaccine-mediated immunotherapy in the treatment of periocular lesions has not been fully evaluated.

SELECTED REFERENCES

Aquino SM. Management of eyelid neoplasms in the dog and cat. *Clin Tech Small Anim Pract*. 2007;**22**(2):46–54. Review.

Finn M, Krohne S, Stiles J. Ocular melanocytic neoplasia. *Compend Contin Educ Vet*. 2008;**30**(1):19–25; quiz 26. Review.

Gwin RM, Alsaker RD, Gelatt KN. Melanoma of the lower eyelid of a dog. *Vet Med Small Anim Clin*. 1976;**71**(7):929–931.

Munger RJ, Gourley IM. Cross lid flap for repair of large upper eyelid defects. *J Am Vet Med Assoc*. 1981;**178**(1):45–48.

Roberts SM, Severin GA, Lavach JD. Prevalence and treatment of palpebral neoplasms in the dog: 200 cases (1975–1983). *J Am Vet Med Assoc*. 1986;**189**(10):1355–1359.

Clinical Atlas of Canine and Feline Ophthalmic Disease, First Edition. Douglas Esson.

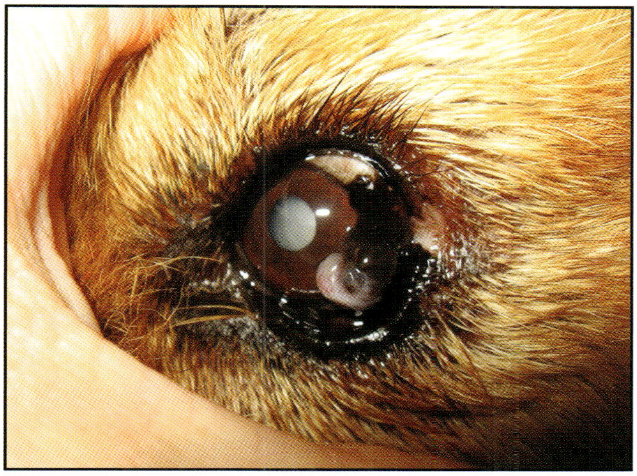

Figure 48.1 Conjunctival melanoma.

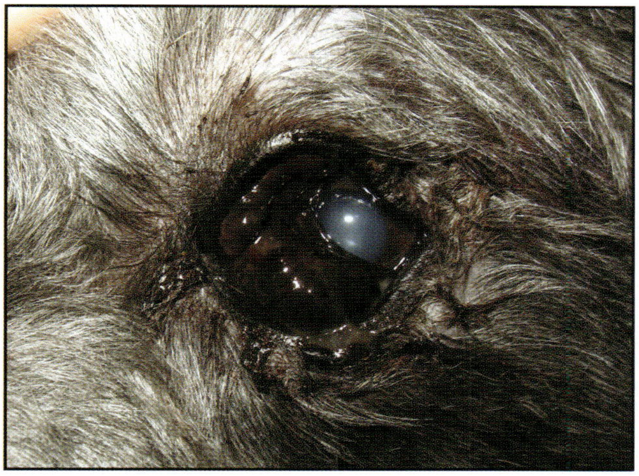

Figure 48.2 Conjunctival melanoma.

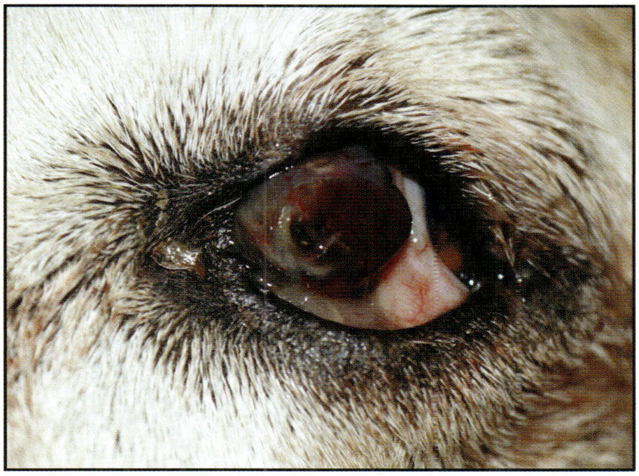

Figure 48.3 Conjunctival melanoma. The lesion affects the palpebral surface of the third eyelid.

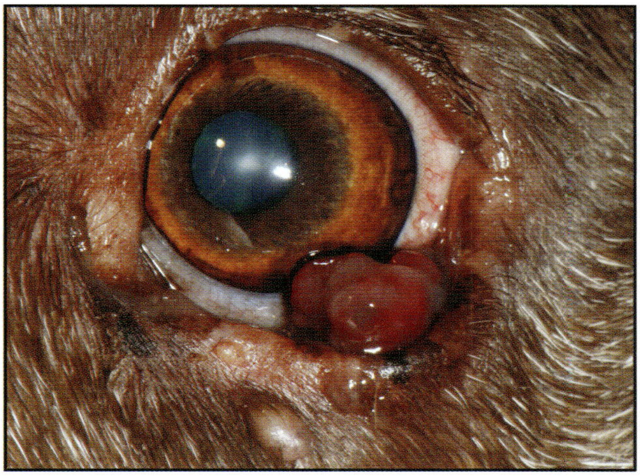

Figure 48.4 Conjunctival melanoma. The lesion represents an amelanotic conjunctival melanoma.

CHAPTER 49
CONJUNCTIVAL HEMANGIOMA/HEMANGIOSARCOMA

PRESENTATION

Tumors of vascular endothelial origin may affect the corneoscleral and/or overlying conjunctival tissues (*see also Corneoscleral Hemangioma/Hemangiosarcoma). These lesions typically present as bright red, smooth, raised, irregular to nodular masses at or near the corneoscleral limbus on the palpebral conjunctival surfaces or on the surfaces of the third eyelid. Tumors enlarge locally and may invade surrounding tissues. Exposure to UV radiation has been proposed to play a role in the development of adnexal hemangioma/hemangiosarcoma. Commonly affected breeds include the Australian Shepherd and the Collie breeds.

DIAGNOSIS AND TREATMENT

A tentative diagnosis of hemangioma/hemangiosarcoma may be made based on the characteristic clinical appearance of these lesions; however, confirmation as well as characterization of malignancy requires incisional or excisional biopsy and histopathology. Systemic health and/or involvement should ideally be evaluated via local lymph node aspiration, three-view radiography, and complete blood count (CBC)/chemistry analysis, although lesions are frequently localized to the adnexal tissues only. Treatment typically encompasses surgical resection where possible (with or without tectonic defect repair using biological or synthetic graft material) and/or the application of adjunctive cryotherapy. Cryotherapy should only be undertaken using an appropriate nitrous-oxide-cooled unit. Focal swelling is common following cryotherapy; however, inflammation rapidly resolves. Postoperative care comprises topical and or systemic anti-inflammatory and/or antimicrobial therapy as appropriate and the use of an Elizabethan collar to prevent self-trauma.

SELECTED REFERENCES

Chandler HL, Newkirk KM, Kusewitt DF, Dubielzig RR, Colitz CM. Immunohistochemical analysis of ocular hemangiomas and hemangiosarcomas in dogs. *Vet Ophthalmol.* 2009;**12**(2):83–90. DOI: 10.1111/j.1463-5224.2008.00684.x.

Hargis AM, Ihrke PJ, Spangler WL, Stannard AA. A retrospective clinicopathologic study of 212 dogs with cutaneous hemangiomas and hemangiosarcomas. *Vet Pathol.* 1992;**29**(4):316–328.

Pirie CG, Knollinger AM, Thomas CB, Dubielzig RR. Canine conjunctival hemangioma and hemangiosarcoma: a retrospective evaluation of 108 cases (1989–2004). *Vet Ophthalmol.* 2006;**9**(4):215–226.

Clinical Atlas of Canine and Feline Ophthalmic Disease, First Edition. Douglas Esson.

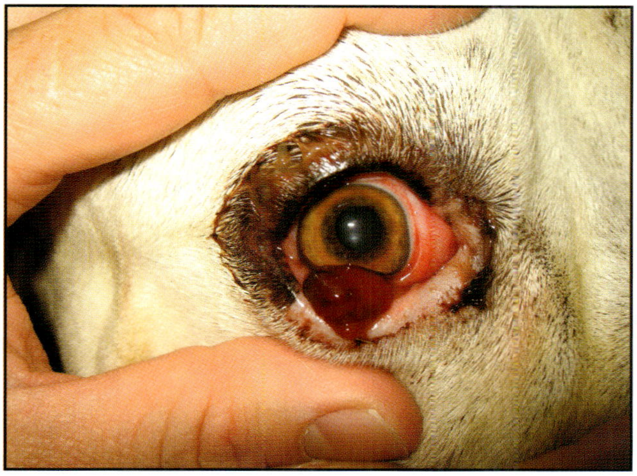

Figure 49.1 Typical presentation associated with conjunctival hemangioma/hemangiosarcoma.

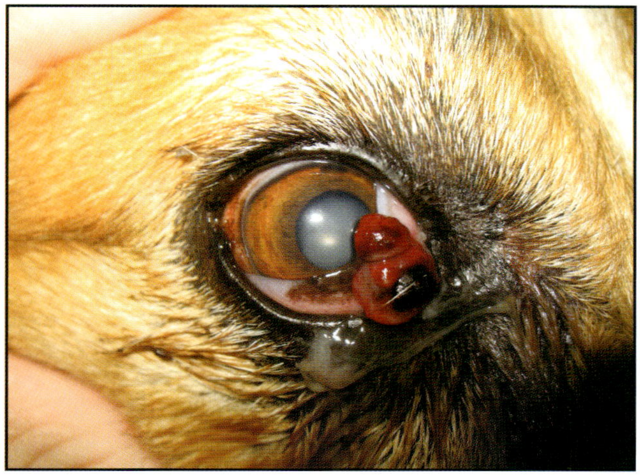

Figure 49.2 Typical presentation associated with conjunctival hemangioma/hemangiosarcoma.

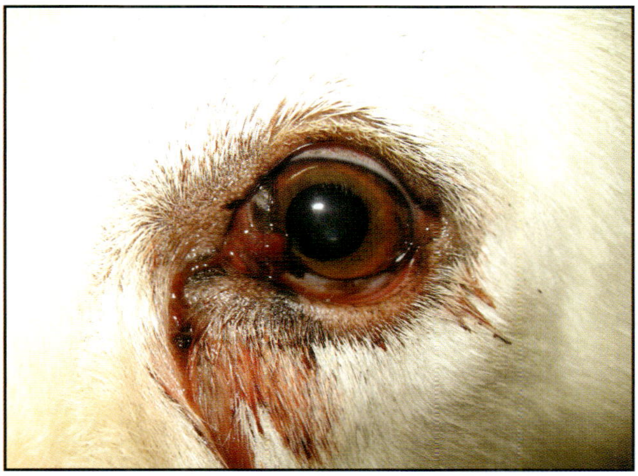

Figure 49.3 Typical presentation associated with conjunctival hemangioma/hemangiosarcoma. Associated hemorrhage is notable.

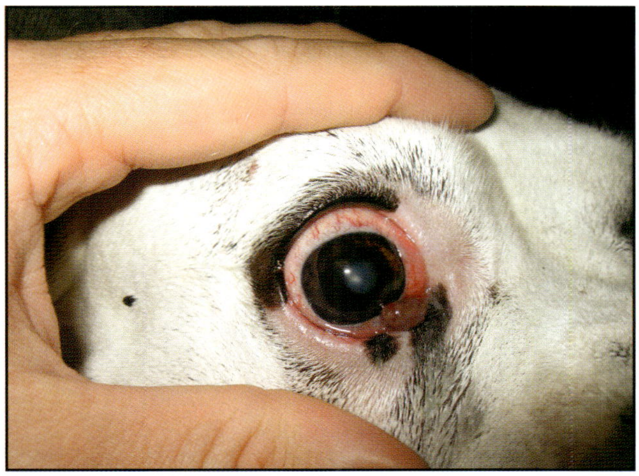

Figure 49.4 Typical presentation associated with conjunctival hemangioma/hemangiosarcoma.

CHAPTER 50
ADENOMA/ADENOCARCINOMA

PRESENTATION

Neoplasia of the third eyelid is not uncommon, the lacrimal gland of the third eyelid frequently representing the site of neoplastic proliferation. These tumors chiefly represent adenoma/adenocarcinoma, the distinction being made histologically. Clinically, neoplasms present as a slowly progressive enlargement, thickening, displacement, and hyperemia of the third eyelid. Secondary conjunctivitis and/or ocular discharge may additionally be present.

DIAGNOSIS AND TREATMENT

The diagnosis is made histologically following incisional or excisional biopsy. Systemic health and/or involvement should ideally be evaluated via local lymph node aspiration, three-view radiography, and complete blood count (CBC)/chemistry analysis, although lesions frequently appear to be localized to the tissues of the third eyelid only. Treatment comprises surgical excision of affected tissue, typically involving removal of the entire third eyelid. Postoperative care comprises routine antimicrobial, anti-inflammatory, and analgesic therapy as well as the use of a protective Elizabethan collar to prevent self-trauma. In addition, an effort should be made to avoid secondary complications associated with decreased corneal protection as well as decreased lacrimal function, potentially including the use of topical cyclosporine or tacrolimus and/or the long-term use of a topical lubricating and protective agent.

Potential Drug-Side-Effects

Potential adverse effects associated with the use of topical cyclosporine and tacrolimus include periocular dermatitis and alopecia.

SELECTED REFERENCES

Komaromy AM, Ramsey DT, Render JA, Clark P. Primary adenocarcinoma of the gland of the nictitating membrane in a cat. *J Am Anim Hosp Assoc*. 1997;**33**(4):333–336.

Schäffer EH, Pfleghaar S, Gordon S, Knödlseder M. Malignant nictitating membrane tumors in dogs and cats. *Tierarztl Prax*. 1994;**22**(4):382–391.

Wang FI, Ting CT, Liu YS. Orbital adenocarcinoma of lacrimal gland origin in a dog. *J Vet Diagn Invest*. 2001;**13**(2):159–161.

Wilcock B, Peiffer R Jr. Adenocarcinoma of the gland of the third eyelid in seven dogs. *J Am Vet Med Assoc*. 1988;**193**(12):1549–1550.

Clinical Atlas of Canine and Feline Ophthalmic Disease, First Edition. Douglas Esson.

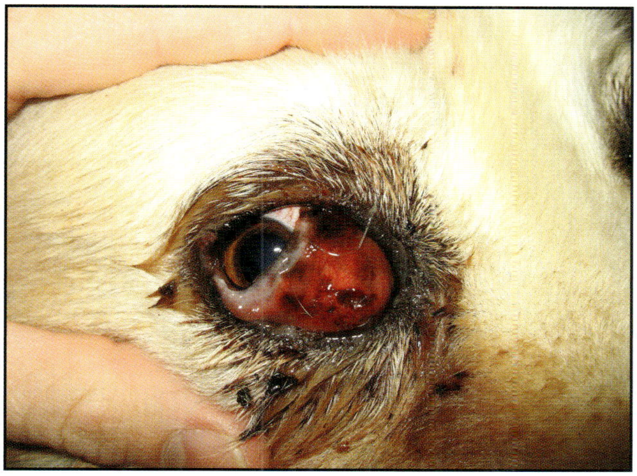

Figure 50.1 Typical presentation associated with conjunctival adenoma/adenocarcinoma.

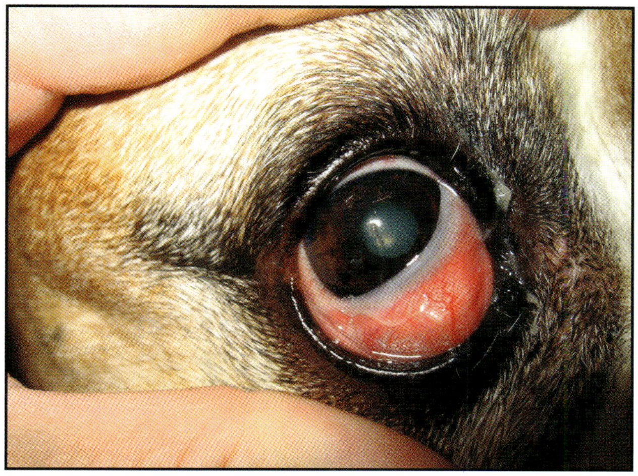

Figure 50.2 Typical presentation associated with conjunctival adenoma/adenocarcinoma.

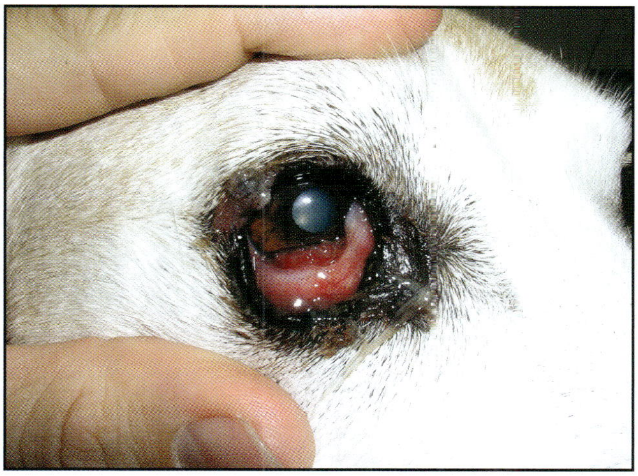

Figure 50.3 Typical presentation associated with conjunctival adenoma/adenocarcinoma. This patient displays the presence of an unrelated (benign), upper eyelid adenoma.

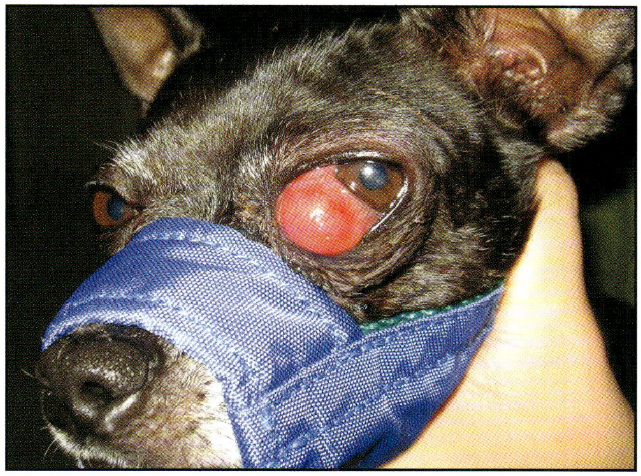

Figure 50.4 Typical presentation associated with conjunctival adenoma/adenocarcinoma.

CHAPTER 51
CONJUNCTIVAL LYMPHOMA

PRESENTATION

Conjunctival/third eyelid (TEL) tissues may be affected by lymphoma (see also Cutaneous Epitheliotropic Lymphoma (CEL), Corneoscleral Lymphoma, Uveal Lymphoma, Chorioretinal Lymphoma, and Retrobulbar Neoplasia). In some cases, ocular and/or adnexal symptoms may be the initial presentation for more generalized disease; however, conjunctival/TEL lymphoma may also represent localized disease. Clinical findings may encompass a spectrum of changes from conjunctival/TEL hyperemia to tissue infiltration and/or nodular and/or diffuse cream-colored mass formation. Both canine and feline species of any breed or crossed breed may be affected.

DIAGNOSIS AND TREATMENT

A diagnosis of conjunctival lymphoma is based on histopathologic interpretation of representative tissue biopsy. Wherever lymphoma is suspected, samples should be harvested before the institution of therapy in order to facilitate the planning of an accurate treatment protocol. Treatment comprises topical anti-inflammatory therapy (typically utilizing a corticosteroid) as well as systemic chemotherapy. Associated ophthalmic changes such as elevated intraocular pressure should be addressed as appropriate. Staging via local lymph node (and/or organ/bone marrow) aspiration, three-view radiography, and complete blood count (CBC)/chemistry analysis is recommended, before initiation of systemic chemotherapy. Diagnostic testing for the presence of infectious viruses, notably FeLV and FIV is additionally recommended in feline patients. Individual chemotherapeutic protocols are most ideally designed by a veterinary oncologist; however, typically include a variable combination of prednisone, vincristine, cyclophosphamide, and/or doxorubicin.

Potential Drug-Side-Effects

Potential adverse effects associated with the use of systemic corticosteroids include polyphagia, polydipsia, polyuria, hair coat changes, weight gain, pancreatitis, gastrointestinal (GI) distress, muscle damage, hepatic impairment, and diabetes. Potential adverse effects associated with the use of vincristine include stomatitis, GI distress, neuropathy, hepatopathy, and myelosuppression. Potential adverse effects associated with the use of cyclophosphamide include GI distress, pancreatitis, hepatotoxicity, and myelosuppression. Potential adverse affects associated with the use of doxorubicin include hypersensitivity, GI distress, cardiac dysfunction, and myelosuppression.

The prognosis varies depending on the extent of disease present before initiating therapy.

SELECTED REFERENCES

Hong IH, Bae SH, Lee SG, Park JK, Ji AR, Ki MR, Han SY, Lee EM, Kim AY, You SY, Kim TH, Jeong KS. Mucosa-associated lymphoid tissue lymphoma of the third eyelid conjunctiva in a dog. *Vet Ophthalmol.* 2011;**14**(1):61–65. doi: 10.1111/j.1463-5224.2010.00843.x.

McCowan C, Malcolm J, Hurn S, O'Reilly A, Hardman C, Stanley R. Conjunctival lymphoma: immunophenotype and outcome in five dogs and three cats. *Vet Ophthalmol.* 2013. doi: 10.1111/vop.12083.

Nola M, Lukenda A, Bollmann M, Kalauz M, Petrovecki M, Bollmann R. Outcome and prognostic factors in ocular adnexal lymphoma. *Croat Med J.* 2004;**45**(3):328–332.

Olbertz L, Lima L, Langohr I, Werner J, Teixeira L, Montiani-Ferreira F. Supposed primary conjunctival lymphoma in a dog. *Vet Ophthalmol.* 2013;**16** Suppl 1:100–104. doi: 10.1111/j.1463-5224.2012.01027.x. Epub 2012 Apr 23.

Clinical Atlas of Canine and Feline Ophthalmic Disease, First Edition. Douglas Esson.

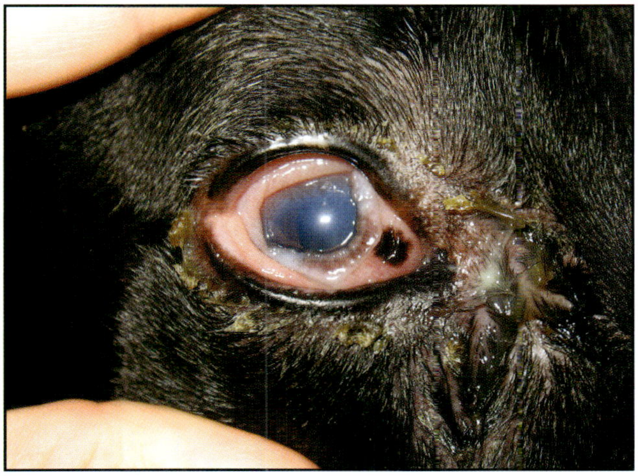

Figure 51.1 Typical presentation associated with conjunctival lymphoma. Notable are perilimbal conjunctival thickening and hyperemia as well as associated corneal changes.

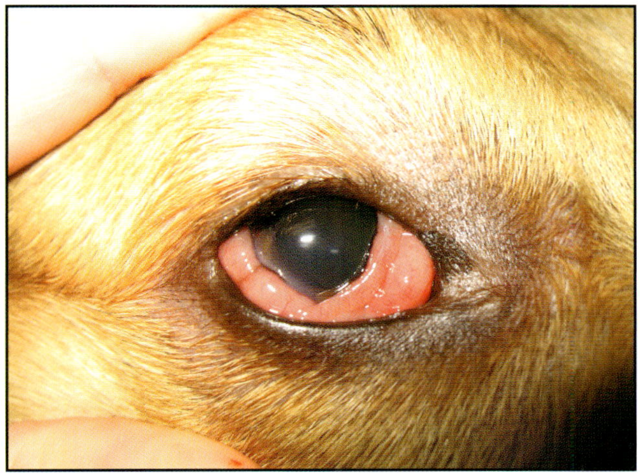

Figure 51.2 Typical presentation associated with conjunctival lymphoma. Notable are perilimbal conjunctival thickening and hyperemia as well as associated corneal changes.

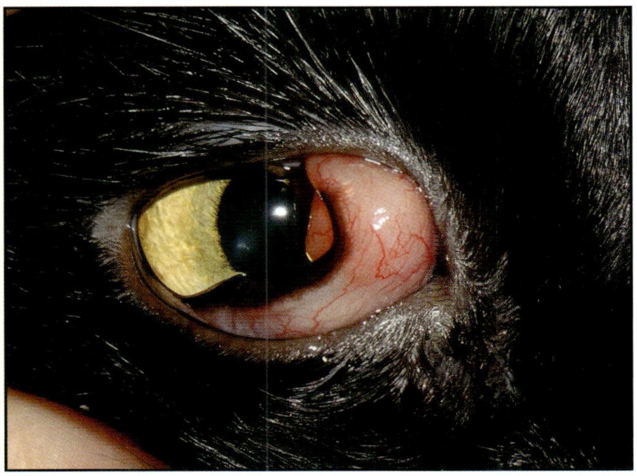

Figure 51.3 Typical presentation associated with conjunctival lymphoma. Conjunctival thickening and hyperemia are predominantly associated with the tissues of the third eyelid.

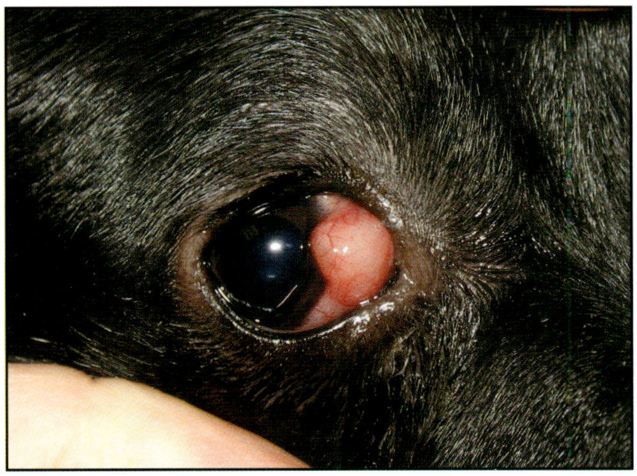

Figure 51.4 Typical presentation associated with conjunctival lymphoma. Conjunctival thickening and hyperemia are predominantly associated with the tissues of the third eyelid.

CHAPTER 52
CONJUNCTIVAL SQUAMOUS CELL CARCINOMA

PRESENTATION

Hereditary factors, exposure to UV sunlight and/or chronic inflammation may contribute to the development of conjunctival and/or third eyelid (TEL) squamous cell carcinoma (SCC), which progress from focal acanthosis through carcinoma *in situ* to outright squamous cell carcinoma with time. Clinically, SCC presents as irregular, pink-colored proliferative to erosive lesions. Commonly affected breeds include the Pug and the English Bulldog.

DIAGNOSIS AND TREATMENT

The diagnosis of SCC is made by histopathology following incisional or excisional biopsy, with SCC frequently appearing clinically similar to (and even encompassing) chronic corneal inflammation/granulation. Systemic health and/or involvement should be evaluated via local lymph node aspiration, three-view radiography, and complete blood count (CBC)/chemistry analysis. Treatment comprises resection of neoplastic tissue where possible, with or without the adjunctive application of cryotherapy and/or radiotherapy. Focal swelling is common postoperatively; however, inflammation rapidly resolves. Postoperative care comprises topical and or systemic anti-inflammatory and/or antimicrobial therapy as appropriate and the use of an Elizabethan collar to prevent self-trauma.

SELECTED REFERENCES

Dreyfus J, Schobert CS, Dubielzig RR. Superficial corneal squamous cell carcinoma occurring in dogs with chronic keratitis. *Vet Ophthalmol.* 2011;**14**(3):161–168. doi: 10.1111/j.1463-5224.2010.00858.x.

Montiani-Ferreira F, Kiupel M, Muzolon P, Truppel J. Corneal squamous cell carcinoma in a dog: a case report. *Vet Ophthalmol.* 2008;**11**(4):269–72. doi: 10.1111/j.1463-5224.2008.00622.x.

Takiyama N, Terasaki E, Uechi M. Corneal squamous cell carcinoma in two dogs. *Vet Ophthalmol.* 2010;**13**(4):266–269. doi: 10.1111/j.1463-5224.2010.00792.x.

Clinical Atlas of Canine and Feline Ophthalmic Disease, First Edition. Douglas Esson.

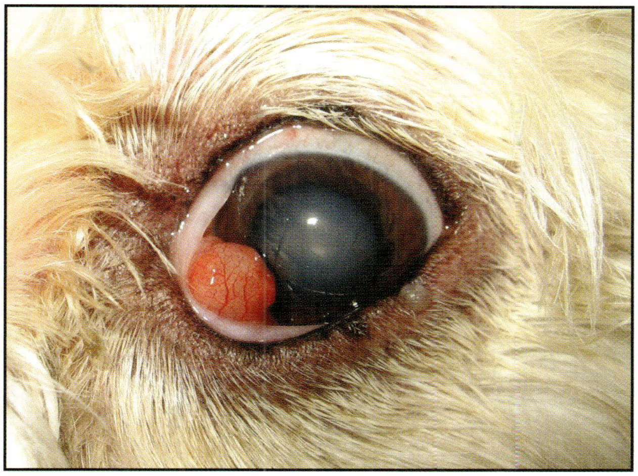

Figure 52.1 Typical presentation associated with conjunctival/TEL squamous cell carcinoma.

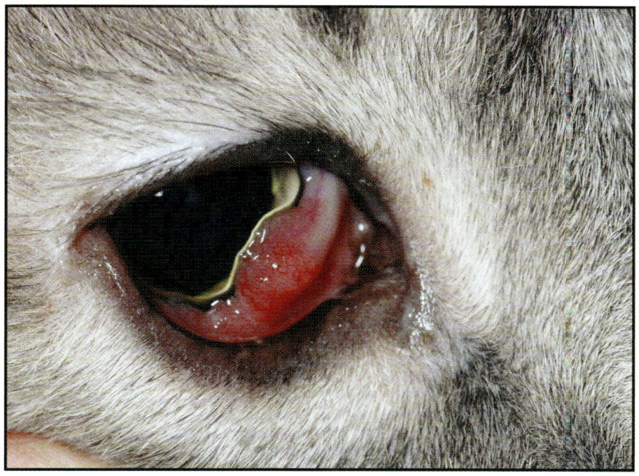

Figure 52.2 Typical presentation associated with conjunctival/TEL squamous cell carcinoma.

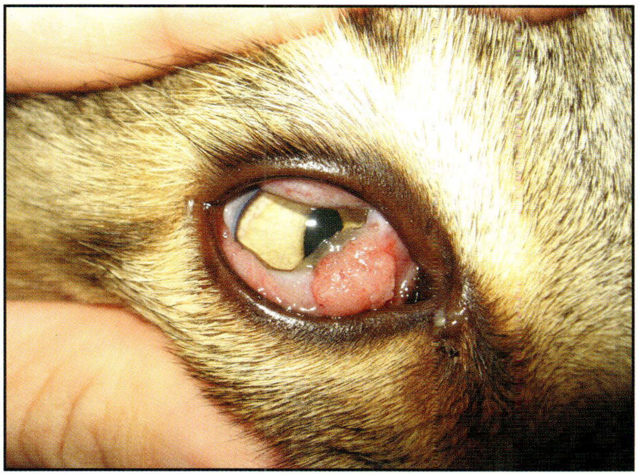

Figure 52.3 Typical presentation associated with conjunctival/TEL squamous cell carcinoma.

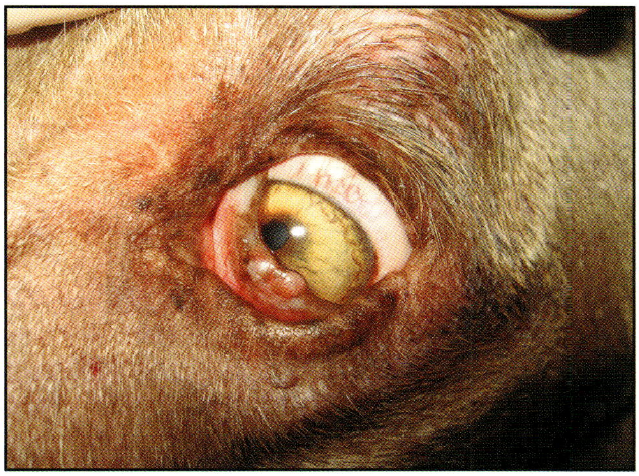

Figure 52.4 Typical presentation associated with conjunctival/TEL squamous cell carcinoma.

Section 4

Corneoscleral Disease

CHAPTER 53
DERMOID

PRESENTATION

A dermoid (also sometimes referred to as a "choristoma") represents an area of normal haired skin in an abnormal location on the eye or adnexal tissue. Lesions may affect the cornea and/or adjacent structures including the limbus, conjunctival surfaces, third eyelid, and/or eyelid. Changes are congenital, so they are typically noted soon after the eyes open at 2 weeks of age. Secondary conjunctivitis and discomfort may manifest as blepharospasm and/or ocular discharge. Commonly affected breeds include the German Shepherd, the Dachshund, and the St Bernard.

DIAGNOSIS AND TREATMENT

The diagnosis of a dermoid is made based on clinical findings. The treatment of choice is surgical excision of the abnormal tissue by superficial peritomy and/or keratectomy. The treatment of choice is surgical excision of the abnormal tissue by superficial peritomy and/or keratectomy. Once excised, these lesions do not recur. The medial and lateral canthal anatomy should be preserved, where possible. Tectonic corneal grafting may or may not be necessary after dermoid removal, based on the depth of the resultant defect. Similarly, resultant eyelid defects may require blepharoplastic reconstruction.

Potential Drug-Side-Effects
Postoperative care comprises routine systemic antimicrobial, anti-inflammatory, and analgesic care.

An Elizabethan collar should be placed in order to prevent self-trauma and corneal health should be frequently monitored until eyelid healing is complete.

SELECTED REFERENCES

Brudenall DK, Bernays ME, Peiffer RL Jr. Central corneal dermoid in a Labrador retriever puppy. *J Small Anim Pract.* 2007;**48**(10):588–590.

Kalpravidh M, Tuntivanich P, Vongsakul S, Sirivaidyapong S. Canine amniotic membrane transplantation for corneal reconstruction after the excision of dermoids in dogs. *Vet Res Commun.* 2009;**33**(8):1003–1012.

Lee JI, Kim MJ, Kim IH, Kim YB, Kim MC. Surgical correction of corneal dermoid in a dog. *J Vet Sci.* 2005;**6**(4):369–370

Clinical Atlas of Canine and Feline Ophthalmic Disease, First Edition. Douglas Esson.

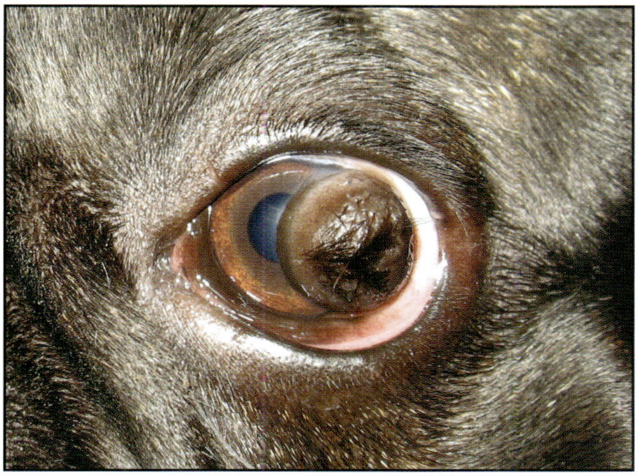

Figure 53.1 Typical presentation associated with a corneoscleral dermoid.

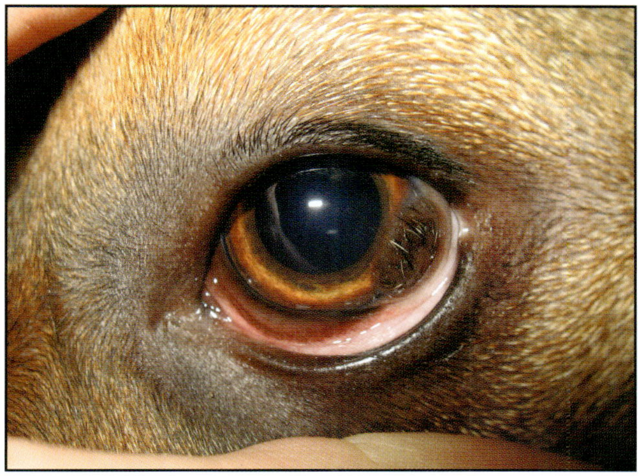

Figure 53.2 Typical presentation associated with a corneoscleral dermoid.

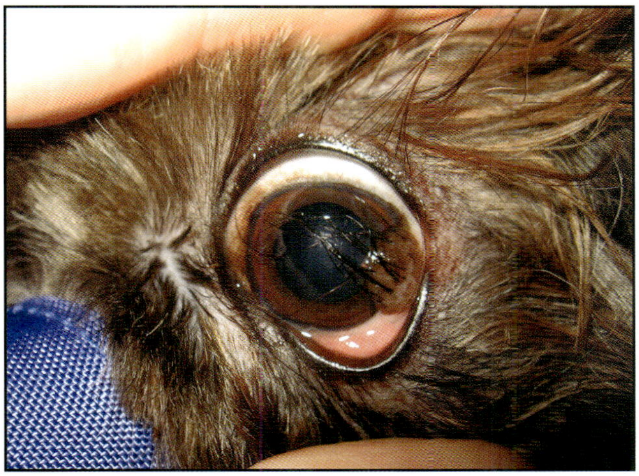

Figure 53.3 Typical presentation associated with a corneoscleral dermoid.

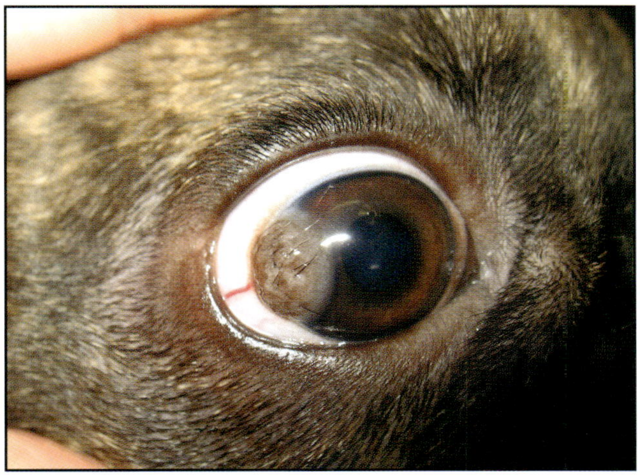

Figure 53.4 Typical presentation associated with a corneoscleral dermoid.

CHAPTER 54
CORNEAL DYSTROPHY

PRESENTATION

Corneal dystrophy describes a group of corneal disorders, likely hereditary in etiology, in which cholesterol, phospholipids, and free fatty acids accumulate within the cornea(s). Lesions appear as subepithelial to stromal gray/white, crystalline, relucencies within the corneal stroma. This disorder is bilateral in presentation (although not always symmetrical) and is not associated with any preexisting or concurrent corneal or ocular inflammation. Multiple patterns of corneal dystrophy have been described, many with breed associations. These may include axial or peripheral, ovoid to circular lesions. Occasionally, corneal dystrophic changes may reflect underlying metabolic storage disease. Commonly affected breeds include the Cavalier King Charles Spaniel, Siberian Husky, Beagle, and Shetland Sheepdog.

DIAGNOSIS AND TREATMENT

The diagnosis of corneal dystrophy is made based on clinical findings. Evaluation of underlying thyroid and adrenocortical function as well as systemic lipid and cholesterol levels, lipoprotein, glucose, calcium, and phosphorus may be indicated in select cases, in order to rule out underlying metabolic abnormalities, which should be addressed as appropriate. Treatment is frequently unnecessary and corticosteroid-based anti-inflammatory medications may exacerbate changes. Keratectomy may be indicated in rare cases of secondary ulceration and/or mineralization associated with epithelial discontinuity and discomfort.

SELECTED REFERENCES

Barsotti G, Pasquini A, Busillo L, Senese M, Cardini G, Guidi G. Corneal crystalline stromal dystrophy and lipidic metabolism in the dog. *Vet Res Commun.* 2008;**32** Suppl 1:S227–S229.

Cooley PL, Dice PF. 2nd. Corneal dystrophy in the dog and cat. *Vet Clin North Am Small Anim Pract*. 1990;**20**(3):681–692.

Crispin SM. Crystalline corneal dystrophy in the dog. *Histochemical and ultrastructural study. Cornea.* 1988;**7**(2):149–161.

Spangler WL, Waring GO, Morrin LA. Oval lipid corneal opacities in beagles. *Vet Pathol.* 1982;**19**(2):150–159.

Clinical Atlas of Canine and Feline Ophthalmic Disease, First Edition. Douglas Esson.

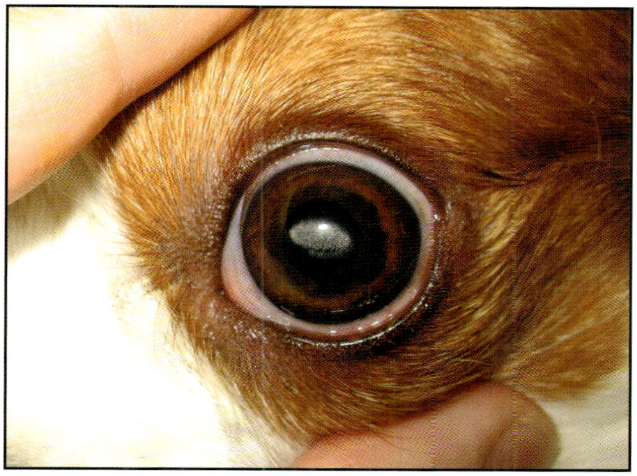

Figure 54.1 Typical presentation of corneal dystrophy. These changes are typically bilateral and are not associated with clinical inflammation.

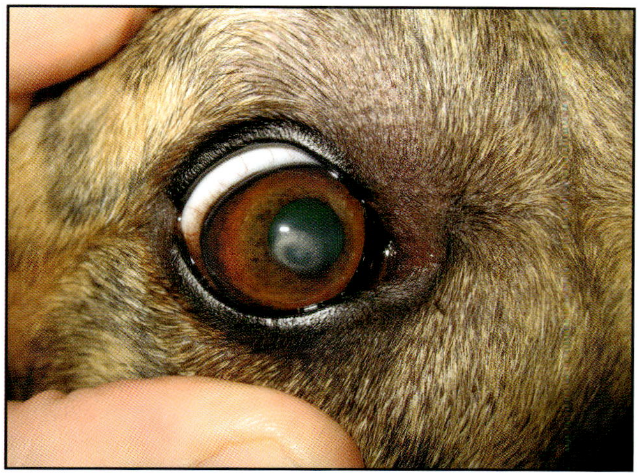

Figure 54.2 Typical presentation of corneal dystrophy. These changes are typically bilateral and are not associated with clinical inflammation.

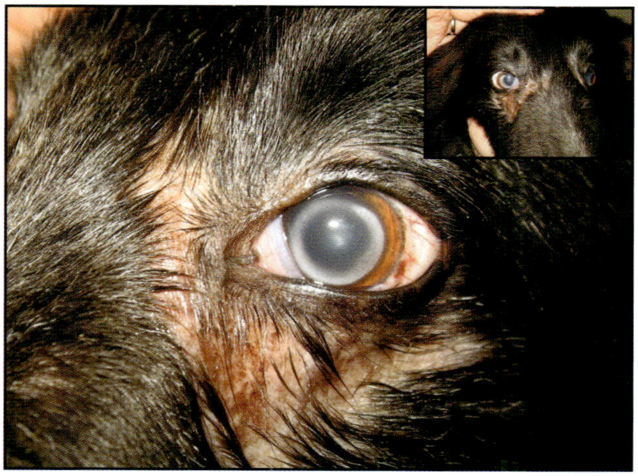

Figure 54.3 Typical presentation of corneal dystrophy. These changes are typically bilateral and are not associated with clinical inflammation.

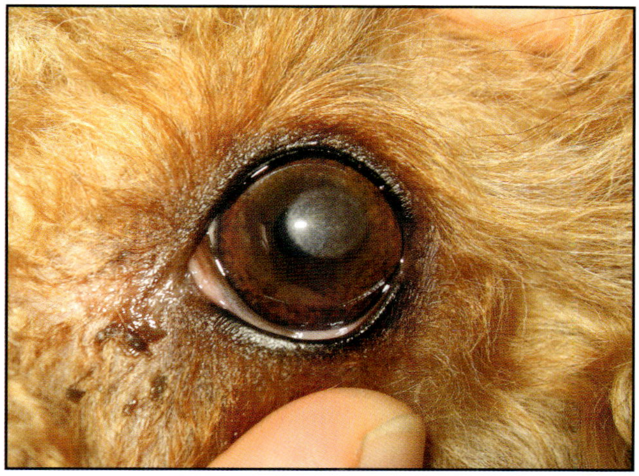

Figure 54.4 Typical presentation of corneal dystrophy. These changes are typically bilateral and are not associated with clinical inflammation.

CHAPTER 55
CORNEAL DEGENERATION

PRESENTATION

Corneal degeneration represents pathological changes occurring in the cornea secondary to preexisting ocular and/or systemic inflammation. Degenerative changes appear as irregular, asymmetric gray/white deposits within the cornea. Lesions may be unilateral or bilateral and are typically associated with neovascularization. Concurrent ulceration and/or secondary infection may additionally be present and unstable regions of degenerative and mineralized tissue may spontaneously slough. Variable discomfort may be manifested by epiphora, blepharospasm, and/or mucoid discharge. Many breeds may be affected, particularly with significantly advanced age.

DIAGNOSIS AND TREATMENT

The diagnosis of corneal degeneration is made based on clinical findings. Evaluation of thyroid and adrenocortical function, complete blood count (CBC)/chemistry values as well as systemic lipid and cholesterol levels is indicated in order to rule out underlying metabolic abnormalities. Mineral deposits may be removed where indicated via diamond-burr keratectomy, chemical keratectomy (using dilute trichloroacetic acid), or surgical keratectomy. Tectonic corneal grafting may or may not be necessary based on the depth of the resultant defect. Exposed mineral may also be partially chelated using topical EDTA solution until reepithelialization is complete. Associated ulceration should be treated medically using topical antimicrobial agents or surgically, if appropriate. In general, topical corticosteroids should be avoided. The use of an Elizabethan collar will prevent self-trauma until corneal healing is complete.

SELECTED REFERENCES

Crispin SM, Barnett KC. Dystrophy, degeneration and infiltration of the canine cornea. *J Small Anim Pract* 1983;**24**:63–83.

Laus JL, dos Santos C, Talieri IC, Oriá AP, Bechara GH. Combined corneal lipid and calcium degeneration in a dog with hyperadrenocorticism: a case report. *Vet Ophthalmol*. 2002;**5**(1):61–64

Ledbetter EC, Kice NC, Matusow RB, Dubovi EJ, Kim SG. The effect of topical ocular corticosteroid administration in dogs with experimentally induced latent canine herpesvirus-1 infection. *Exp Eye Res*. 2010;**90**(6):711–717. doi: 10.1016/j.exer.2010.03.001. Epub 2010 Mar 16.

Sansom J, Blunden T. Calcareous degeneration of the canine cornea. *Vet Ophthalmol*. 2010;**13**(4):238–243.

Clinical Atlas of Canine and Feline Ophthalmic Disease, First Edition. Douglas Esson.

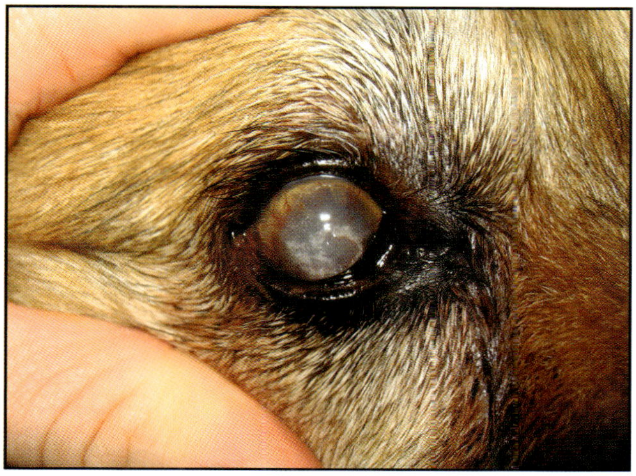

Figure 55.1 Typical presentation associated with corneal degeneration. Active inflammation as well as ulcerative keratitis are present.

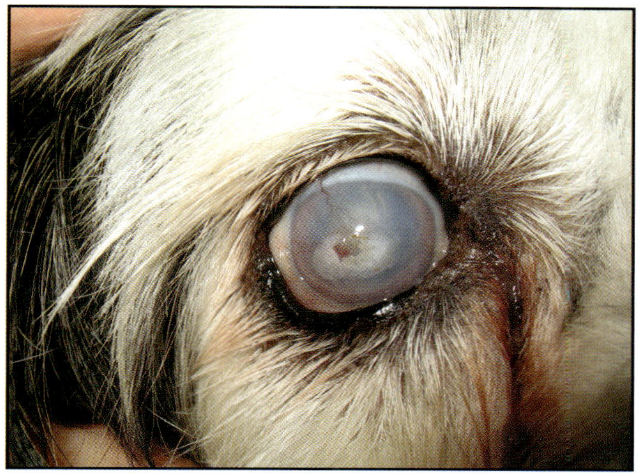

Figure 55.2 Typical presentation associated with corneal degeneration. Active inflammation as well as ulcerative keratitis are present.

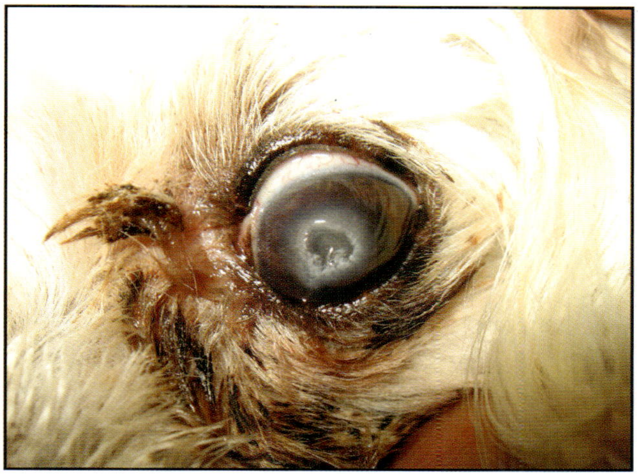

Figure 55.3 Typical presentation associated with corneal degeneration. Active inflammation as well as ulcerative keratitis are present.

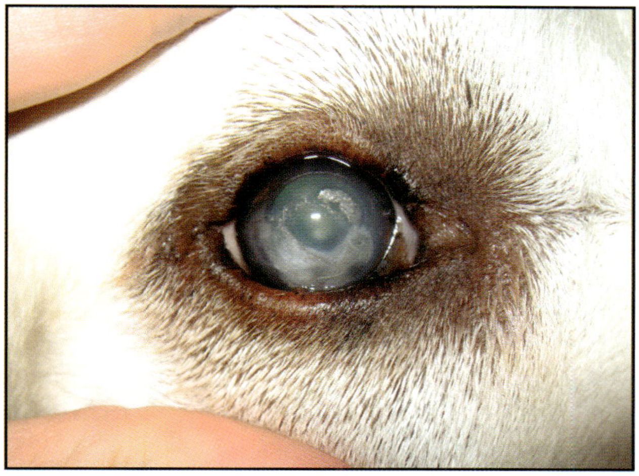

Figure 55.4 Typical presentation associated with corneal degeneration.

CHAPTER 56
CORNEAL ENDOTHELIAL DECOMPENSATION

PRESENTATION

Corneal endothelial decompensation represents a progressive loss of corneal endothelial cell function and density and results in slowly progressive corneal edema. Corneal endothelial cells do not regenerate and have only a limited ability to compensate. Clinically, this disease presents as progressive, avascular, corneal edema, marked by blue/gray discoloration, and corneal thickening. Changes typically begin within the superotemporal corneal quadrant. The disease is bilateral, although not always symmetrical. Initially, changes do not result in significant visual disturbance or discomfort; however, with progression, a cycle of painful bullous and/or ulcerative keratopathy may develop. Commonly affected breeds include the Boston Terrier, the Dachshund, Chihuahua, and the Miniature Poodle.

DIAGNOSIS AND TREATMENT

When indicated, definitive surgical treatment includes limited thermo- or CO_2 laser keratoplasty, the placement of a "Gunderson" conjunctival pedicle graft, or, ultimately, penetrating keratoplasty. The palliative use of sodium chloride ointment has been reported to increase patient comfort; however, will not adequately address underlying endothelial dysfunction. The palliative use of topical anti-inflammatory agents has also been advocated by some authors.

SELECTED REFERENCES

Cooley PL, Dice PF. 2nd. Corneal dystrophy in the dog and cat. *Vet Clin North Am Small Anim Pract*. 1990;**20**(3):681–692.

Gwin R, Pollack F, Warren J, *et al*. Primary canine corneal endothelial cell dystrophy: specular microscopic evaluation, diagnosis and therapy. *J Am Anim Hosp Assoc*. 1982;**18**:471–479.

Martin C, Dice P. Corneal endothelial dystrophy in the dog. *J Am Anim Hosp Assoc*. 1982;**18**:327–336.

Michau TM, Gilger BC, Maggio F, Davidson MG. Use of thermokeratoplasty for treatment of ulcerative keratitis and bullous keratopathy secondary to corneal endothelial disease in dogs: 13 cases (1994–2001). *J Am Vet Med Assoc*. 2003;**222**(5):607–612.

Clinical Atlas of Canine and Feline Ophthalmic Disease, First Edition. Douglas Esson.

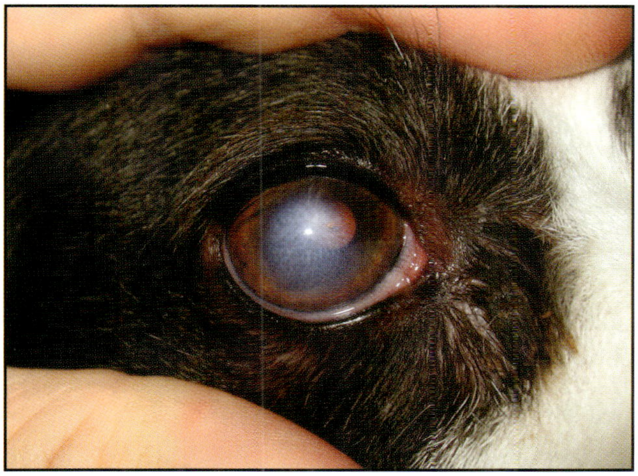

Figure 56.1 Typical presentation associated with corneal endothelial decompensation and secondary corneal edema.

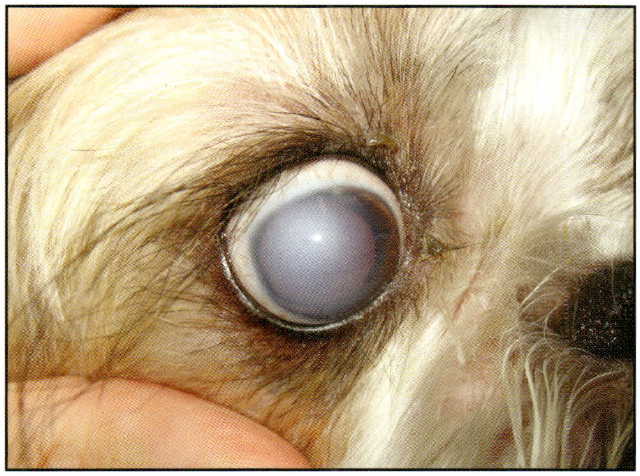

Figure 56.2 Typical presentation associated with corneal endothelial decompensation and secondary corneal edema.

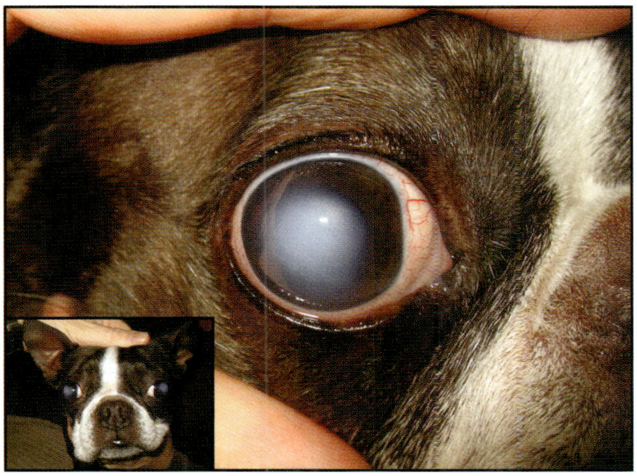

Figure 56.3 Typical presentation associated with corneal endothelial decompensation and secondary corneal edema. Inset demonstrates the bilateral nature of the disease.

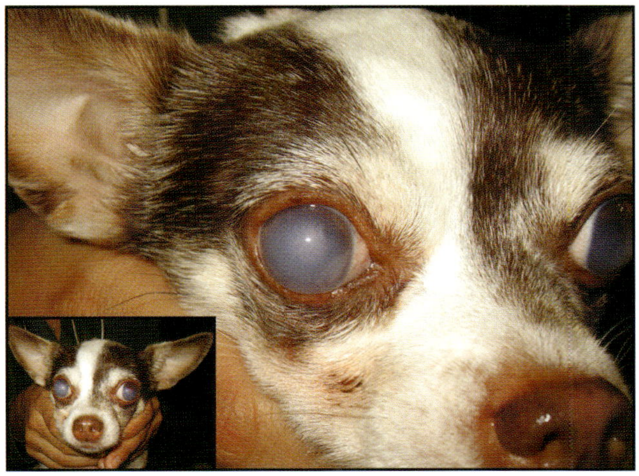

Figure 56.4 Typical presentation associated with corneal endothelial decompensation and secondary corneal edema. Inset demonstrates the bilateral nature of the disease.

CHAPTER 57
SCLERITIS

PRESENTATION

Scleritis describes a primary inflammatory disorder of the canine scleral and/or episcleral tissues, which is thought to be immune-mediated in origin. Clinically, this condition presents as an inflammatory infiltrate around part or all of the corneoscleral limbus, affecting one or both eyes. Associated discomfort may be manifested by blepharospasm and/or ocular discharge. Adjacent structures including the uveal tract may be involved and demonstrate clinical inflammation, extending in rare cases to necrotic scleral lesions, uveitis, retinal detachment, and/or glaucoma. Commonly affected breeds include the Cocker Spaniel and Boston Terrier.

DIAGNOSIS AND TREATMENT

The diagnosis of scleritis is made based on clinical findings, confirmed if necessary by tissue biopsy and histopathology, which typically reveals a significant lymphoplasmacytic infiltrate. Systemic screening for immune-mediated disorders may be indicated in severe cases. Treatment comprises topical and/or systemic immune-modulatory therapy using corticosteroids and or adjunctive agents such as azathioprine, chlorambucil, and cyclosporine.

Potential Drug-Side-Effects

Potential adverse effects associated with the use of topical corticosteroids include impaired wound healing and corneal degeneration. Potential adverse effects associated with the use of systemic cortiocosteroids include polyphagia, polydipsia, polyuria, hair coat changes, weight gain, pancreatitis, gastrointestinal (GI) distress, muscle damage, hepatic impairment, and diabetes. Potential adverse effects associated with the use of systemic azathioprine and chlorambucil include GI distress, pancreatitis, hepatotoxicity, and myelosuppression. Potential adverse affects associated with the use of cyclosporine include hypersensitivity and GI distress.

Scleritis can typically be managed; however, in most cases, ongoing therapy is required in order to maintain the patient in a disease-free state.

SELECTED REFERENCES

Breaux CB, Sandmeyer LS, Grahn BH. Immunohistochemical investigation of canine episcleritis. *Vet Ophthalmol*. 2007;**10**(3):168–172.

Denk N, Sandmeyer LS, Lim CC, Bauer BS, Grahn BH. A retrospective study of the clinical, histological, and immunohistochemical manifestations of 5 dogs originally diagnosed histologically as necrotizing scleritis. *Vet Ophthalmol*. 2012;**15**(2):102–109. doi: 10.1111/j.1463-5224.2011.00948.x. Epub 2011 Sep 29.

Grahn BH, Sandmeyer LS. Canine episcleritis, nodular episclerokeratitis, scleritis, and necrotic scleritis. *Vet Clin North Am Small Anim Pract*. 2008;**38**(2):291–308, vi. doi: 10.1016/j.cvsm.2007.11.003.

Sandmeyer LS, Breaux CB, Grahn BH. What are your clinical diagnosis, differential diagnoses, therapeutic plan, and prognosis? Diffuse episcleritis of the right eye. *Can Vet J*. 2008;**49**(1):89–90.

Clinical Atlas of Canine and Feline Ophthalmic Disease, First Edition. Douglas Esson.

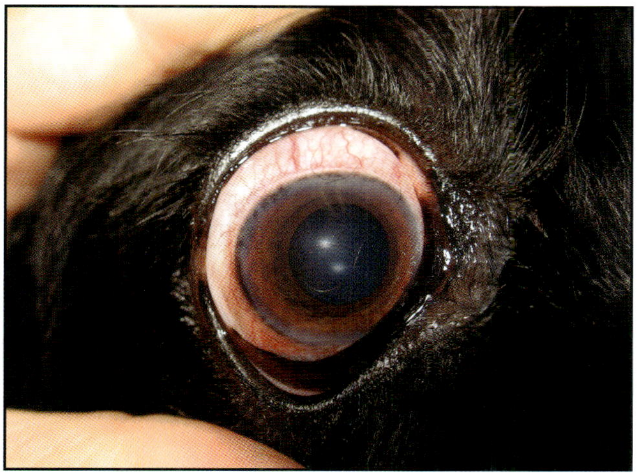

Figure 57.1 Typical presentation associated with primary scleritis. Limbal infiltration is visible.

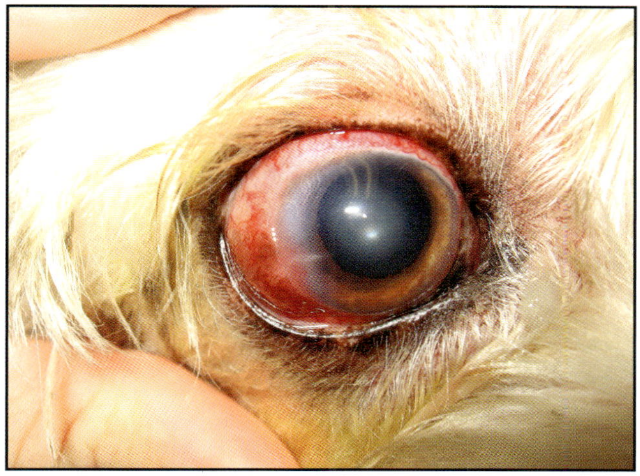

Figure 57.2 Typical presentation associated with primary scleritis. Limbal infiltration is visible.

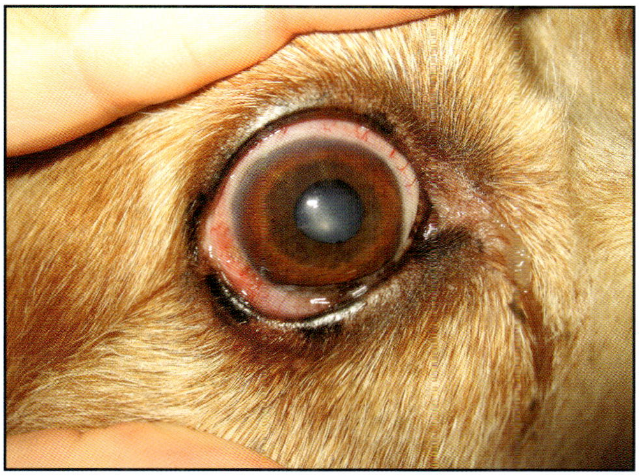

Figure 57.3 Typical presentation associated with primary scleritis. Limbal infiltration is visible.

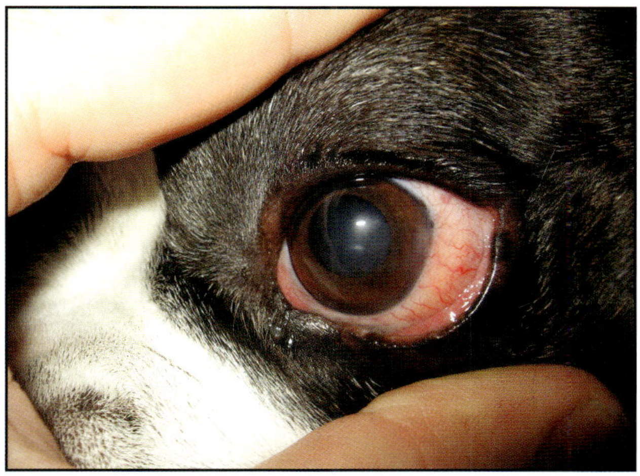

Figure 57.4 Typical presentation associated with primary scleritis. Limbal infiltration is visible.

CHAPTER 58
NODULAR GRANULOMATOUS EPISCLERITIS

PRESENTATION

Nodular granulomatous episcleritis (NGE) describes a proliferative inflammatory disorder of the canine scleral and/or episcleral tissues and is thought be immune-mediated in origin. Multiple terms have been used to describe this condition, including nodular fasciitis, fibrous histiocytoma, pseudotumor, and collie-granuloma. Clinically, affected patients display one or more smooth, firm, mass(es) affecting the corneoscleral limbus of one or both eyes, arising most commonly in the superotemporal region. Associated discomfort may be manifested by blepharospasm and/or ocular discharge. Commonly affected breeds include the Collie breeds, Spaniel breeds, and Terrier breeds.

DIAGNOSIS AND TREATMENT

The diagnosis of NGE is made on the basis of clinical findings, confirmed where indicated by tissue biopsy and histopathology, which typically reveals a proliferation of fibroblasts and a significant infiltration of lymphocytes, plasma cells, and histiocytes. Treatment comprises topical and/or systemic immune-modulatory therapy using corticosteroids and or adjunctive agents such as azathioprine, chlorambucil, and cyclosporine.

Potential Drug-Side-Effects

Potential adverse effects associated with the use of topical corticosteroids include impaired wound healing and corneal degeneration. Potential adverse effects associated with the use of systemic corticosteroids include polyphagia, polydipsia, polyuria, hair coat changes, weight gain, pancreatitis, gastrointestinal (GI) distress, muscle damage, hepatic impairment, and diabetes. Potential adverse effects associated with the use of systemic azathioprine and chlorambucil include GI distress, pancreatitis, hepatotoxicity, and myelosuppression. Potential adverse affects associated with the use of cyclosporine include hypersensitivity and GI distress.

In severe cases, lesions may initially be managed by the injection of repository corticosteroids, surgical resection, cryotherapy, and/or the application of B-irradiation. NGE can typically be managed; however, in most cases, ongoing therapy is required in order to maintain the patient in a disease-free state.

SELECTED REFERENCES

Barnes LD, Pearce JW, Berent LM, Fox DB, Giuliano EA. Surgical management of orbital nodular granulomatous episcleritis in a dog. *Vet Ophthalmol.* 2010;**13**(4):251–258. doi: 10.1111/j.1463-5224.2010.00781.x.

Day MJ, Mould JR, Carter WJ. An immunohistochemical investigation of canine idiopathic granulomatous scleritis. *Vet Ophthalmol.* 2008;**11**(1):11–17. doi: 10.1111/j.1463-5224.2007.00592.x.

Grahn BH, Sandmeyer LS. Canine episcleritis, nodular episclerokeratitis, scleritis, and necrotic scleritis. *Vet Clin North Am Small Anim Pract.* 2008;**38**(2):291–308, vi. doi: 10.1016/j.cvsm.2007.11.003. Review.

Clinical Atlas of Canine and Feline Ophthalmic Disease, First Edition. Douglas Esson.

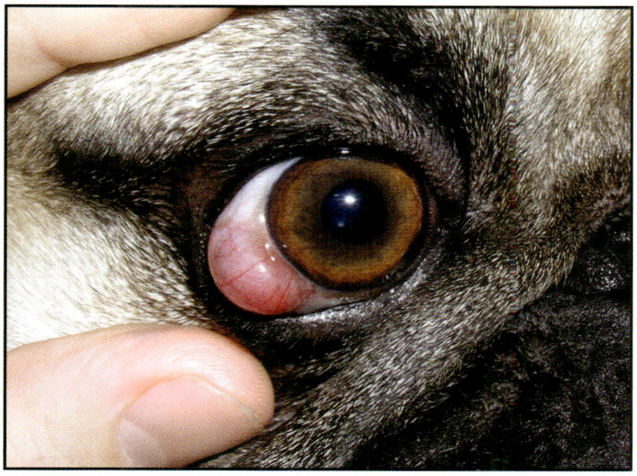

Figure 58.1 Typical presentation associated with nodular granulomatous episcleritis (NGE).

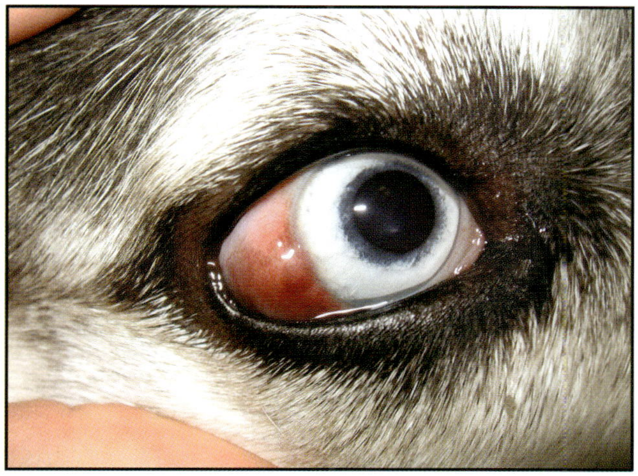

Figure 58.2 Typical presentation associated with nodular granulomatous episcleritis (NGE).

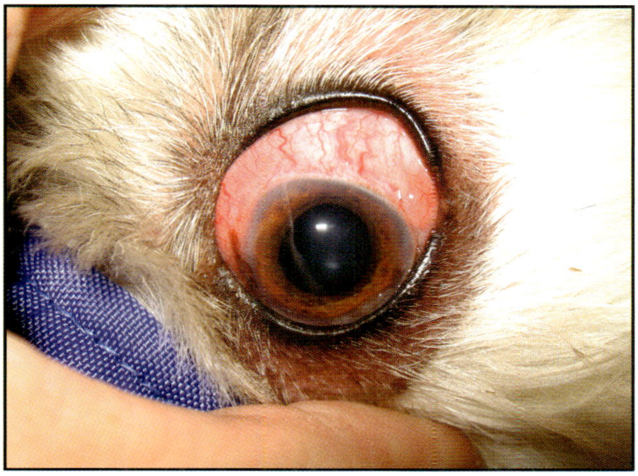

Figure 58.3 Typical presentation associated with nodular granulomatous episcleritis (NGE).

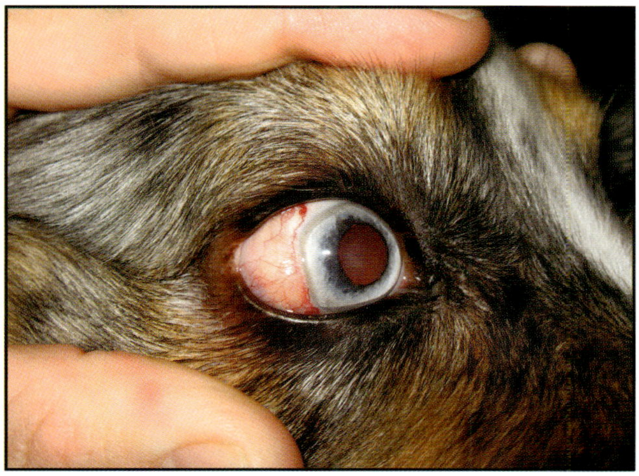

Figure 58.4 Typical presentation associated with nodular granulomatous episcleritis (NGE).

CHAPTER 59
CHRONIC SUPERFICIAL KERATITIS (CSK)

PRESENTATION

Chronic superficial keratitis (CSK) describes a (typically) bilateral inflammatory condition, which predominantly affects the corneal tissues. Changes encompass vascular proliferation, inflammatory cell infiltration, and secondary pigment deposition. Cellular infiltration comprises lymphocytes, plasma cells, neutrophils, and melanocytes. These changes most commonly arise from the lateral limbal region and progress across the central corneas. Adjacent eyelid margin, conjunctival and third eyelid inflammation are frequently associated with this process. Secondary corneal degeneration and mineralization may ensue in chronic and severe cases. This disease has been also referred to as "pannus" and "Uberreiter's syndrome." CSK is considered to represent an immune-mediated process with an underlying hereditary basis. Exposure to UV sunlight likely exacerbates clinical symptoms. Commonly affected breeds include the German Shepherd, Belgian Malinois, and Greyhound.

DIAGNOSIS AND TREATMENT

The diagnosis of CSK is made on the basis of clinical findings, supported if necessary by tissue biopsy. Untreated, CSK has the potential to result in blindness. In addition, chronic corneal inflammation may be risk a factor for the development of corneal squamous cell carcinoma. Inflammatory changes typically respond to topical anti-inflammatory therapy using corticosteroids (± topical immune-suppressive agents including cyclosporine and/or tacrolimus). Occasionally, repository subconjunctival corticosteroids may be indicated. In severe cases, systemic therapy using corticosteroids and/or azathioprine additionally may be required.

Potential Drug-Side-Effects

Potential adverse effects associated with the use of topical corticosteroids include impaired wound healing and corneal degeneration. Potential adverse effects associated with the use of systemic corticosteroids include polyphagia, polydipsia, polyuria, hair coat changes, weight gain, pancreatitis, gastrointestinal (GI) distress, muscle damage, hepatic impairment, and diabetes. Potential adverse effects associated with the use of systemic azothioprine include GI distress, pancreatitis, hepatotoxicity, and myelosuppression Potential adverse effects associated with the use of topical cyclosporine and tacrolimus include periocular dermatitis and alopecia.

CSK is easily controlled in most cases; however, ongoing topical therapy is typically required in order to prevent a recurrence of symptoms. In unusually severe and chronic cases, surgical superficial keratectomy ± the use of adjunctive B-radiation may be indicated.

SELECTED REFERENCES

Allgoewer I, Hoecht S. Radiotherapy for canine chronic superficial keratitis using soft X-rays (15 kV). *Vet Ophthalmol.* 2010;**13**(1):20–25. doi: 10.1111/j.1463-5224.2009.00750.x.

Balicki I. Clinical study on the application of tacrolimus and DMSO in the treatment of chronic superficial keratitis in dogs. *Pol J Vet Sci.* 2012;**15**(4):667–676.

Peiffer RL Jr, Gelatt KN, Gwin RM. Chronic superficial keratitis. *Vet Med Small Anim Clin.* 1977;**72**(1):35–37. No abstract available.

Williams DL. Histological and immunohistochemical evaluation of canine chronic superficial keratitis. *Res Vet Sci.* 1999;**67**(2):191–195.

Clinical Atlas of Canine and Feline Ophthalmic Disease, First Edition. Douglas Esson.

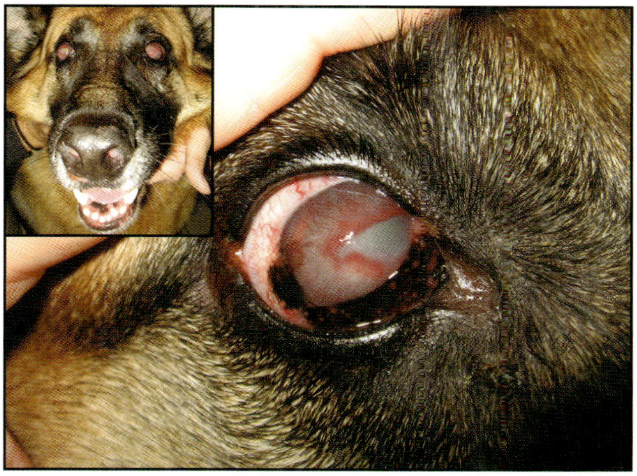

Figure 59.1 Typical presentation associated with chronic superficial keratitis. Associated infiltration of third eyelid tissues is notable. Inset demonstrates the typically bilateral presentation of the condition.

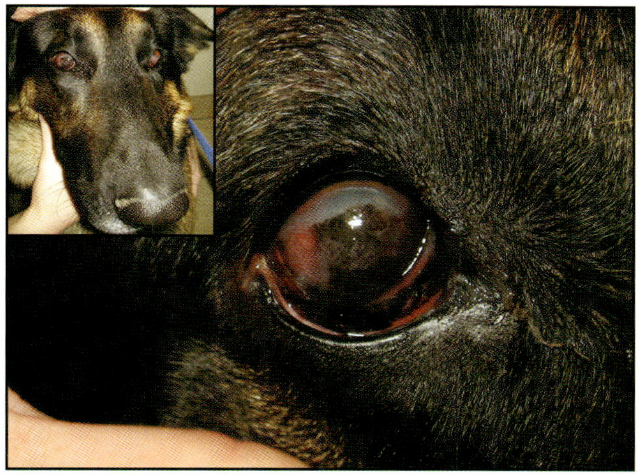

Figure 59.2 Typical presentation associated with chronic superficial keratitis. Secondary corneal pigmentation is notable. Inset demonstrates the typically bilateral presentation of the condition.

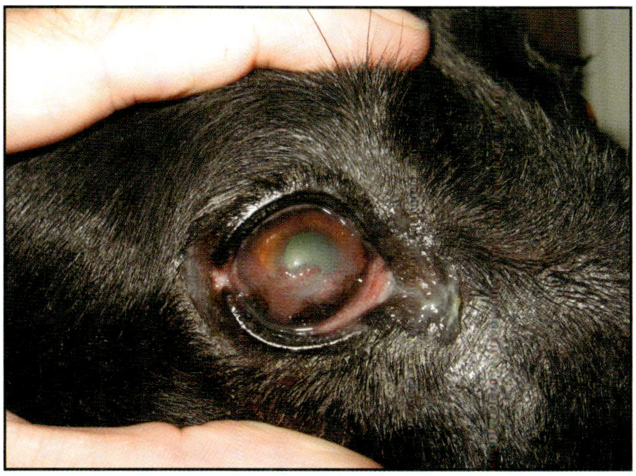

Figure 59.3 Typical presentation associated with chronic superficial keratitis.

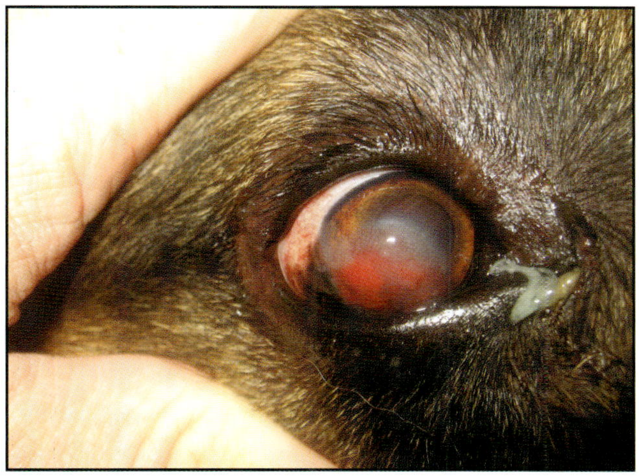

Figure 59.4 Typical presentation associated with chronic superficial keratitis.

CHAPTER 60
EOSINOPHILIC KERATOCONJUNCTIVITIS

PRESENTATION

Eosinophilic keratoconjunctivitis (EKC) describes a feline condition comprising infiltration of the corneal and/or conjunctival tissues with an eosinophil-rich inflammatory infiltrate. Clinically, affected cats display a variable degree of cream- to white-colored infiltration and "plaque-like" deposition, frequently in association with vascular keratitis. Changes typically originate from the corneoscleral limbus and may be unilateral or bilateral. Associated discomfort may be manifested by blepharospasm and/or ocular discharge.

DIAGNOSIS AND TREATMENT

The diagnosis of EKC is confirmed by the cytologic or histopathologic evaluation of samples harvested from affected tissues. Treatment comprises topical and/or systemic anti-inflammatory therapy, typically comprising corticosteroids. Adjunctive cyclosporine therapy may also be beneficial in selected cases. In severe cases, a prompt clinical response is typically noted following the institution of systemic megestrol acetate therapy; however, the significant potential adverse effects that may be associated with its use dictate clinical caution and close monitoring of treated patients. Finally, the relationship between feline herpesviral disease and EKC remains unclear and topical and/or systemic antiviral therapy may additionally be warranted in selected cases.

Potential Drug-Side-Effects

Potential adverse effects associated with the use of systemic corticosteroids include polyphagia, polydipsia, polyuria, hair coat changes, weight gain, pancreatitis, gastrointestinal (GI) distress, muscle damage, hepatic impairment, and diabetes. Potential adverse effects associated with the use of topical corticosteroids include impaired wound healing and corneal degeneration. Potential adverse effects associated with the use of topical cyclosporine include periocular dermatitis and alopecia. Potential adverse affects associated with the use of megestrol acetate include the development of diabetes mellitus, mammary hyperplasia, and neoplasia.

EKC is easily controlled in most cases; however, ongoing therapy is typically required in order to control the condition and prevent a recurrence of symptoms.

SELECTED REFERENCES

Andrew SE. Immune-mediated canine and feline keratitis. *Vet Clin North Am Small Anim Pract*. 2008;**38**(2):269–290, vi. doi: 10.1016/j.cvsm.2007.11.007.

Dean E, Meunier V. Feline eosinophilic keratoconjunctivitis: a retrospective study of 45 cases (56 eyes). *Feline Med Surg*. 2013;**15**(8):661–666. doi: 10.1177/1098612X12472181. Epub 2013 Jan 15.

Nasisse MP, Glover TL, Moore CP, Weigler BJ. Detection of feline herpesvirus 1 DNA in corneas of cats with eosinophilic keratitis or corneal sequestration. *Am J Vet Res*. 1998;**59**(7):856–858.

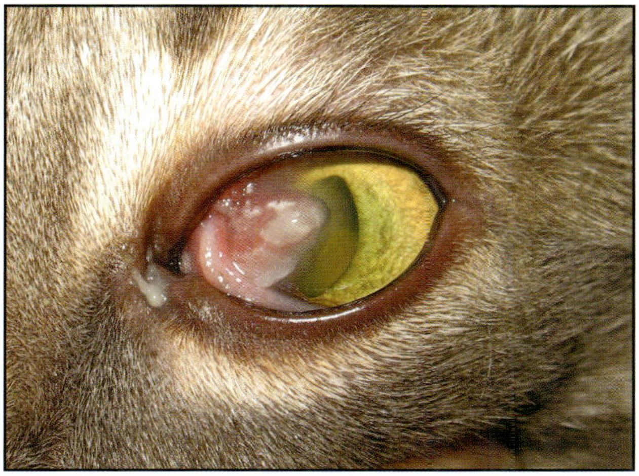

Figure 60.1 Typical presentation associated with eosinophilic keratoconjunctivitis, comprising cream-colored corneal infiltration and vascular changes.

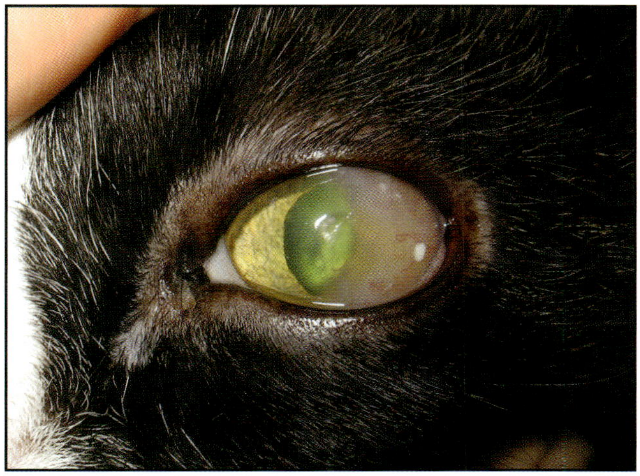

Figure 60.2 Typical presentation associated with eosinophilic keratoconjunctivitis, comprising cream-colored corneal infiltration and vascular changes.

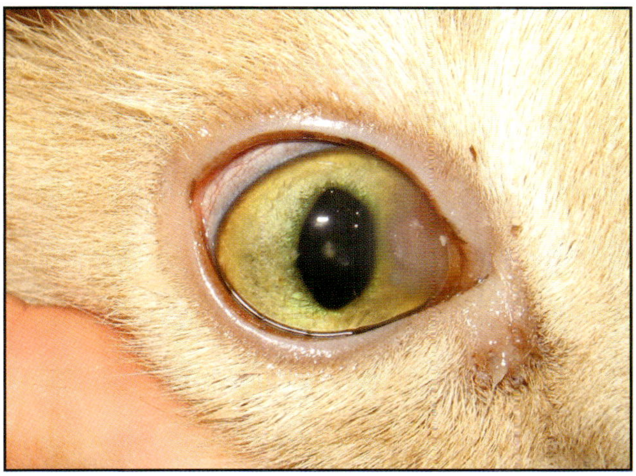

Figure 60.3 Typical presentation associated with Eosinophilic keratoconjunctivitis, comprising cream-colored corneal infiltration and vascular changes.

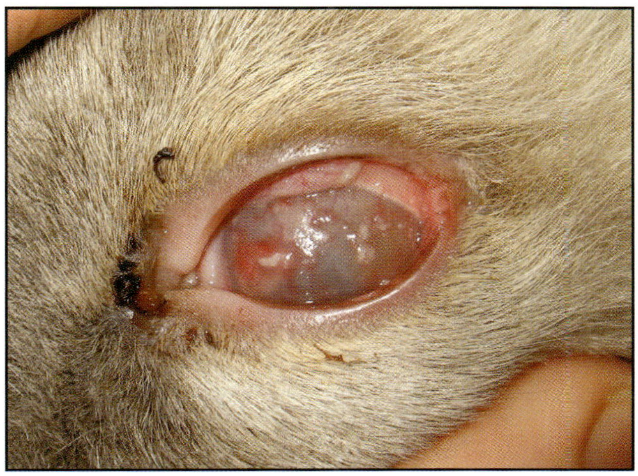

Figure 60.4 Typical presentation associated with eosinophilic keratoconjunctivitis, comprising cream-colored corneal infiltration and vascular changes.

CHAPTER 61
HERPESVIRAL-ASSOCIATED KERATITIS

PRESENTATION

Feline herpes virus-1 (FHV-1) is a widespread and prevalent cause of ophthalmic disease, affecting both kittens and mature cats (particularly shelter animals and those from multi-cat households). Initial infection occurs via contact with the virus (typically through cat-to-cat contact) or contaminated fomites. Once infected, cats become latent carriers of the disease, which may recrudesce under conditions of physiologic or pharmacologic immunosuppression. Symptoms may include pyrexia, lethargy, inappetance, signs of upper respiratory disease (such as coughing or sneezing), conjunctivitis, chemosis, symblepharon, and dendritic, superficial or stromal ulcerative keratitis (see also Herpesviral-Associated Conjunctivitis). Discomfort may be manifested as blepharospasm and/or ocular discharge. Symptoms may be unilateral or bilateral.

DIAGNOSIS AND TREATMENT

Accurate testing for the presence of FHV-1 and its correlation with ophthalmic disease is problematic; however, polymerase-chain-reaction assays, based on tissue samples, are currently considered most reliable. Ultimately, healthy cats recover spontaneously from outbreaks over the course of several weeks; however, treatment is frequently indicated. Topical and/or systemic antiviral agents may be administered, including trifluorothymidine, idoxuridine, cidofovir, ganciclovir, and/or famciclovir.

Potential Drug-Side-Effects

Potential complications associated with the use of topical antiviral agents include local irritation. Potential complications associated with the use of systemic antiviral medications include gastrointestinal (GI) distress, myelosuppression, and/or hepatopathy.

The concurrent administration of systemic L-lysine may decrease the severity of symptoms, potentially via the inhibition of herpesviral metabolism. Caution is indicated when considering the use of anti-inflammatory therapy to treat herpesviral-associated disease. Nonsteroidal agents are generally considered less likely to result in complication and the use of corticosteroids generally considered contraindicated in most cases. Corneal ulcers should be treated medically or surgically, as indicated. Herpesviral-associated conjunctivitis may be complicated by underlying systemic disease (such as FeLV and FIV), concurrent viral pathogens (such as calicivirus) and/or secondary infection with *Chlamydophila*, *Mycoplasma*, and/or bacterial pathogens.

SELECTED REFERENCES

Drazenovich TL, Fascetti AJ, Westermeyer HD, Sykes JE, Bannasch MJ, Kass PH, Hurley KF, Maggs DJ. Effects of dietary lysine supplementation on upper respiratory and ocular disease and detection of infectious organisms in cats within an animal shelter. *Am J Vet Res*. 2009;**70**(11):1391–1400. doi: 10.2460/ajvr.70.11.1391.

Fontenelle JP, Powell CC, Veir JK, Radecki SV, Lappin MR. Effect of topical ophthalmic application of cidofovir on experimentally induced primary ocular feline herpesvirus-1 infection in cats. *Am J Vet Res*. 2008;**69**(2):289–293. doi: 10.2460/ajvr.69.2.289.

Maggs DJ. Update on pathogenesis, diagnosis, and treatment of feline herpesvirus type 1. *Clin Tech Small Anim Pract*. 2005;**20**(2):94–101.

Maggs DJ. Antiviral therapy for feline herpesvirus infections. *Vet Clin North Am Small Anim Pract*. 2010;**40**(6):1055–1062. doi: 10.1016/j.cvsm.2010.07.010.

Thomasy SM, Lim CC, Reilly CM, Kass PH, Lappin MR, Maggs DJ. Evaluation of orally administered famciclovir in cats experimentally infected with feline herpesvirus type-1. *Am J Vet Res*. 2011;**72**(1):85–95. doi: 10.2460/ajvr.72.1.85.

Clinical Atlas of Canine and Feline Ophthalmic Disease, First Edition. Douglas Esson.

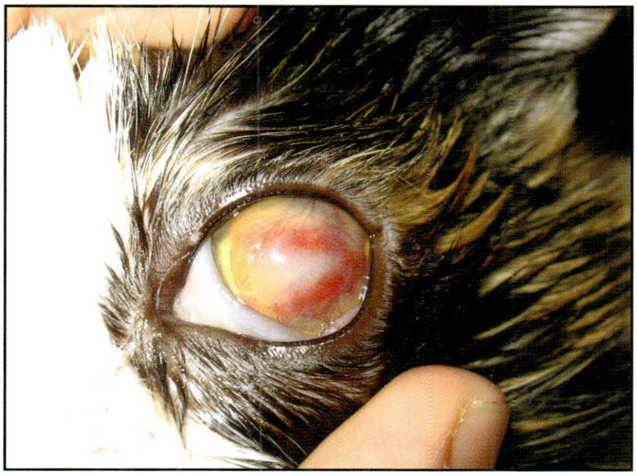

Figure 61.1 Vascular keratitis secondary to herpes-viral-associated infection.

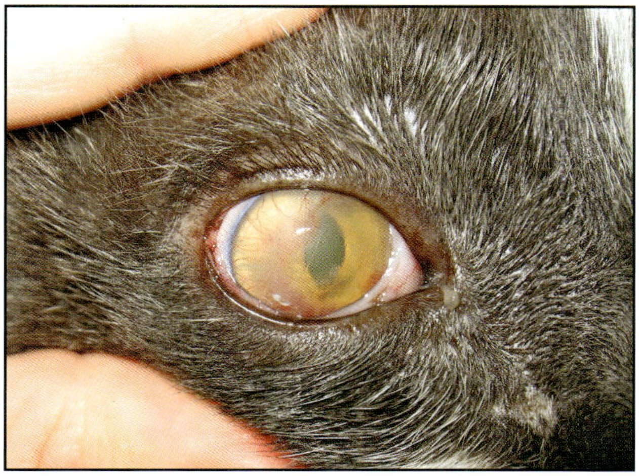

Figure 61.2 Vascular keratitis secondary to herpes-viral-associated infection.

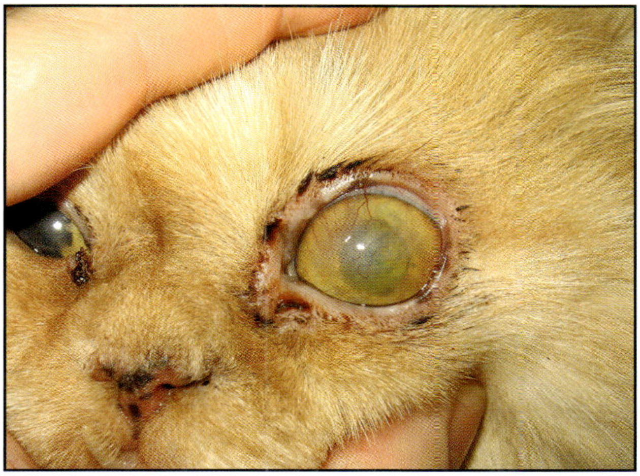

Figure 61.3 Vascular keratitis secondary to herpes-viral-associated infection.

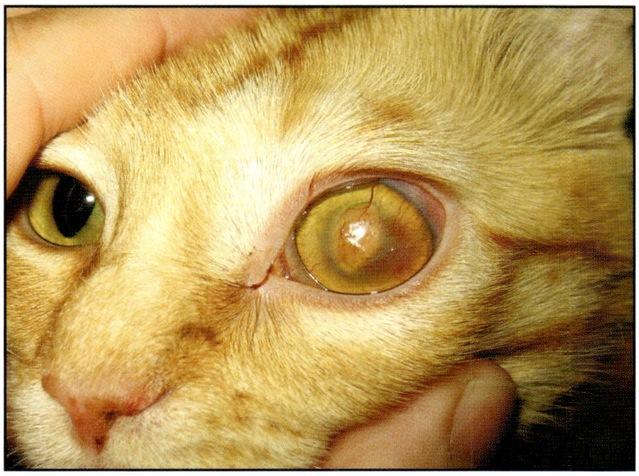

Figure 61.4 Vascular keratitis secondary to herpes-viral-associated infection.

As a consequence, tetracyclines, azithromycin, and fluoroquinolones represent appropriate antimicrobial choices when treating potentially complicated cases.

Potential Drug-Side-Effects

Potential adverse effects associated with tetracyclines and azithromycin include gastrointestinal (GI) distress, photosensitivity, and hepatic damage. Potential adverse effects associated with fluoroquinolones include GI distress, hepatic disease, neurologic disease, and/or retinal toxicity.

CHAPTER 62
CANINE MULTIFOCAL IMMUNE-MEDIATED PUNCTATE KERATITIS (MIPK)

PRESENTATION

Multifocal immune-mediated punctate keratitis (MIPK) describes a canine condition that results in multiple sites of discrete corneal inflammation and/or ulceration and which is suspected to be immune-mediated in etiology. Lesions are typically oval to circular, well-defined and may be associated with an arborizing vascular response. Secondary infection may result in rapid progression of these lesions. Commonly affected breeds include the Shetland Sheepdog and Dachshund.

DIAGNOSIS AND TREATMENT

The diagnosis of immune-mediated punctate keratitis is made on the basis of clinical findings. Ulcerative keratitis, thought to be immune-mediated in origin, should be managed with a cautious combination of topical (± systemic) antimicrobial as well as anti-inflammatory therapy. Appropriate anti-inflammatory agents may include NSAIDS, glucocorticoids and/or cyclosporine.

Potential Drug-Side-Effects

Potential adverse effects associated with the use of topical corticosteroids include impaired wound healing and corneal degeneration. Potential adverse effects associated with the use of topical cyclosporine and tacrolimus include periocular dermatitis and alopecia. Potential adverse effects associated with the use of systemic prednisone include polyphagia, polydipsia, polyuria, hair coat changes, weight gain, pancreatitis, gastrointestinal (GI) distress, muscle damage, hepatic impairment, and diabetes.

The potential for acute clinical deterioration is initially high and patients should be frequently monitored until corneal inflammation is adequately controlled. The prognosis for controlling this disease is generally good; however, many cases require long-term, low-dose maintenance therapy in order to prevent a recurrence of symptoms.

SELECTED REFERENCES

Andrew SE. Immune-mediated canine and feline keratitis. *Vet Clin North Am Small Anim Pract*. 2008;**38**(2):269–290, vi. doi: 10.1016/j.cvsm.2007.11.007. Review.

Clerc C, Jegou J. Superficial punctuate keratitis. *Can Pract*. 1996;**21**:6–11.

Dice PF 2nd. Primary corneal disease in the dog and cat. *Vet Clin North Am Small Anim Pract*. 1980;**10**(2):339–356.

Clinical Atlas of Canine and Feline Ophthalmic Disease, First Edition. Douglas Esson.

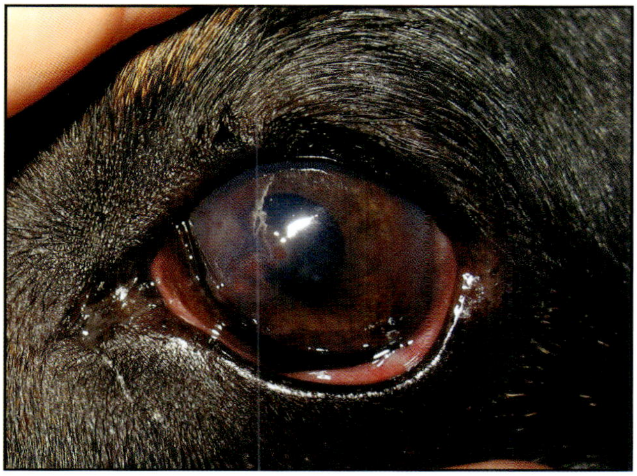

Figure 62.1 Typical presentation associated with canine multifocal immune-mediated punctate keratitis.

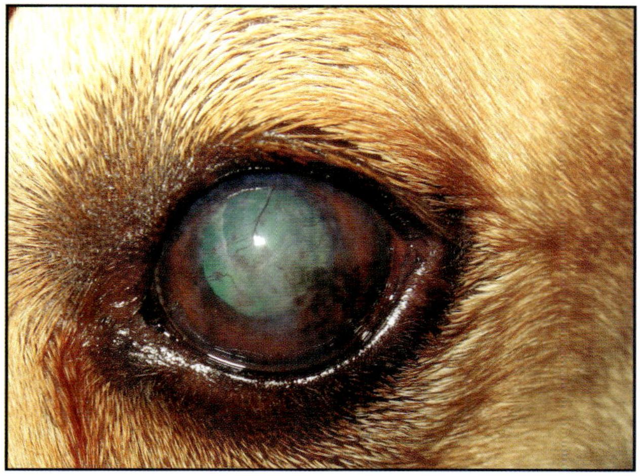

Figure 62.2 Typical presentation associated with canine multifocal immune-mediated punctate keratitis.

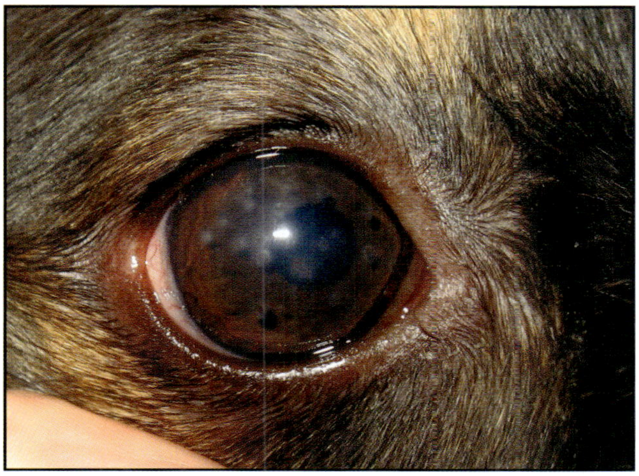

Figure 62.3 Typical presentation associated with canine multifocal immune-mediated punctate keratitis.

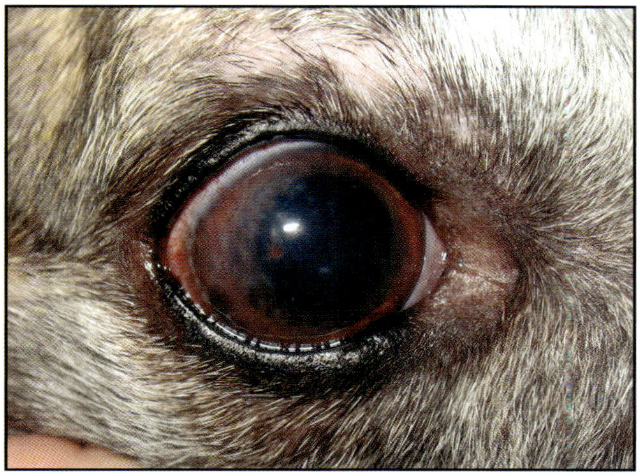

Figure 62.4 Typical presentation associated with canine multifocal immune-mediated punctate keratitis.

CHAPTER 63
ENDOTHELIITIS

PRESENTATION

Uveitis, infection with canine adenovirus type-1 (CAV-1) and/or vaccination with modified live CAV-1 strains may be associated with endothelitis (see also Vaccine-Associated Uveitis). Ocular symptoms may include the presence of aqueous flare, pupillary miosis, and/or corneal edema (sometimes described as "blue eye") secondary to endothelial cell dysfunction. Potential sequela include bullous keratopathy, ulcerative keratitis, and/or secondary glaucoma. The Afghan hound has been described as being at increased risk.

DIAGNOSIS AND TREATMENT

The diagnosis of endotheliitis is made on the basis of clinical findings in conjunction with history (including that of recent vaccination), routine complete blood count (CBC)/chemistry analysis, and/or testing for the presence of infectious organisms. Treatment typically encompasses the administration of topical and systemic (steroidal) anti-inflammatory therapy (unless contraindicated). In many cases, symptoms will resolve if appropriately treated early in the course of the disease. Secondary pathologies including corneal ulceration and/or glaucoma should be managed as appropriate if present (see also Secondary (Post-Inflammatory) Glaucoma).

Potential Drug-Side-Effects

Potential adverse effects associated with the use of topical corticosteroids include impaired wound healing and corneal degeneration. Potential adverse effects associated with the use of systemic prednisone include polyphagia, polydipsia, polyuria, hair coat changes, weight gain, pancreatitis, gastrointestinal (GI) distress, muscle damage, hepatic impairment, and diabetes.

SELECTED REFERENCES

Aguirre G, Carmichael L, Bistner S. Corneal endothelium in viral induced anterior uveitis. Ultrastructural changes following canine adenovirus type 1 infection. *Arch Ophthalmol*. 1975;**93**(3):219–224.

Curtis R, Barnett KC. Canine adenovirus-induced ocular lesions in the Afghan hound. *Cornell Vet*. 1981;**71**(1):85–95.

Curtis R, Barnett KC. The 'blue eye' phenomenon. *Vet Rec*. 1983;**112**(15):347–353.

Clinical Atlas of Canine and Feline Ophthalmic Disease, First Edition. Douglas Esson.

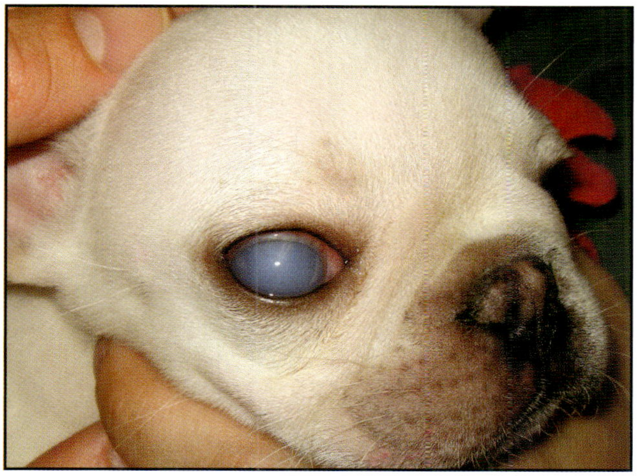

Figure 63.1 Endotheliitis secondary to a vaccine-associated reaction.

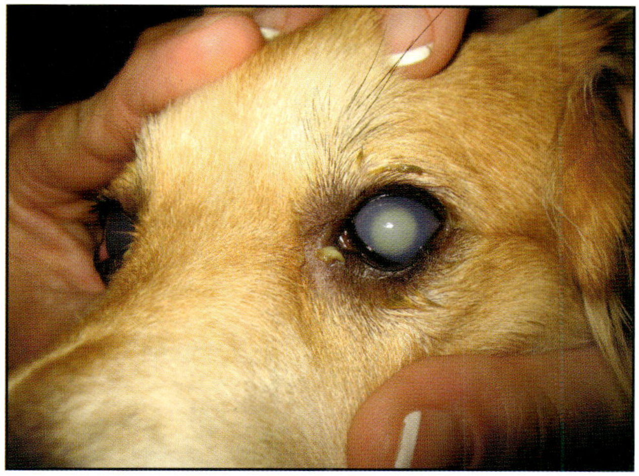

Figure 63.2 Endotheliitis secondary to a vaccine-associated reaction.

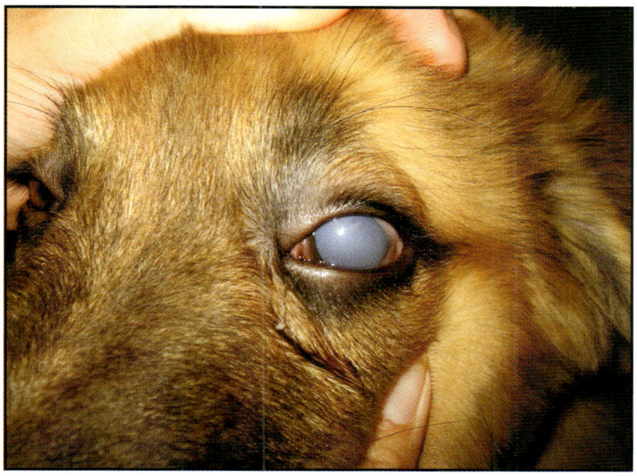

Figure 63.3 Endotheliitis secondary to a vaccine-associated reaction.

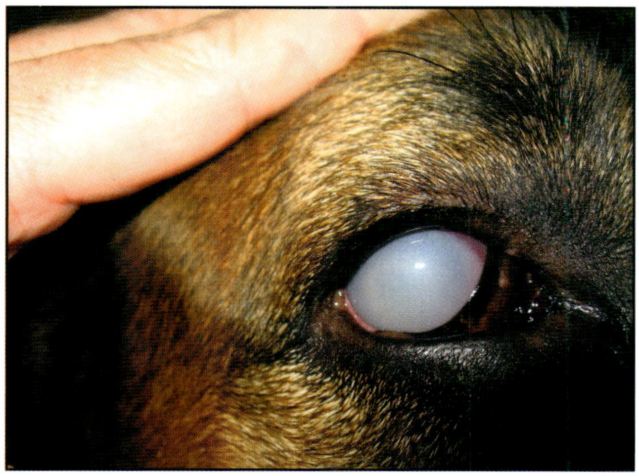

Figure 63.4 Endotheliitis secondary to a vaccine-associated reaction.

CHAPTER 64
BULLOUS KERATOPATHY

PRESENTATION

Bullous keratopathy describes an acute decompensation of corneal stromal tissue. Severe, acute, focal, or generalized corneal edema may lead to the development of one or more large, unstable corneal bullae (see also Keratomalacia (Melting Ulcers)). Changes may develop extremely rapidly (typically within 24–48 h), coalesce, and/or rupture. Clinically, this condition appears as grossly distorted edematous corneal tissue, which typically bulges forward. This process is mediated by proteolytic enzymes that may derive from corneal cells, inflammatory cells, and/or bacterial pathogens and may or may not be associated with preexisting corneal inflammation and/or ulceration. Bullous keratopathy may occur in canine and feline species of any breed or crossed breed; however, brachycephalic animals are frequently affected.

DIAGNOSIS AND TREATMENT

Bullous keratopathy is diagnosed on the basis of clinical findings. Treatment comprises the stabilization of the metalloprotease enzymes that mediate this process. Appropriate topical therapeutic agents include serum (fresh or frozen), tetracyclines, EDTA solution, and/or *N*-acetyl cysteine. Topical anti-collagenases should be applied frequently. The use of corticosteroids is generally contraindicated. Secondary bacterial infection may be treated using appropriate antimicrobials. In severe cases, or those associated with existing or impending corneal rupture, surgical resection of diseased tissue, and/or tectonic corneal grafting procedures may be indicated. The use of an Elizabethan collar will prevent self-trauma during the healing process.

SELECTED REFERENCES

Cooley PL, Dice PF 2nd. Corneal dystrophy in the dog and cat. *Vet Clin North Am Small Anim Pract*. 1990;**20**(3):681–692. Review.

Moore PA. Feline corneal disease. *Clin Tech Small Anim Pract*. 2005;**20**(2):83–93. Review.

Ollivier FJ, Gilger BC, Barrie KP, Kallberg ME, Plummer CE, O'Reilly S, Gelatt KN, Brooks DE. Proteinases of the cornea and preocular tear film. *Vet Ophthalmol*. 2007;**10**(4):199–206. Review.

Pattullo K. Acute bullous keratopathy in a domestic shorthair. *Can Vet J*. 2008;**49**(2):187–189.

Clinical Atlas of Canine and Feline Ophthalmic Disease, First Edition. Douglas Esson.

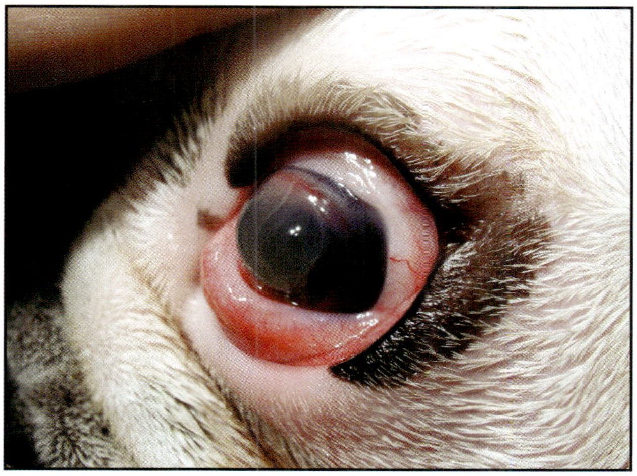

Figure 64.1 Bullous keratopathy as a result of keratitis and uncontrolled protease-mediated tissue destruction.

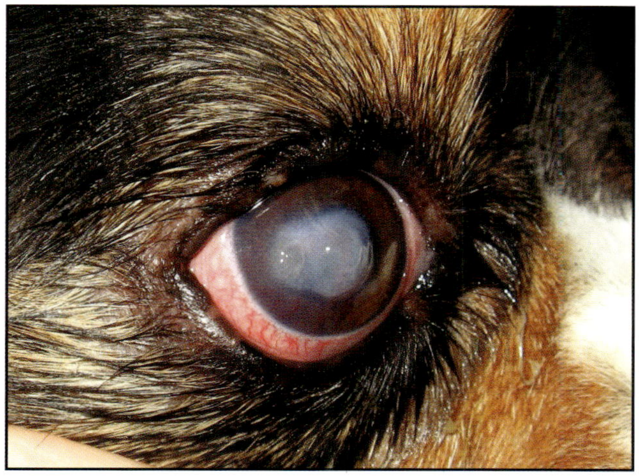

Figure 64.2 Bullous keratopathy as a result of keratitis and uncontrolled protease-mediated tissue destruction.

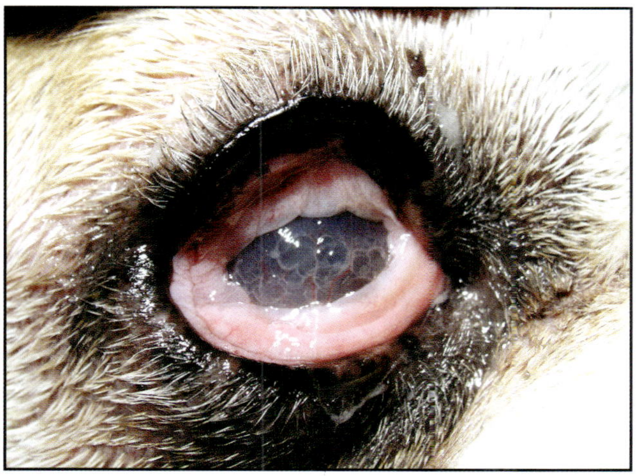

Figure 64.3 Bullous keratopathy as a result of keratitis and uncontrolled protease-mediated tissue destruction.

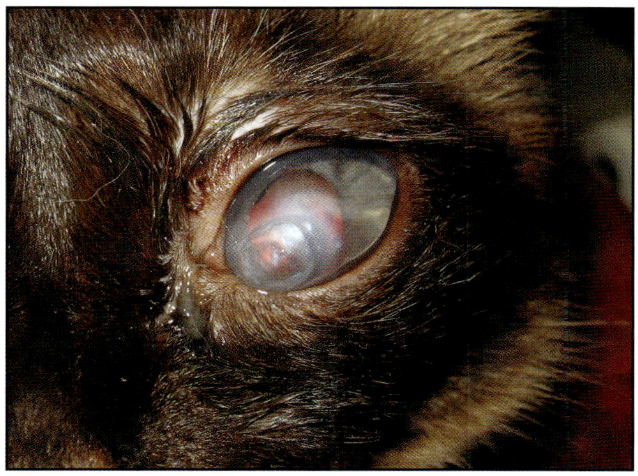

Figure 64.4 Bullous keratopathy as a result of keratitis and uncontrolled protease-mediated tissue destruction.

CHAPTER 65
FELINE CORNEAL SEQUESTRUM

PRESENTATION

The feline corneal sequestrum represents a localized region of corneal necrosis and associated inflammation. Clinically, corneal sequestra appear as tan to brown regions of corneal discoloration. Lesions may vary significantly in both size and depth and may or may not be associated with concurrent ulceration. The condition may be unilateral or bilateral. Associated discomfort may be manifested as blepharospasm and/or ocular discharge. Chronic preexisting keratitis, corneal ulceration, the performing of inappropriate "grid keratotomies," and/or the presence of FHV-1 as well as breed predispositions are potential contributory factors. Commonly affected breeds include the Persian and Himalayan.

DIAGNOSIS AND TREATMENT

The diagnosis of feline corneal sequestrum is made based on clinical findings. The treatment of choice for corneal sequsetra is excision via surgical keratectomy, facilitated by operating microscopy. The size and depth of keratectomy is determined by the extent of the lesion and tectonic corneal grafting may or may not additionally be warranted following the removal of diseased tissue. Topical and/or systemic antimicrobial as well as topical and/or systemic antiviral agents may or may not be indicated on a case-by-case basis. The routine use of an Elizabethan collar postoperatively will prevent self-trauma.

SELECTED REFERENCES

Cullen CL, Wadowska DW, Singh A, Melekhovets Y. Ultrastructural findings in feline corneal sequestra. *Vet Ophthalmol.* 2005;**8**(5):295–303.

Featherstone HJ, Sansom J. Feline corneal sequestra: a review of 64 cases (80 eyes) from 1993 to 2000. *Vet Ophthalmol.* 2004;**7**(4):213–227.

Grahn BH, Sisler S, Storey E. Qualitative tear film and conjunctival goblet cell assessment of cats with corneal sequestra. *Vet Ophthalmol.* 2005;**8**(3):167–170.

Volopich S, Benetka V, Schwendenwein I, Möstl K, Sommerfeld-Stur I, Nell B. Cytologic findings, and feline herpesvirus DNA and Chlamydophila felis antigen detection rates in normal cats and cats with conjunctival and corneal lesions. *Vet Ophthalmol.* 2005;**8**(1):25–32.

Clinical Atlas of Canine and Feline Ophthalmic Disease, First Edition. Douglas Esson.

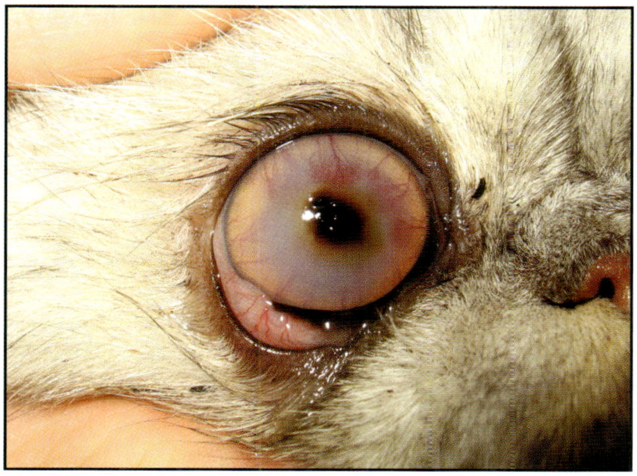

Figure 65.1 Typical presentation associated with a feline corneal sequestrum.

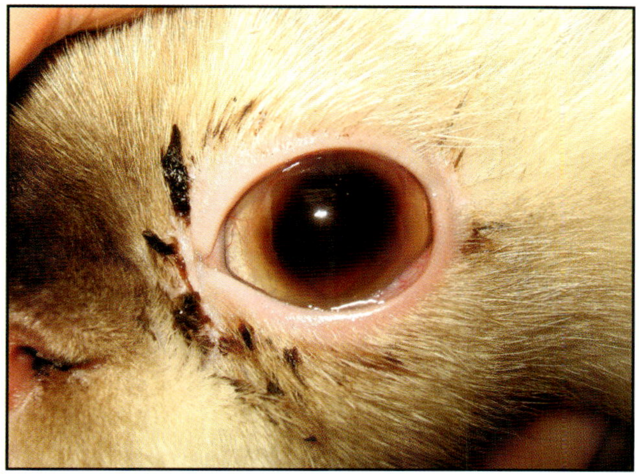

Figure 65.2 Typical presentation associated with a feline corneal sequestrum.

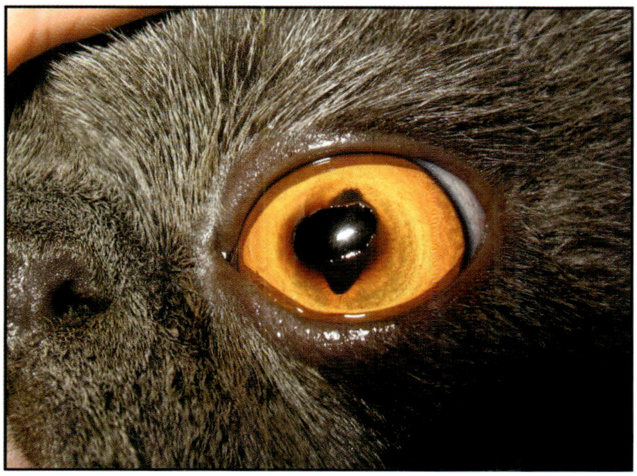

Figure 65.3 Typical presentation associated with a feline corneal sequestrum.

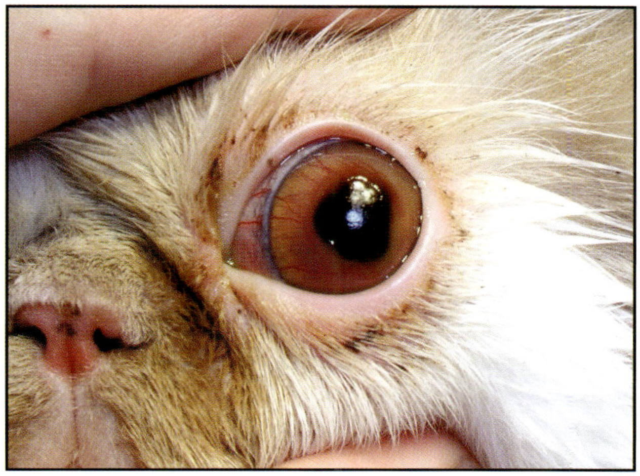

Figure 65.4 Typical presentation associated with a feline corneal sequestrum.

CHAPTER 66
PIGMENTARY KERATITIS

PRESENTATION

Pigmentary keratitis describes a relatively common presentation comprising the progressive deposition of pigment on the corneal and associated conjunctival surface(s). Clinically, this process is apparent as a smooth to irregular brown opacification, affecting a variable surface area. Concurrent inflammatory keratitis, marked by neovascularization, may additionally be present. Severe cases may exhibit complete pigmentary keratitis resulting in significant visual impairment or even functional blindness. Contributing factors may include exposure as a result of conformational lagophthalmos, chronic or severe keratitis, quantitative and/or qualitative tear film disorders, trichiasis and/or genetic factors. Commonly affected breeds include the Pug, the Pekingese, Shih Tzu, and Lhasa Apso.

DIAGNOSIS AND TREATMENT

The diagnosis of pigmentary keratitis is made based on clinical findings. Treatment comprises addressing any underlying disorders including corneal inflammation and/or tear film disorders, typically using topical corticosteroids, cyclosporine, tacrolimus, and/or tear film replacements/stabilizers. Long-term medication may be required in order to minimize progression of disease.

Potential Drug-Side-Effects

Potential adverse effects associated with the use of topical corticosteroids include impaired wound healing and corneal degeneration. Potential adverse effects associated with the use of topical cyclosporine and tacrolimus include periocular dermatitis and alopecia.

In addition, increased corneal protection and tear film coverage via reduction of the palpebral fissure through limited medial and/or lateral canthoplasty may help palliate progression of disease. Multiple techniques to decrease the size of palpebral fissure have been described, including the generally appropriate Roberts/Jensen medial pocket canthoplasty. Although corneal pigment is readily removed via keratectomy, the likelihood of its recurrence is high. The judicious application of cryotherapy or B-radiation may help limit recurrence in selected cases.

SELECTED REFERENCES

Azoulay T. Adjunctive cryotherapy for pigmentary keratitis in dogs: a study of 16 corneas. *Vet Ophthalmol*. 2013. doi: 10.1111/vop.12089. [Epub ahead of print]

Bedford PG. Technique of lateral canthoplasty for the correction of macropalpebral fissure in the dog. *J Small Anim Pract*. 1998;**39**(3):117–120.

Labelle AL, Dresser CB, Hamor RE, Allender MC, Disney JL. Characteristics of, prevalence of, and risk factors for corneal pigmentation (pigmentary keratopathy) in Pugs. *J Am Vet Med Assoc*. 2013;**243**(5):667–674. doi: 10.2460/javma.243.5.667.

van der Woerdt A. Adnexal surgery in dogs and cats. *Vet Ophthalmol*. 2004;**7**(5):284–290. Review.

Clinical Atlas of Canine and Feline Ophthalmic Disease, First Edition. Douglas Esson.

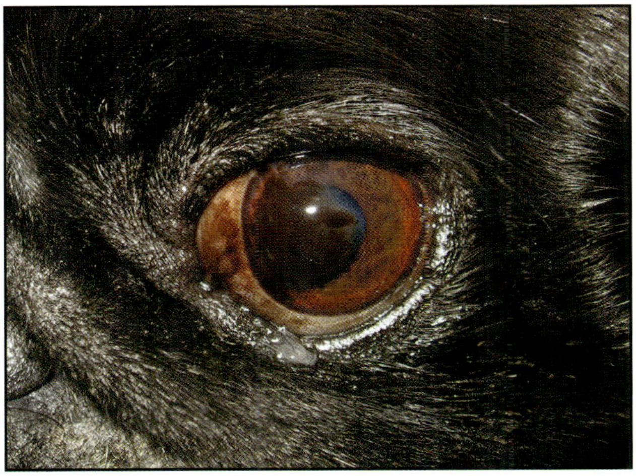

Figure 66.1 Pigmentary keratitis.

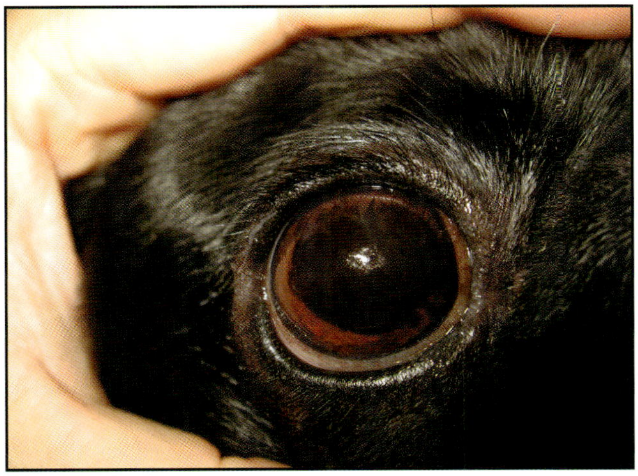

Figure 66.2 Pigmentary keratitis.

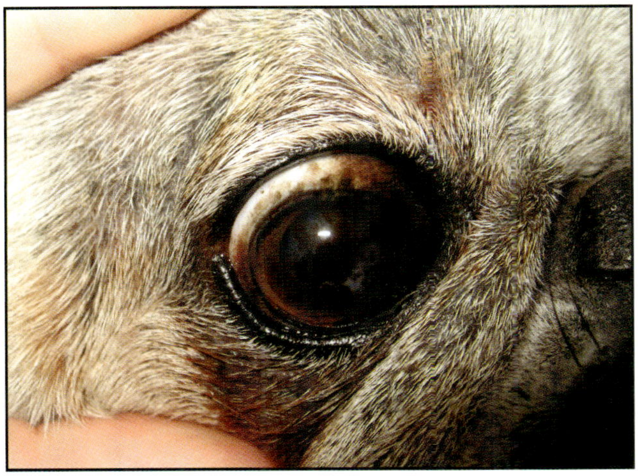

Figure 66.3 Pigmentary keratitis.

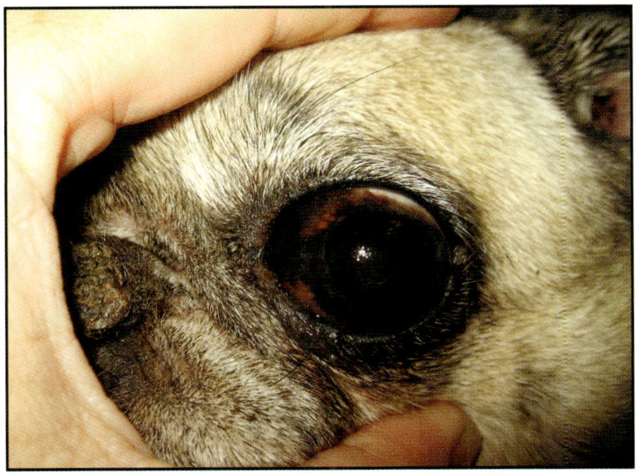

Figure 66.4 Pigmentary keratitis.

CHAPTER 67
CORNEAL ABSCESSATION

PRESENTATION

A corneal abscess may form following a breakdown in the epithelial (or rarely endothelial) barrier, allowing bacterial and/or fungal organisms entry into the corneal stroma, resulting in the formation of a nidus of infectious and/or inflammatory material. Clinically, this condition presents as a variably sized, focal tan to yellow area of stromal corneal discoloration, which is typically associated with intense discomfort as well as an aggressive vascular response. Fluorescein staining frequently fails to demonstrate concurrent corneal ulceration. Discomfort may be manifested as blepharospasm and/or ocular discharge.

DIAGNOSIS AND TREATMENT

The diagnosis of corneal abscessation is made on the basis of clinical findings. Treatment includes the exposure and removal of the infective focus via debridement/curettage as well as the institution of aggressive systemic and/or topical antimicrobial therapy. Intact epithelial surfaces and/or accumulations of biologic material are significant impediments to antimicrobial penetration and healing. Ideally, therapy should be based on cytological interpretation and Gram's staining as well as the subsequent culture and sensitivity testing of microbial samples. Concurrent topical and/or systemic (nonsteroidal) anti-inflammatory therapy may be indicated in selected cases. Affected corneas should be monitored closely and repeatedly during the healing process. The routine use of an Elizabethan collar postoperatively will prevent self-trauma.

SELECTED REFERENCES

Ledbetter EC, Munger RJ, Ring RD, Scarlett JM. Efficacy of two chondroitin sulfate ophthalmic solutions in the therapy of spontaneous chronic corneal epithelial defects and ulcerative keratitis associated with bullous keratopathy in dogs. *Vet Ophthalmol*. 2006;**9**(2):77–87.

Ollivier FJ. Bacterial corneal diseases in dogs and cats. *Clin Tech Small Anim Pract*. 2003;**18**(3):193–198.

Sherman A, Daniels JB, Wilkie DA, Lutz E. Actinomyces bowdenii ulcerative keratitis in a dog. *Vet Ophthalmol*. 2013;**16**(5):386–391. doi: 10.1111/vop.12001. Epub 2012 Nov 4.

Clinical Atlas of Canine and Feline Ophthalmic Disease, First Edition. Douglas Esson.

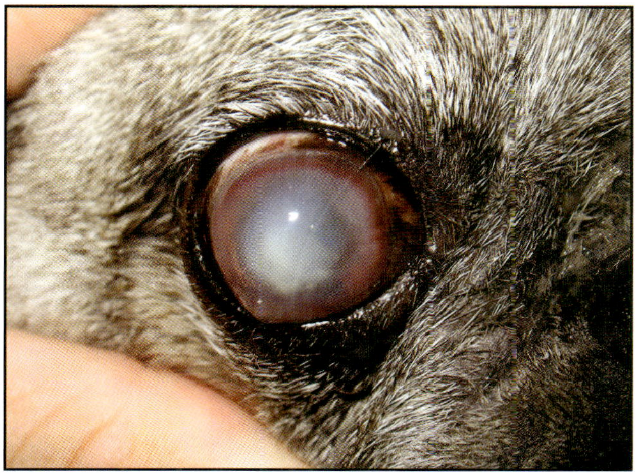

Figure 67.1 Typical presentation associated with corneal abscessation.

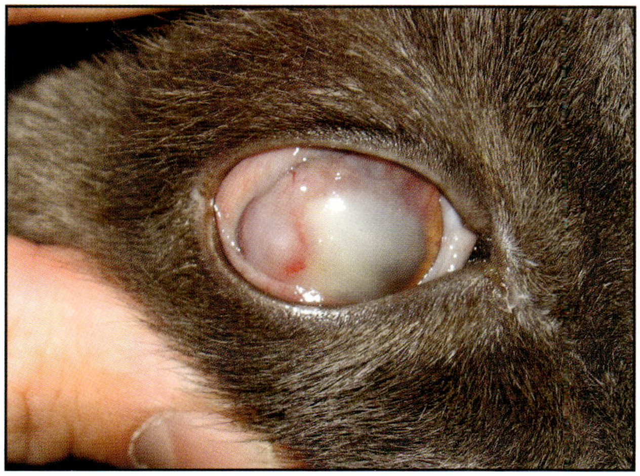

Figure 67.2 Typical presentation associated with corneal abscessation.

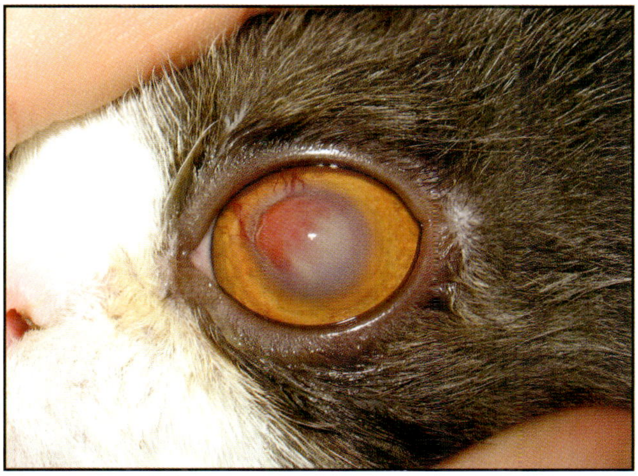

Figure 67.3 Typical presentation associated with corneal abscessation.

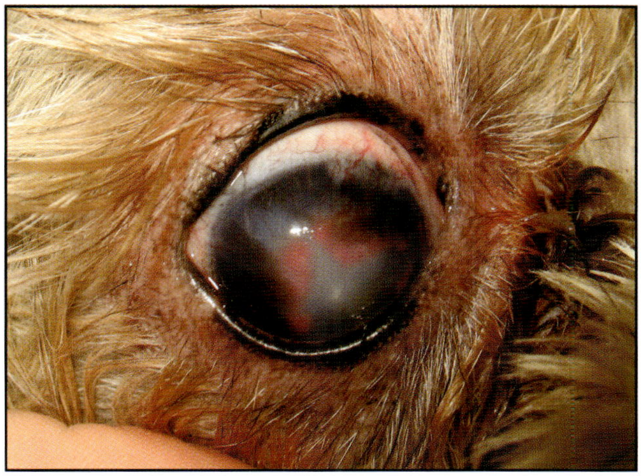

Figure 67.4 Typical presentation associated with corneal abscessation.

CHAPTER 68
CORNEAL HEMORRHAGE

PRESENTATION

Intracorneal hemorrhage may occasionally result in association with the presence of corneal blood vessels. Clinically, this condition presents as variable red to tan discoloration, arising in a fanlike pattern from an adjacent corneal vessel, occurring at any depth within the cornea and typically affecting one eye only.

DIAGNOSIS AND TREATMENT

The diagnosis of intracorneal hemorrhage is made on the basis of clinical findings. Most cases of discrete corneal hemorrhage will resolve spontaneously. The presence of underlying coagulopathy/vasculopathy, metabolic disease, and/or hypertension should be ruled out in affected cases. Neoplastic vasculopathies represent the most important differential diagnosis (see also Corneoscleral Hemangioma/Hemangiosarcoma). In addition, the abnormal presence of blood vessels within the cornea should be evaluated, specifically identifying and treating associated surface or intraocular disease. Topical steroidal or non-steroidal agents will help speed the resorption of blood; however, discoloration may be present for months to years and some degree or permanent opacification may remain at the site of hemorrhage following its resorption, particularly in cases of deep stromal hemorrhage.

Potential Drug-Side-Effects

Potential adverse effects associated with the use of topical corticosteroids include impaired wound healing and corneal degeneration.

SELECTED REFERENCES

Matas M, Donaldson D, Newton RJ. Intracorneal hemorrhage in 19 dogs (22 eyes) from 2000 to 2010: a retrospective study. *Vet Ophthalmol.* 2012;**15**(2):86–91. doi: 10.1111/j.1463-5224.2011.00944.x. Epub 2011 Nov 29.

McDonnell PJ, Green WR, Stevens RE, Bargeron CB, Riquelme JL. Blood staining of the cornea. Light microscopic and ultrastructural features. *Ophthalmology.* 1985;**92**(12):1668–1674.

Swanson JF. Ocular manifestations of systemic disease in the dog and cat. Recent developments. *Vet Clin North Am Small Anim Pract.* 1990;**20**(3):849–867.

Clinical Atlas of Canine and Feline Ophthalmic Disease, First Edition. Douglas Esson.

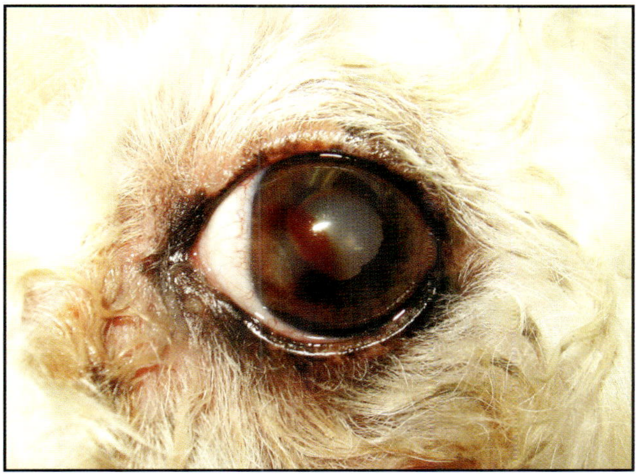

Figure 68.1 Typical presentation associated with the presence of intracorneal hemorrhage.

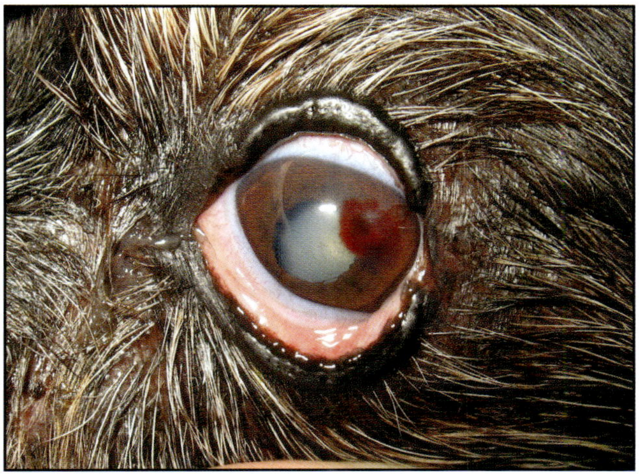

Figure 68.2 Typical presentation associated with the presence of intracorneal hemorrhage.

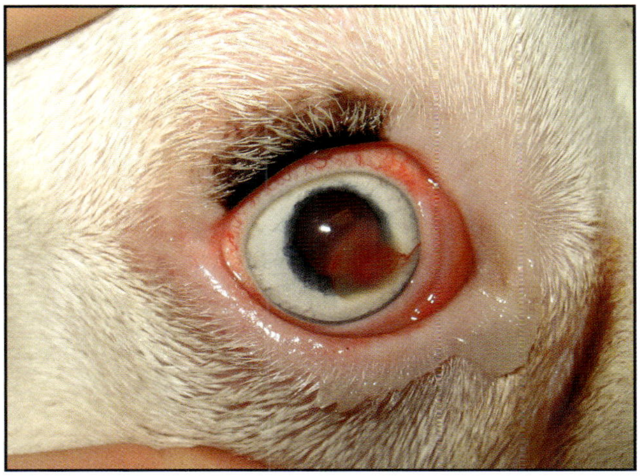

Figure 68.3 Typical presentation associated with the presence of intracorneal hemorrhage.

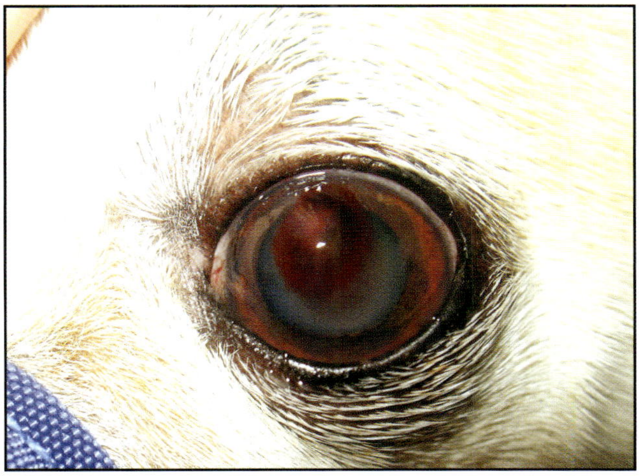

Figure 68.4 Typical presentation associated with the presence of intracorneal hemorrhage.

CHAPTER 69
CORNEOSCLERAL LACERATION

PRESENTATION

Traumatic corneoscleral laceration is relatively commonly encountered and constitutes an ocular emergency. Cat-claw injuries are frequently the cause of these injuries. Corneal laceration is typically marked by extreme discomfort, blepharospasm, ocular discharge, hemorrhage, the accumulation of fibrin/mucous at the wound site, anterior chamber shallowing or collapse, and/or the prolapse of uveal tissue.

DIAGNOSIS AND TREATMENT

The diagnosis of corneoscleral laceration is made on the basis of clinical findings in conjunction with clinical history. Lacerated globes are tectonically fragile and affected patients should be handled with extreme caution in order to minimize the risk of further intraocular pathology including iris prolapse and/or retinal detachment. The mechanical manipulation of tissue, including attempted debridement or "wiping away" of accumulated fibrin, before surgical repair is contraindicated. Systemic (steroidal or nonsteroidal) anti-inflammatory and/or antimicrobial therapy are generally appropriate. Surgical repair should be performed as soon as possible, with a variety of techniques described. The use of an Elizabethan collar will prevent self-trauma before referral and postoperatively. An important consideration is the potential that lenticular structures may also have been damaged. Failure to identify and address this potential complication will significantly increase the risk of potentially catastrophic, secondary pathology including glaucoma as a result of uncontrolled phacoclastic uveitis (see also Phacoclastic Uveitis and FPTS).

SELECTED REFERENCES

Giuliano EA. Feline ocular emergencies. *Clin Tech Small Anim Pract*. 2005;**20**(2):135–141.

Mandell DC. Ophthalmic emergencies. *Clin Tech Small Anim Pract*. 2000;**15**(2):94–100. Review.

Paulsen ME, Kass PH. Traumatic corneal laceration with associated lens capsule disruption: a retrospective study of 77 clinical cases from 1999 to 2009. *Vet Ophthalmol*. 2012;**15**(6):355–368.

Clinical Atlas of Canine and Feline Ophthalmic Disease, First Edition. Douglas Esson.

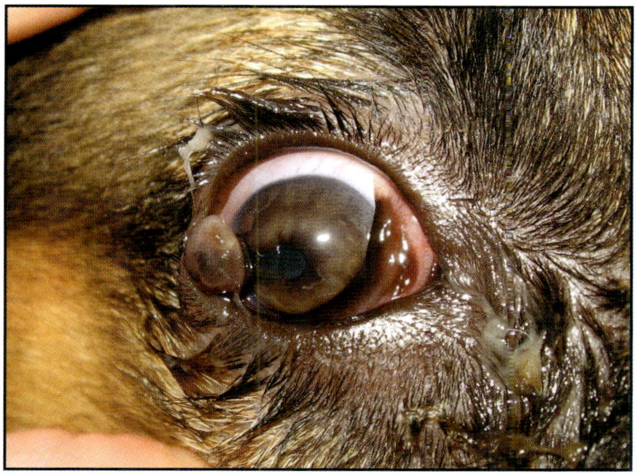

Figure 69.1 Typical presentation associated with corneoscleral laceration. Pupillary dyscoria in association with iris prolapse is present.

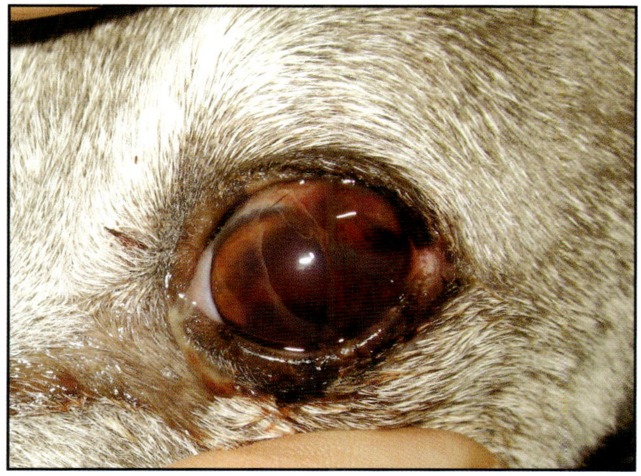

Figure 69.2 Typical presentation associated with corneoscleral laceration. Hyphema in association with limbal iris prolapse is present.

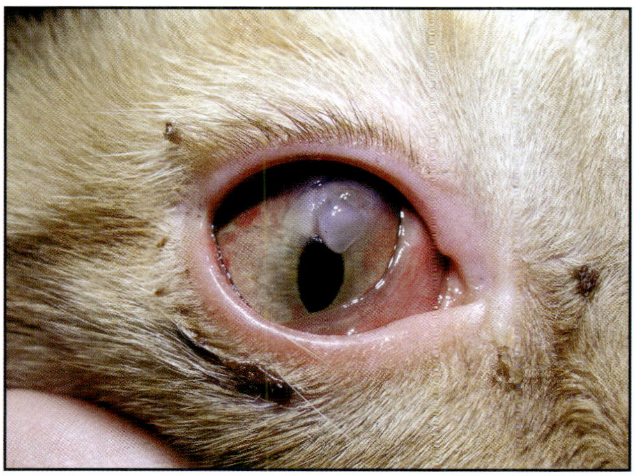

Figure 69.3 Typical presentation associated with corneal laceration. Iritis as well as the presence of "flap" of lacerated corneal tissue, typical of a cat-claw injury, is present.

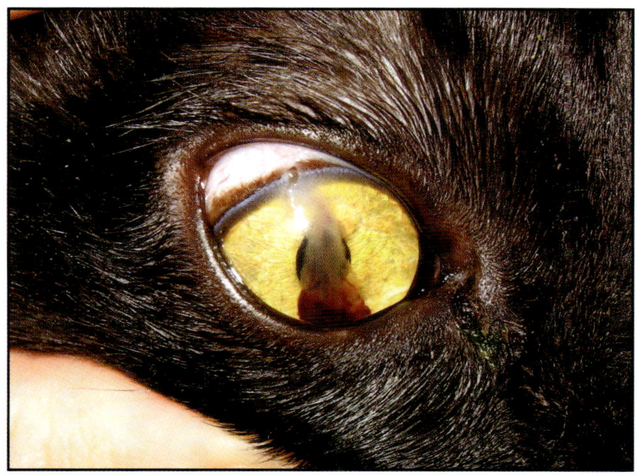

Figure 69.4 Typical presentation associated with corneal laceration. Intracameral hemorrhage and fibrin are present.

CHAPTER 70
SPONTANEOUS CHRONIC CORNEAL EPITHELIAL DEFECTS (SCCEDs)

PRESENTATION

Spontaneous chronic corneal epithelial defects (SCCEDs) are a relatively common cause of canine corneal pathology. These lesions are frequently described as "indolent" or "Boxer" ulcers. SCCEDs likely arise as a result of corneal micro-trauma in association with preexisting structural and/or physiological corneal abnormalities. Clinically, SCCEDs present as chronic superficial corneal ulcerations, typically surrounded by a visible rim of poorly adherent epithelial tissue, which is easily under-run by fluorescein dye, creating a "halo" effect following corneal staining. Significant associated corneal inflammation, vascularization, and/or granulation may develop in association with long-standing lesions. Discomfort is marked by blepharospasm and/or ocular discharge. Commonly affected breeds include the Boxer, Boston Terrier, French Bulldog, and Labrador Retriever.

DIAGNOSIS AND TREATMENT

The diagnosis of a SCCED is made on the basis of its typical clinical appearance and staining pattern. SCCEDs are treated by physical debridement of both loose superficial epithelial tissue as well as the underlying stromal surface. Medical therapy alone is unlikely to result in corneal healing. Similarly, the placement of a "third eyelid flap" is unlikely to address underlying pathology and result in adequate healing. Debridement may be performed using sterile cotton-tipped applicators, a sterile spatula, a scalpel blade, or a diamond-tipped burr. A linear or punctate keratotomy may additionally be performed following corneal debridement. In challenging or refractory cases, a superficial keratectomy may ultimately be required. Routine topical antimicrobial therapy is indicated pending corneal healing and the postoperative use of an Elizabethan collar will prevent self-trauma. Dogs with a history of SCCEDs are prone to the development of similar lesions within the contralateral eye.

SELECTED REFERENCES

Bentley E. Spontaneous chronic corneal epithelial defects in dogs: a review. *J Am Anim Hosp Assoc*. 2005;**41**(3):158–165. Review.

Bentley E, Abrams GA, Covitz D, Cook CS, Fischer CA, Hacker D, Stuhr CM, Reid TW, Murphy CJ. Morphology and immunohistochemistry of spontaneous chronic corneal epithelial defects (SCCED) in dogs. *Invest Ophthalmol Vis Sci*. 2001;**42**(10):2262–2269.

Cutler TJ. Corneal epithelial disease. *Vet Clin North Am Equine Pract*. 2004 Aug;**20**(2):319–343, vi.

Gosling AA, Labelle AL, Breaux CB. Management of spontaneous chronic corneal epithelial defects (SCCEDs) in dogs with diamond burr debridement and placement of a bandage contact lens. *Vet Ophthalmol*. 2013;**16**(2):83–88.

Clinical Atlas of Canine and Feline Ophthalmic Disease, First Edition. Douglas Esson.

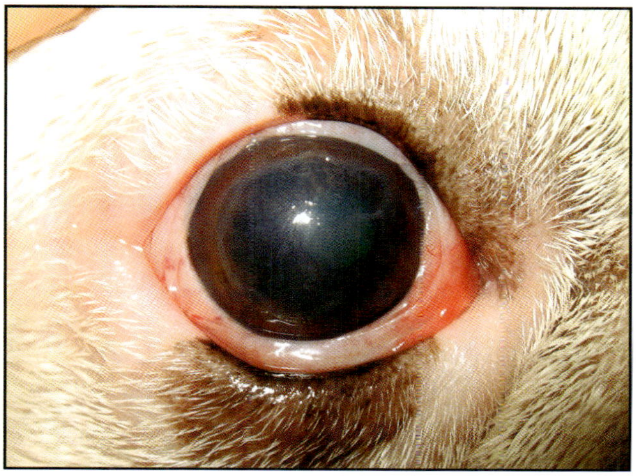

Figure 70.1 Typical presentation associated with a spontaneous chronic corneal epithelial defect. A rim of poorly adherent epithelial tissue is noted to surround the lesion.

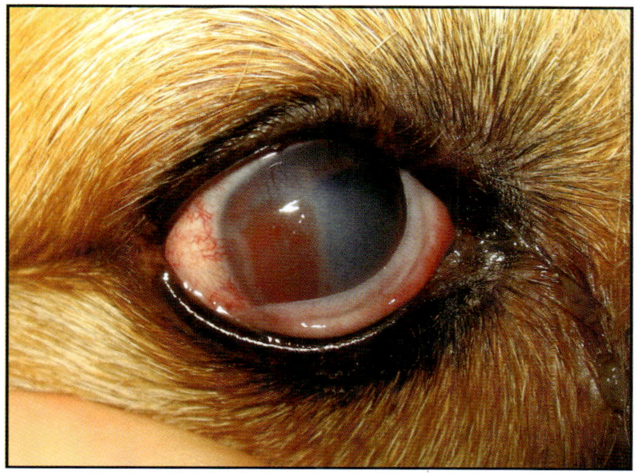

Figure 70.2 Typical presentation associated with a spontaneous chronic corneal epithelial defect. A rim of poorly adherent epithelial tissue is noted to surround the lesion.

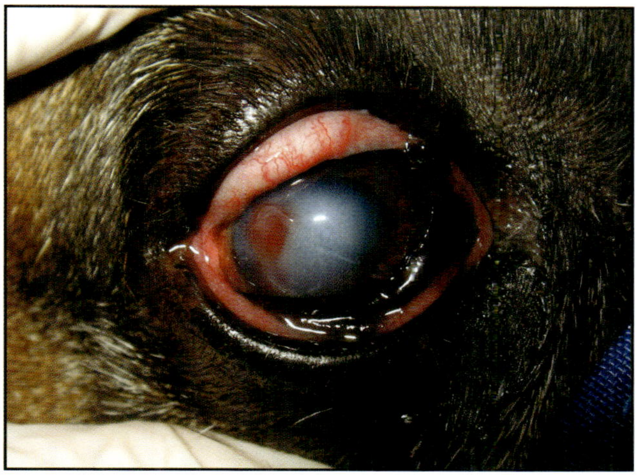

Figure 70.3 Typical presentation associated with a spontaneous chronic corneal epithelial defect. A rim of poorly adherent epithelial tissue is noted to surround the lesion.

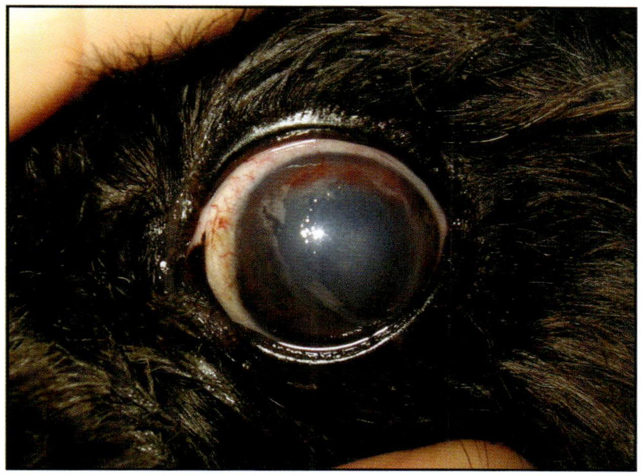

Figure 70.4 Typical presentation associated with a spontaneous chronic corneal epithelial defect. A rim of poorly adherent epithelial tissue is noted to surround the lesion.

CHAPTER 71
STROMAL ULCERATIVE KERATITIS

PRESENTATION

Corneal ulceration may arise secondary to a multitude of etiologies including conformational abnormalities, tear film deficiencies (quantitative and/or qualitative), neurological dysfunction, trauma, and/or microbial contamination. Stromal ulcers are identified as deep defects of variable size in the cornea, which stain positive with fluorescein dye and which may be associated with edema as well as a variable vascular response. Discomfort may be marked by blepharospasm and/or mucoid ocular discharge. Commonly affected breeds include the Shih Tzu, Pug, Lhasa Apso, and Boston Terrier.

DIAGNOSIS AND TREATMENT

The diagnosis of stromal ulcerative keratitis is made based on clinical findings. Bacterial keratitis should be treated using appropriate antimicrobial therapy. Ideally, treatment should be based on cytological interpretation and Gram's staining as well as the subsequent culture and sensitivity testing of microbial samples. In cases of deep stromal ulceration, or those associated with existing or impending corneal rupture, surgical tectonic corneal grafting may be indicated. A variety of appropriate techniques have been described including the placement of a conjunctival pedicle graft (CPG), conjunctival island graft (CIG), or the advancement of a corneoscleral transposition (CCT), facilitated by operating microscopy. The use of corticosteroids is generally contraindicated in the management of stromal ulcerative keratitis. The use of an Elizabethan collar will prevent self-trauma during the healing process.

SELECTED REFERENCES

Kern TJ. Ulcerative keratitis. *Vet Clin North Am Small Anim Pract*. 1990;**20**(3):643–666.

Ollivier FJ. Bacterial corneal diseases in dogs and cats. *Clin Tech Small Anim Pract*. 2003;**18**(3):193–198.

Scagliotti RH. Tarsoconjunctival island graft for the treatment of deep corneal ulcers, desmetocoeles, and perforations in 35 dogs and 6 cats. *Semin Vet Med Surg (Small Anim)*. 1988;**3**(1):69–76.

Wilkie DA, Whittaker C. Surgery of the cornea. *Vet Clin North Am Small Anim Pract*. 1997;**27**(5):1067–1107.

Clinical Atlas of Canine and Feline Ophthalmic Disease, First Edition. Douglas Esson.

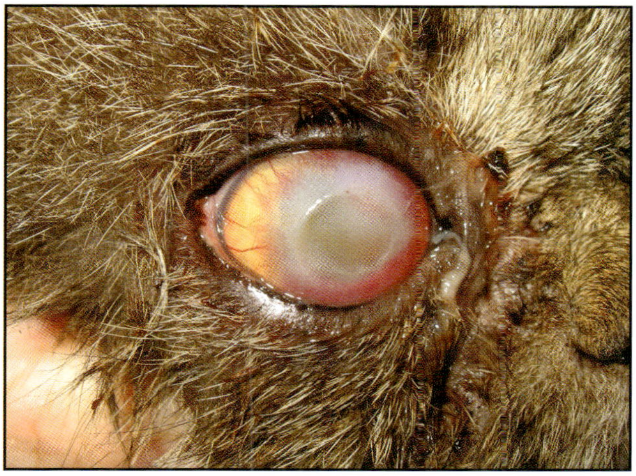

Figure 71.1 Stromal ulcerative keratitis.

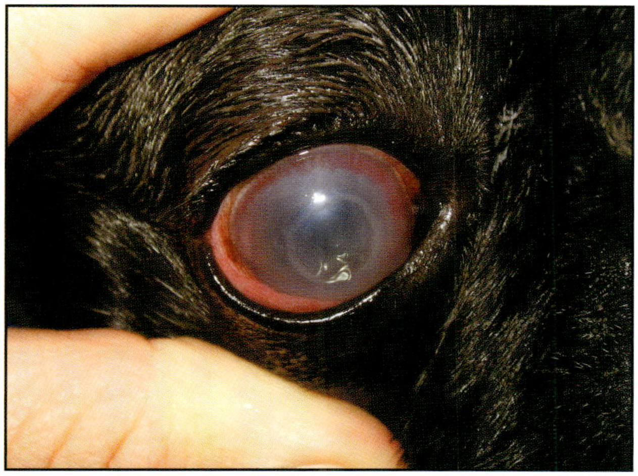

Figure 71.2 Stromal ulcerative keratitis.

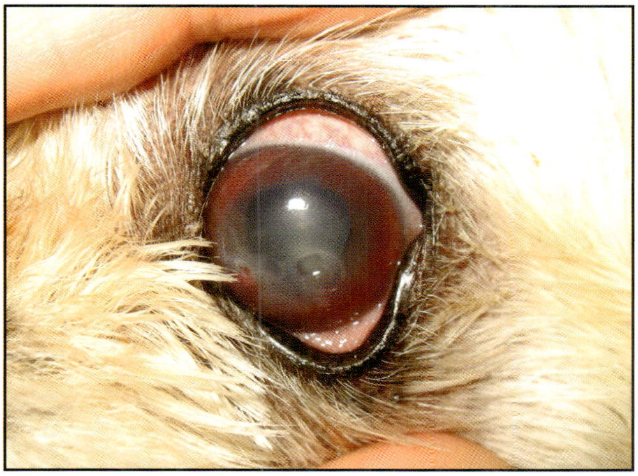

Figure 71.3 Stromal ulcerative keratitis

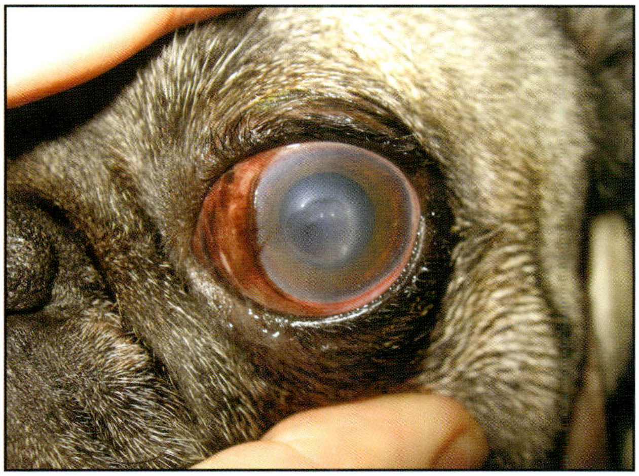

Figure 71.4 Stromal ulcerative keratitis.

CHAPTER 72
DESCEMETOCELE

PRESENTATION

A descemetocele describes a deep corneal ulcer in which the overlying epithelium and stroma are no longer present so that only descemet's membrane prevents globe rupture. This thin layer may be appreciated to be bulging forward in the center of the ulcerative lesion. The presence of a descemetocele is typically marked by discomfort, blepharospasm, and/or ocular discharge.

DIAGNOSIS AND TREATMENT

A descemetocele may be diagnosed as a corneal ulcer, the center of which fails to retain fluorescein dye. Copiously irrigating deep corneal lesions following fluorescein staining will differentiate deep stromal ulcers from descemetoceles because stain will not be rinsed away from exposed corneal stroma in the absence of a descemetocele. Affected globes are tectonically fragile and affected patients should be handled with extreme caution in order to minimize the risk of globe rupture. Covering a descemetocele with a "third eyelid flap" does not provide significant wound support and is generally contraindicated. Surgical repair should be performed as soon as possible. A variety of appropriate techniques have been described including the placement of a conjunctival pedicle graft (CPG), conjunctival island graft (CIG), or the advancement of a corneoscleral transposition (CCT), facilitated by operating microscopy. Antimicrobial and/or analgesic therapy should be administered as indicated post-operatively. The use of an Elizabethan collar will prevent self-trauma.

SELECTED REFERENCES

Brightman AH, McLaughlin SA, Brogdon JD. Autogenous lamellar corneal grafting in dogs. *J Am Vet Med Assoc*. 1989;**195**(4):469–475.

Hansen PA, Guandalini A. A retrospective study of 30 cases of frozen lamellar corneal graft in dogs and cats. *Vet Ophthalmol*. 1999;**2**(4):233–241.

Mandell DC. Ophthalmic emergencies. *Clin Tech Small Anim Pract*. 2000;**15**(2):94–100.

Wilkie DA, Whittaker C. Surgery of the cornea. *Vet Clin North Am Small Anim Pract*. 1997;**27**(5):1067–1107.

Clinical Atlas of Canine and Feline Ophthalmic Disease, First Edition. Douglas Esson.

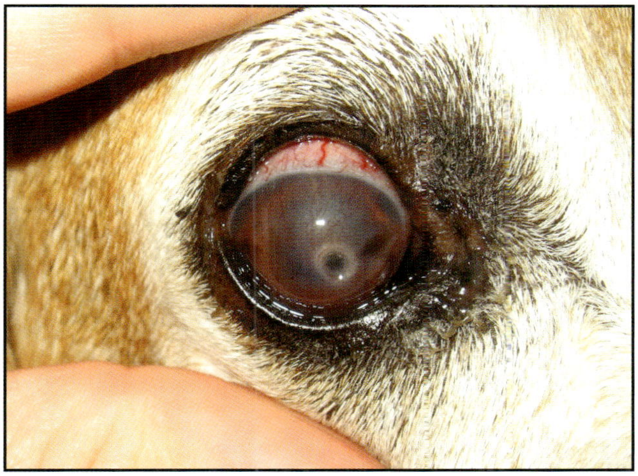

Figure 72.1 Typical presentation associated with a corneal descemetocele.

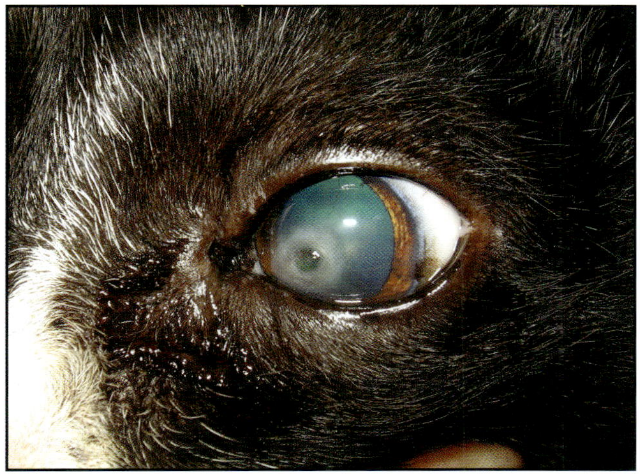

Figure 72.2 Typical presentation associated with a corneal descemetocele.

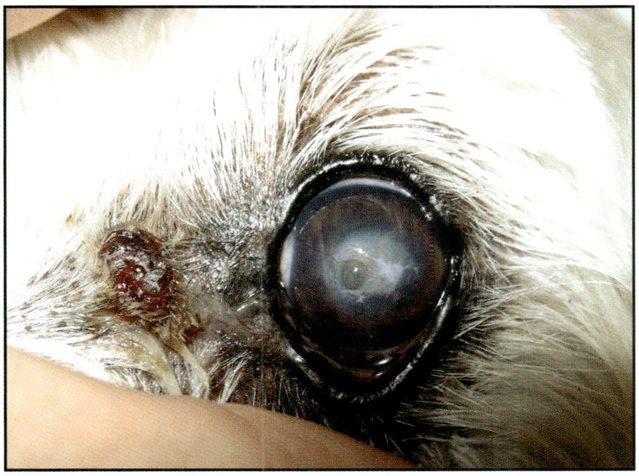

Figure 72.3 Typical presentation associated with a corneal descemetocele.

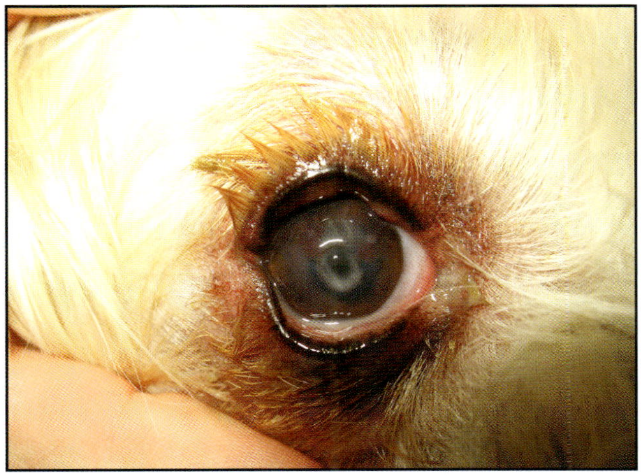

Figure 72.4 Typical presentation associated with a corneal descemetocele.

CHAPTER 73
KERATOMALACIA (MELTING ULCERS)

PRESENTATION

Corneal ulceration may arise secondary to a multitude of etiologies including conformational abnormalities, tear film deficiencies (quantitative and/or qualitative), neurological dysfunction, trauma, and/or microbial contamination. Tissue dissolution through the action of enzymatic proteases is a normal part of corneal metabolism as well as the healing and remodeling process; however, uncontrolled lysis or "melting" of corneal tissue as a result of excessive protease activity has the potential to result in significant pathology (see also Bullous Keratopathy). Excessive enzymatic activity may stem from corneal or inflammatory cells as well pathological microorganisms. Affected tissue becomes edematous and soft, manifesting as corneal thickening and gray discoloration. An associated corneal vascular response may additionally be present. Keratomalacia is frequency complicated by severe secondary bacterial infection. Discomfort may be marked by blepharospasm and/or mucoid ocular discharge. Commonly affected breeds include the Shih Tzu, Pug, Lhasa Apso, and Boston Terrier.

DIAGNOSIS AND TREATMENT

The diagnosis of keratomalacia is made on the basis of clinical findings. Treatment comprises the stabilization of the metalloprotease enzymes that mediate this process. Appropriate topical therapeutic agents include serum (fresh or frozen), tetracyclines, EDTA solution, and/or *N*-acetylcysteine. Anticollagenases should be applied frequently. Bacterial keratitis should be treated using appropriate antimicrobial agents. Ideally, therapy should be based on cytological interpretation and Gram' staining as well as the subsequent culture and sensitivity testing of microbial samples. In severe cases, or those associated with existing or impending corneal rupture, surgical resection of diseased tissue, and/or tectonic corneal grafting procedures may be indicated. The use of corticosteroids is generally contraindicated. The use of an Elizabethan collar will prevent self-trauma during the healing process.

SELECTED REFERENCES

Ollivier FJ, Brooks DE, Kallberg ME, Komaromy AM, Lassaline ME, Andrew SE, Gelatt KN, Stevens GR, Blalock TD, van Setten GB, Schultz GS. Evaluation of various compounds to inhibit activity of matrix metalloproteinases in the tear film of horses with ulcerative keratitis. *Am J Vet Res*. 2003;**64**(9):1081–1087.

Ollivier FJ, Gilger BC, Barrie KP, Kallberg ME, Plummer CE, O'Reilly S, Gelatt KN, Brooks DE. Proteinases of the cornea and preocular tear film. *Vet Ophthalmol*. 2007;**10**(4):199–206.

Wang L, Pan Q, Xue Q, Cui J, Qi C. Evaluation of matrix metalloproteinase concentrations in precorneal tear film from dogs with Pseudomonas aeruginosa-associated keratitis. *Am J Vet Res*. 2008;**69**(10):1341–1345.

Clinical Atlas of Canine and Feline Ophthalmic Disease, First Edition. Douglas Esson.

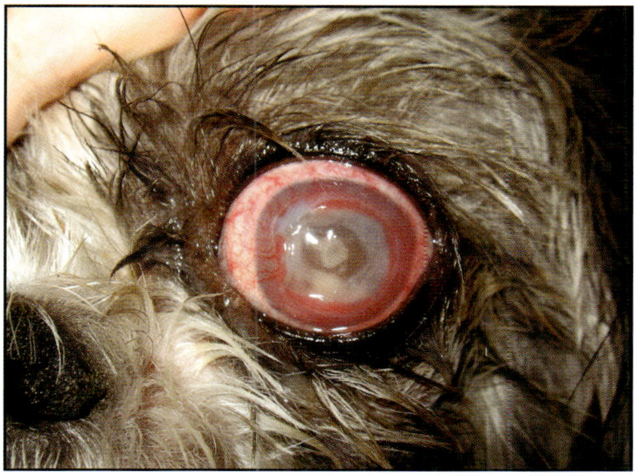

Figure 73.1 Typical presentation of corneal ulceration in association with keratomalacia.

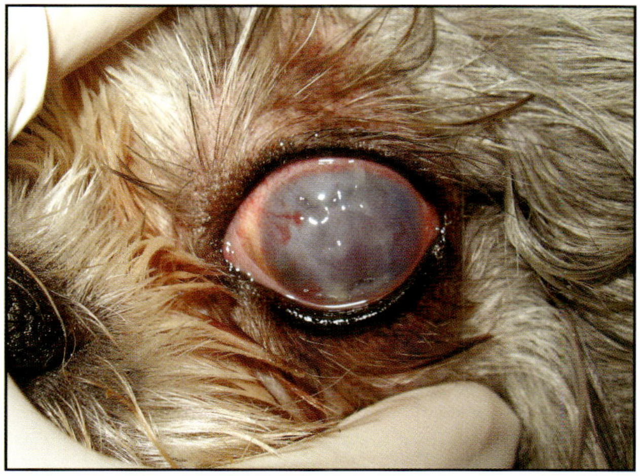

Figure 73.2 Typical presentation of corneal ulceration in association with keratomalacia.

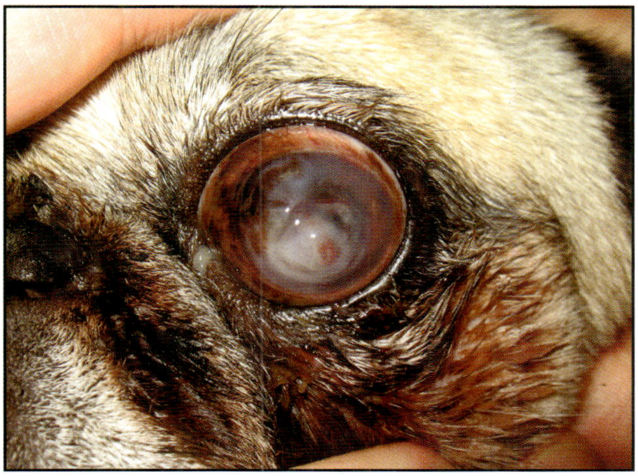

Figure 73.3 Typical presentation of corneal ulceration in association with keratomalacia.

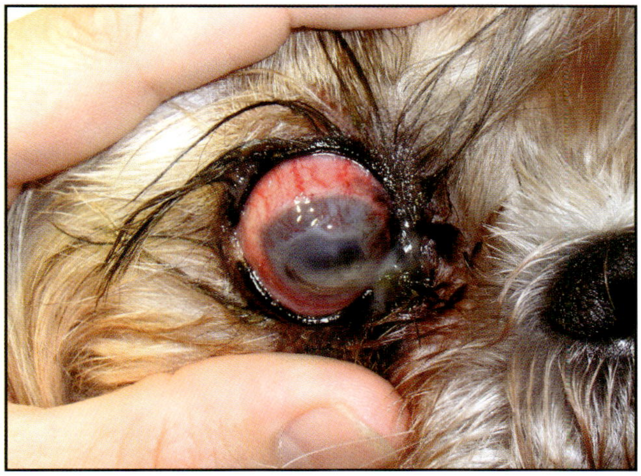

Figure 73.4 Typical presentation of corneal ulceration in association with keratomalacia.

CHAPTER 74
CORNEAL PERFORATION

PRESENTATION

Corneal perforation as a result of trauma, severe, progressive corneal ulceration or a ruptured descemetocele, constitutes an ocular emergency. Corneal perforation is typically marked by extreme discomfort, blepharospasm, discharge, hemorrhage, anterior chamber shallowing or collapse, and the accumulation of fibrin/mucous at the wound site.

DIAGNOSIS AND TREATMENT

The diagnosis of corneal perforation is made based on clinical findings. Perforated globes are tectonically fragile and affected patients should be handled with extreme caution to minimize the risk of further intraocular pathology including iris prolapse and/or retinal detachment. The mechanical manipulation of tissue, including attempted of accumulated fibrin debridement, is contraindicated until surgical repair can be performed. Covering a perforated cornea with a "third eyelid flap" does not provide significant wound support and is generally contraindicated. Surgical repair should be performed as soon as possible, with a variety of techniques described. Antimicrobial and/or analgesic therapy should be administered as indicated post-operatively. Systemic (steroidal or nonsteroidal) anti-inflammatory therapy is generally indicated The use of an Elizabethan collar will prevent self-trauma before referral and postoperatively.

SELECTED REFERENCES

Mandell DC. Ophthalmic emergencies. *Clin Tech Small Anim Pract*. 2000;**15**(2):94–100. Review.

Ollivier FJ. Bacterial corneal diseases in dogs and cats. *Clin Tech Small Anim Pract*. 2003;**18**(3):193–198.

Scagliotti RH. Tarsoconjunctival island graft for the treatment of deep corneal ulcers, desmetocoeles, and perforations in 35 dogs and 6 cats. *Semin Vet Med Surg (Small Anim)*. 1988;**3**(1):69–76.

Wilkie DA, Whittaker C. Surgery of the cornea. *Vet Clin North Am Small Anim Pract*. 1997;**27**(5):1067–1107.

Clinical Atlas of Canine and Feline Ophthalmic Disease, First Edition. Douglas Esson.

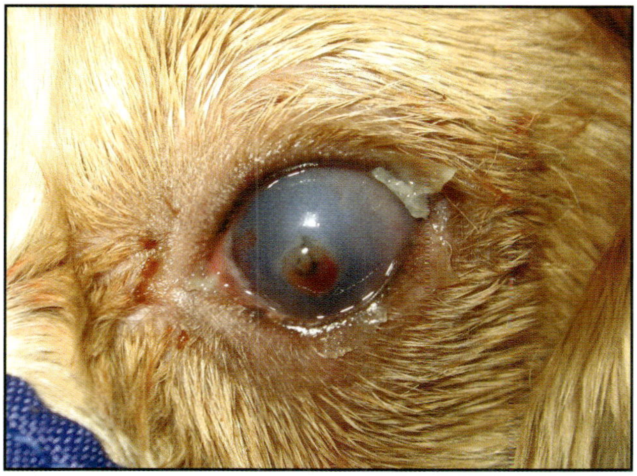

Figure 74.1 Presentation associated with corneal perforation. An organized fibrin "plug" is visible at the site of the lesion.

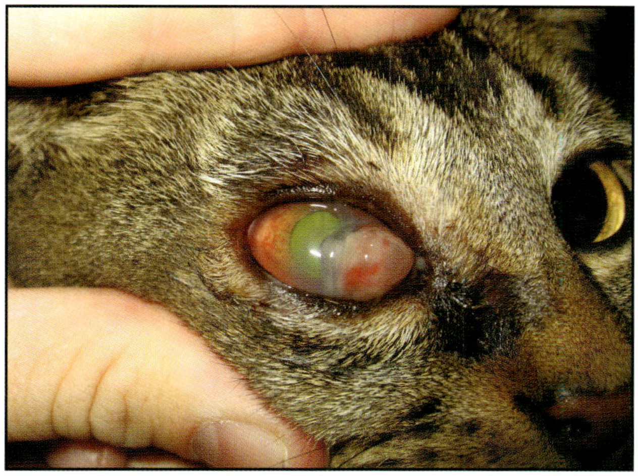

Figure 74.2 Presentation associated with corneal perforation. An organized fibrin "plug" is visible at the site of the lesion.

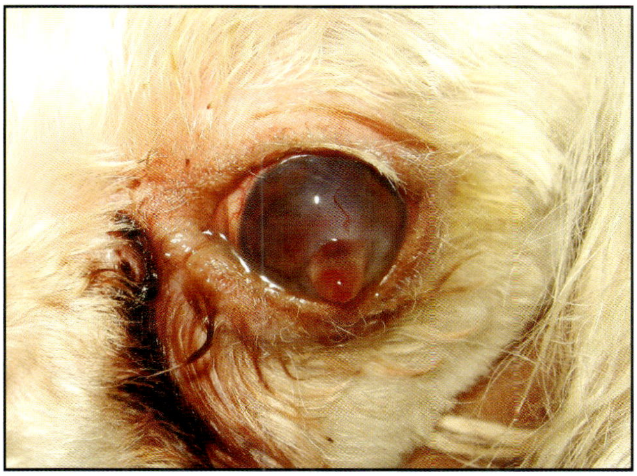

Figure 74.3 Presentation associated with corneal perforation. An organized fibrin "plug" is visible at the site of the lesion.

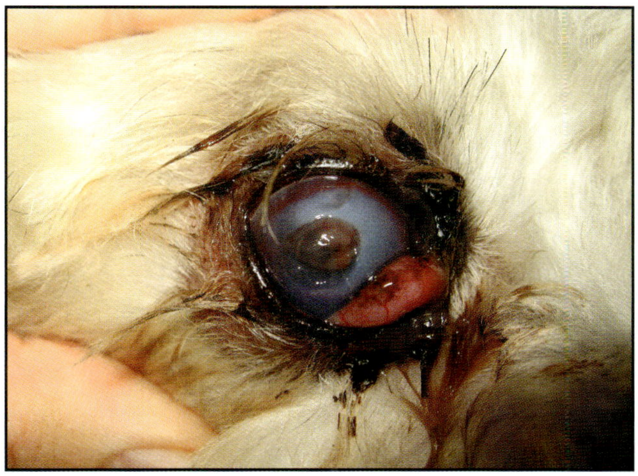

Figure 74.4 Presentation associated with corneal perforation. An organized fibrin "plug" is visible at the site of the lesion.

CHAPTER 75
EPITHELIAL INCLUSION CYSTS

PRESENTATION

Occasionally, following corneal healing, epithelial cells may become trapped beneath the epithelial surface and organize into small cysts, which gradually enlarge as they accumulate proteinaceous debris. Clinically, these lesions appear as one or more focal, relatively well-circumscribed, smooth, raised yellow to tan swellings, protruding from the corneal surface at the site of prior trauma. A mild superficial vascular response is typically associated with the presence of inclusion cysts. These lesions do not, however, result in significant discomfort.

DIAGNOSIS AND TREATMENT

The diagnosis of epithelial inclusion cysts is made on the basis of clinical findings. If problematic or significantly progressive, these lesions may be removed either by surgical keratectomy or more simply by CO_2 laser ablation. Postoperative topical antimicrobial and anti-inflammatory therapy is indicated and the use of a protective Elizabethan collar will prevent self-trauma during corneal healing.

SELECTED REFERENCES

Choi US, Labelle P, Kim S, Kim J, Cha J, Lee KC, Lee HB, Kim NS, Kim MS. Successful treatment of an unusually large corneal epithelial inclusion cyst using equine amniotic membrane in a dog. *Vet Ophthalmol.* 2010;**13**(2):122–125.

Cullen CL, Grahn BH. Diagnostic ophthalmology. Epithelial inclusion cyst of the right cornea. *Can Vet J.* 2001;**42**(3):230–231.

Simonazzi B, Castania M, Bosco V, Giudice C, Rondena M. A case of multiple unilateral corneal epithelial inclusion cysts in a dog. *J Small Anim Pract*. 2009;**50**(7):373–376.

Clinical Atlas of Canine and Feline Ophthalmic Disease, First Edition. Douglas Esson.

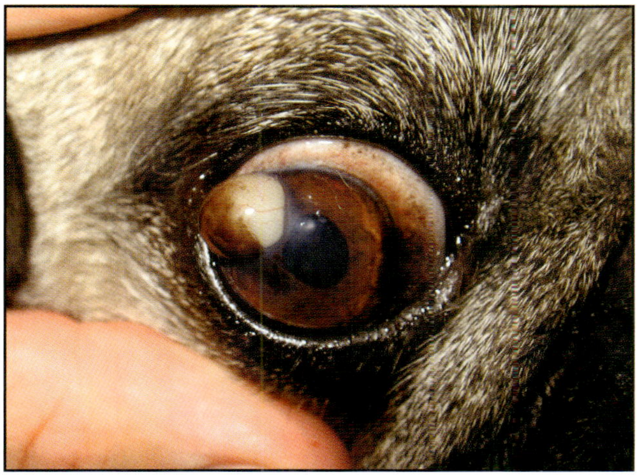

Figure 75.1 Typical presentation associated with the presence of a corneal epithelial inclusion cyst.

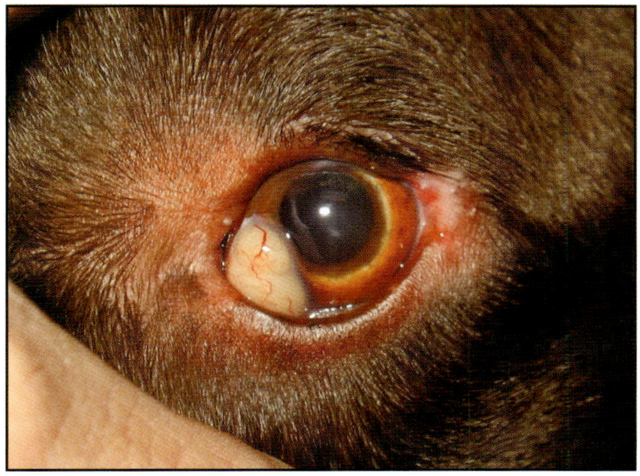

Figure 75.2 Typical presentation associated with the presence of a corneal epithelial inclusion cyst.

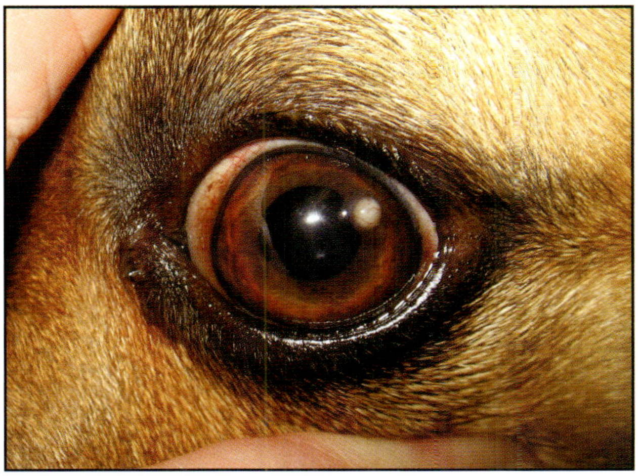

Figure 75.3 Typical presentation associated with the presence of a corneal epithelial inclusion cyst.

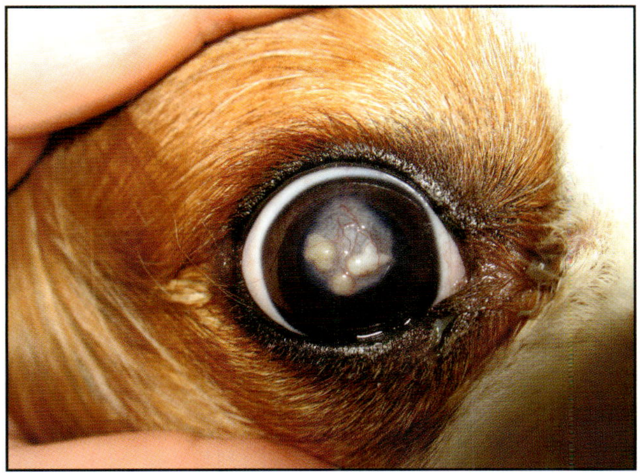

Figure 75.4 Typical presentation associated with the presence of corneal epithelial inclusion cysts.

CHAPTER 76
CORNEAL FOREIGN BODY

PRESENTATION

The potential presence of foreign material should always be considered when evaluating a painful eye. Foreign material is commonly plant-based in origin. Foreign bodies may affect either the corneoscleral surface (where they may become deeply embedded as a result of enzymatic activity) or the bulbar fornix behind the eyelid or third eyelid. Ocular foreign bodies typically result in significant blepharospasm, chemosis, conjunctivitis, and/or ocular discharge.

DIAGNOSIS AND TREATMENT

The diagnosis of a corneal foreign body is made on the basis of clinical findings. The application of topical anesthesia may facilitate the identification of foreign material, however, painful cases may require sedation or even anesthesia in order to facilitate thorough examination. Appropriate treatment comprises the removal of foreign material. Care should be taken to ensure complete removal to prevent the loss of biologic material into the anterior chamber (which may lead to endophthalmitis) and also to medically manage and/or tectonically repair any defects which remain following foreign body removal. The postoperative use of a protective Elizabethan collar will prevent self-trauma until corneal healing is complete.

SELECTED REFERENCES

Cullen CL, Grahn BH. Diagnostic ophthalmology. Right corneal foreign body, secondary ulcerative keratitis, and anterior uveitis. *Can Vet J*. 2005;**46**(11):1054–1055.

Gelatt KN. Organic corneal foreign bodies in the dog. *Vet Med Small Anim Clin*. 1974;**69**(11):1423–1428.

Rebhun WC. Conjunctival and corneal foreign bodies. *Vet Med Small Anim Clin*. 1973;**68**(8):874–877.

Clinical Atlas of Canine and Feline Ophthalmic Disease, First Edition. Douglas Esson.

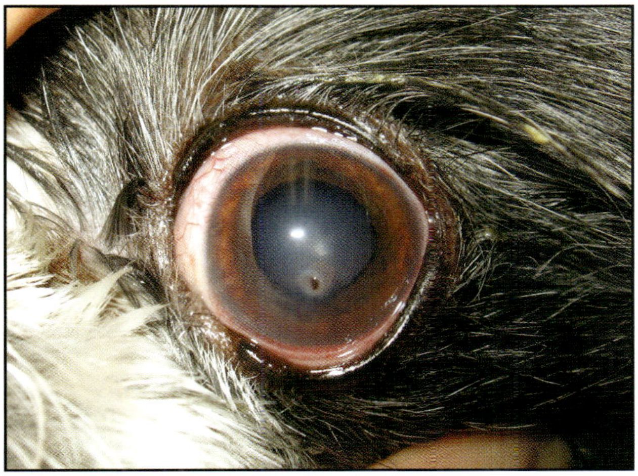

Figure 76.1 Typical presentation associated with the presence of a plant-based corneal foreign body.

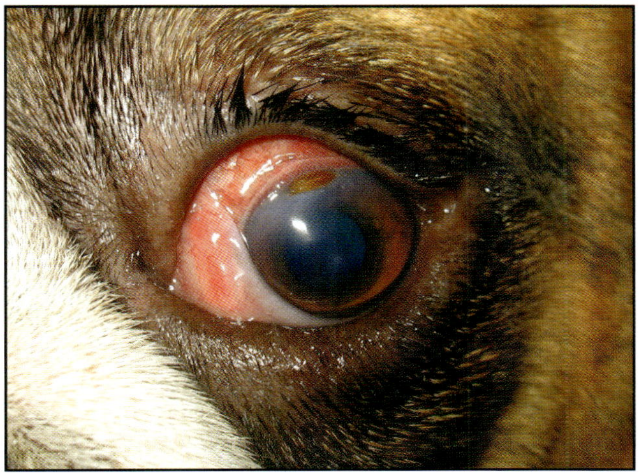

Figure 76.2 Typical presentation associated with the presence of a plant-based corneal foreign body.

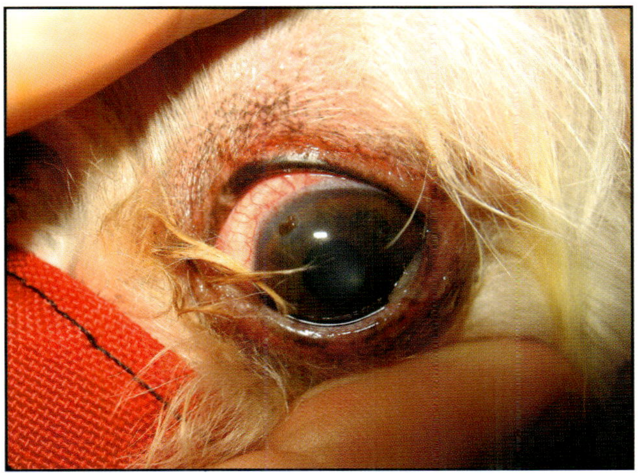

Figure 76.3 Typical presentation associated with the presence of a plant-based corneal foreign body.

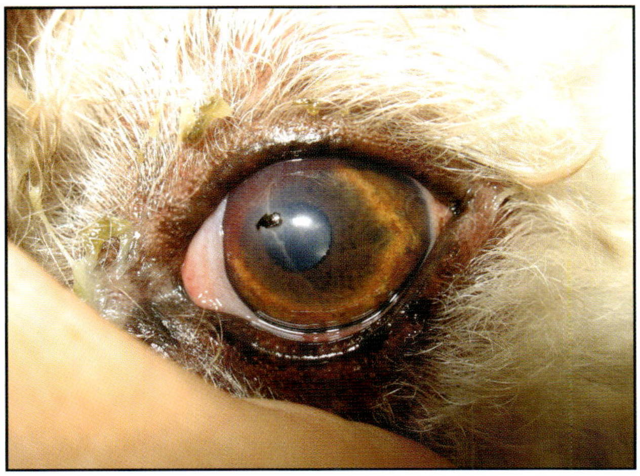

Figure 76.4 Typical presentation associated with the presence of a plant-based corneal foreign body.

CHAPTER 77
LIMBAL MELANOCYTOMA

PRESENTATION

Limbal (epibulbar) melanocytomas represent a relatively common neoplastic proliferation of melanocytic cells at the corneoscleral limbus and may affect dogs or cats. In rare instances, these lesions may display malignant characteristics including significant anaplasia and/or metastasis. Lesions typically present as well-defined, raised, and pigmented masses with a smooth surface. Progressive enlargement typically results in corneoscleral and/or intraocular invasion and may ultimately lead to glaucoma and/or retinal detachment. Limbal melanocytomas should be differentiated from extension of more malignant uveal melanomas. Commonly affected breeds include the Labrador Retriever, Golden Retriever, and German Shepherd.

DIAGNOSIS AND TREATMENT

The diagnosis of melanocytoma is made on the basis of clinical findings, supported by histopathology, following incisional or excisional biopsy. These lesions are typically relatively benign and frequently appear to be localized to ocular tissues only. Nevertheless, the evaluation of systemic health and/or involvement via local lymph node aspiration, three-view radiography, and complete blood count (CBC)/chemistry analysis, is recommended. Treatment typically encompasses surgical resection where possible (with or without adjunctive tectonic grafting procedures using either biologic or synthetic materials). Pigment-rich melanocytomas are also relatively susceptible to the application of cryotherapy. The prognosis following prompt surgical intervention is generally good; however, recurrence is possible.

SELECTED REFERENCES

Cooley PL, Dice PF 2nd. Corneal dystrophy in the dog and cat. *Vet Clin North Am Small Anim Pract*. 1990;**20**(3):681–692.

Donaldson D, Sansom J, Adams V. Review Canine limbal melanoma: 30 cases (1992–2004). Part 2. Treatment with lamellar resection and adjunctive strontium-90beta plesiotherapy—efficacy and morbidity. *Vet Ophthalmol*. 2006;**9**(3):179–185.

Norman JC, Urbanz JL, Calvarese ST. Penetrating keratoscleroplasty and bimodal grafting for treatment of limbal melanocytoma in a dog. *Vet Ophthalmol*. 2008;**11**(5):340–345. doi: 10.1111/j.1463-5224.2008.00645.x.

Spangler WL, Kass PH. The histologic and epidemiologic bases for prognostic considerations in canine melanocytic neoplasia. *Vet Pathol*. 2006;**43**(2):136–149.

Wilkie DA, Wolf ED. Treatment of epibulbar melanocytoma in a dog, using full-thickness eyewall resection and synthetic graft. *J Am Vet Med Assoc*. 1991;**198**(6):1019–1022.

Clinical Atlas of Canine and Feline Ophthalmic Disease, First Edition. Douglas Esson.

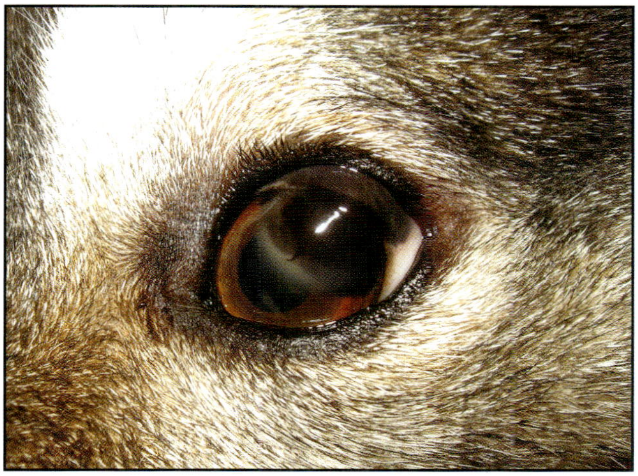

Figure 77.1 Typical presentation associated with the presence of limbal melanocytoma.

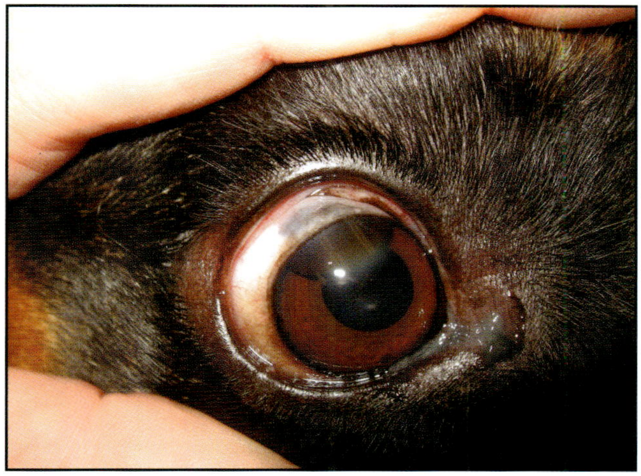

Figure 77.2 Typical presentation associated with the presence of limbal melanocytoma.

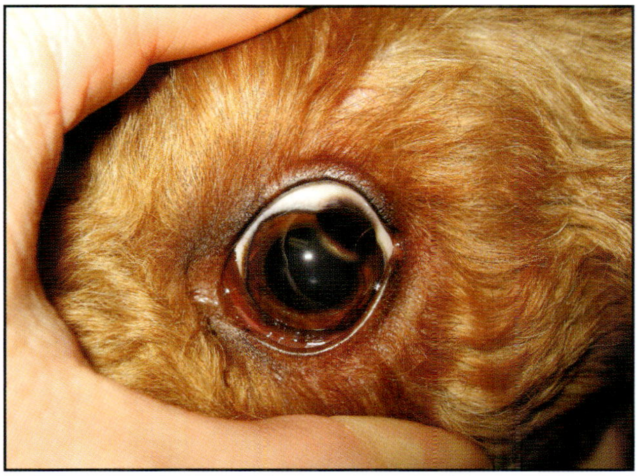

Figure 77.3 Typical presentation associated with the presence of limbal melanocytoma.

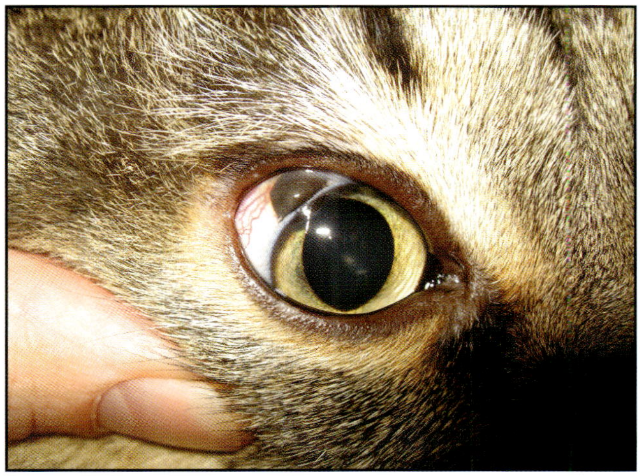

Figure 77.4 Typical presentation associated with the presence of limbal melanocytoma.

CHAPTER 78
FUNGAL KERATITIS

PRESENTATION

Fungal keratitis is relatively uncommon in dogs and cats. Environmental contamination, commensal overgrowth, epithelial trauma, and/or immunosuppression (notably using antibiotic/corticosteroid combinations) may facilitate the entry of fungal organisms, which may include *penicillium, fusarium, cladosporium, curvularia, aspergillus,* and *candida* sp. Lesions may be ulcerative or nonulcerative, often resulting in the presence of raised, gray- to tan-colored corneal plaques with an irregular surface. Discomfort is typically manifested by blepharospasm and/or epiphora. Progressive keratitis, keratomalacia, and/or secondary bacterial contamination may ultimately result in corneal perforation.

DIAGNOSIS AND TREATMENT

The diagnosis of fungal keratitis is made on the basis of clinical findings, supported by cytological or histological interpretation of representative material as well as ancillary diagnostics including microbial culture and sensitivity, serologic, and/or polymerase chain reaction (PCR) testing. Medical therapy comprises the topical and/or systemic administration of antifungal agents including natamycin, fluconazole, miconazole, and/or voriconazole. The adjunctive use of antibiotics and/or anti-inflammatory agents may also be indicated in some cases. In some cases, surgical resection of affected tissue and the introduction of a vascular supply via conjunctival grafting, may be indicated.

Potential Drug-Side-Effects

Potential adverse effects associated with the use of antifungal agents include local irritation as well as gastrointestinal (GI) distress and/or hepatopathy.

SELECTED REFERENCES

Ben-Shlomo G, Plummer C, Barrie K, Brooks D. Curvularia keratomycosis in a dog. *Vet Ophthalmol.* 2010;**13**(2):126–130.

Grundon RA, O'Reilly A, Muhlnickel C, Hardman C, Stanley RG. Keratomycosis in a dog treated with topical 1% voriconazole solution. *Vet Ophthalmol.* 2010;**13**(5):331–335.

Pucket JD, Allbaugh RA, Rankin AJ. Treatment of dematiaceous fungal keratitis in a dog. *J Am Vet Med Assoc.* 2012;**240**(9):1104–1108.

Scott EM, Carter RT. Canine keratomycosis in 11 dogs: a case series (2000–2011). *J Am Anim Hosp Assoc.* 2014;**50**(2):112–8. doi: 10.5326/JAAHA-MS-6012. Epub 2014 Jan 20.

Clinical Atlas of Canine and Feline Ophthalmic Disease, First Edition. Douglas Esson.

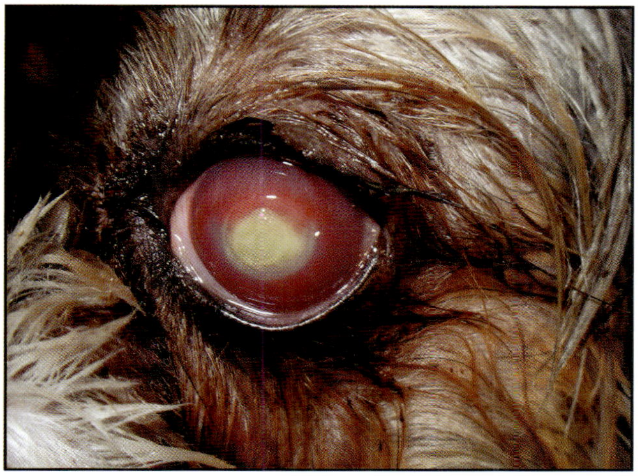

Figure 78.1 Typical presentation associated with fungal keratitis.

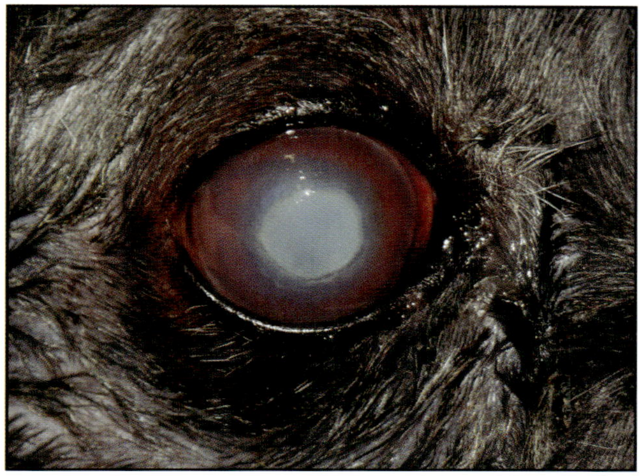

Figure 78.2 Typical presentation associated with fungal keratitis.

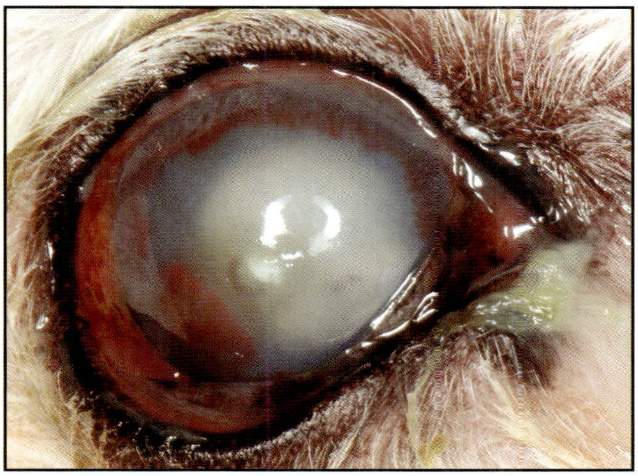

Figure 78.3 Typical presentation associated with fungal keratitis.

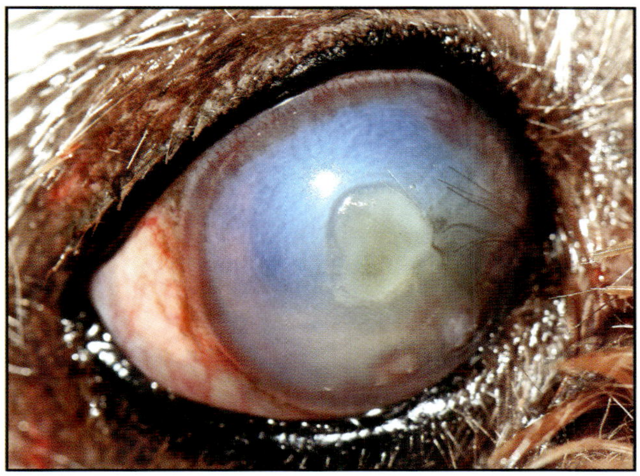

Figure 78.4 Typical presentation associated with fungal keratitis.

CHAPTER 79
CORNEOSCLERAL HEMANGIOMA/HEMANGIOSARCOMA

PRESENTATION

Tumors of vascular endothelial origin may affect the corneoscleral tissues and/or overlying conjunctival tissues (see also Conjunctival Hemangioma/Hemangiosarcoma). These lesions typically present as bright red, smooth, raised, irregular to nodular masses at or near the corneoscleral limbus. Tumors enlarge locally and may invade surrounding tissues. Exposure to UV radiation has been proposed to play a factor in the development of adnexal hemangioma/ hemangiosarcoma. Commonly affected breeds include the Australian Shepherd and the Collie breeds.

DIAGNOSIS AND TREATMENT

A tentative diagnosis of hemangioma/hemangiosarcoma may be made on the basis of the characteristic clinical appearance of these lesions; however confirmation as well as characterization of malignancy requires incisional or excisional biopsy and histopathology. Systemic health and/or involvement should be evaluated via local lymph node aspiration, three-view radiography, and complete blood count (CBC)/chemistry analysis, although lesions are frequently localized to the adnexal tissues only. Treatment typically encompasses surgical resection where possible and/or the application of adjunctive cryotherapy. Cryotherapy should only be undertaken using an appropriate nitrous oxide–cooled unit. Focal swelling is common following cryotherapy; however, inflammation rapidly resolves. Postoperative care comprises topical and or systemic anti-inflammatory and/or antimicrobial therapy as appropriate and the use of an Elizabethan collar to prevent self-trauma.

SELECTED REFERENCES

Chandler HL, Newkirk KM, Kusewitt DF, Dubielzig RR, Colitz CM. Immunohistochemical analysis of ocular hemangiomas and hemangiosarcomas in dogs. *Vet Ophthalmol.* 2009;**12**(2):83–90. doi: 10.1111/j.1463-5224.2008.00684.x.

Hargis AM, Ihrke PJ, Spangler WL, Stannard AA. A retrospective clinicopathologic study of 212 dogs with cutaneous hemangiomas and hemangiosarcomas. *Vet Pathol.* 1992;**29**(4):316–328.

Pirie CG, Knollinger AM, Thomas CB, Dubielzig RR. Canine conjunctival hemangioma and hemangiosarcoma: a retrospective evaluation of 108 cases (1989–2004). *Vet Ophthalmol.* 2006;**9**(4):215–226.

Clinical Atlas of Canine and Feline Ophthalmic Disease, First Edition. Douglas Esson.

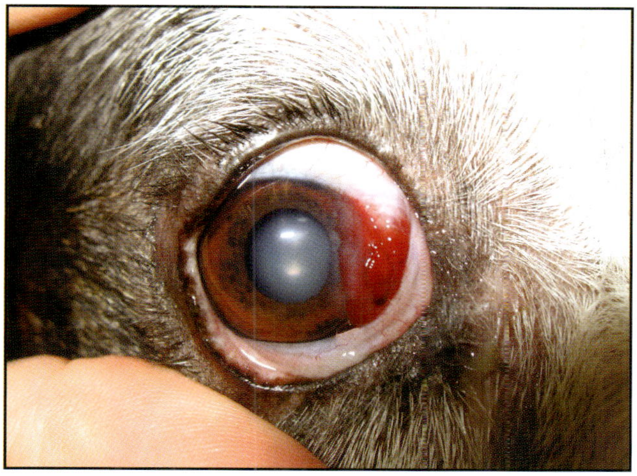

Figure 79.1 Typical presentation associated with corneoscleral hemangioma/hemangiosarcoma.

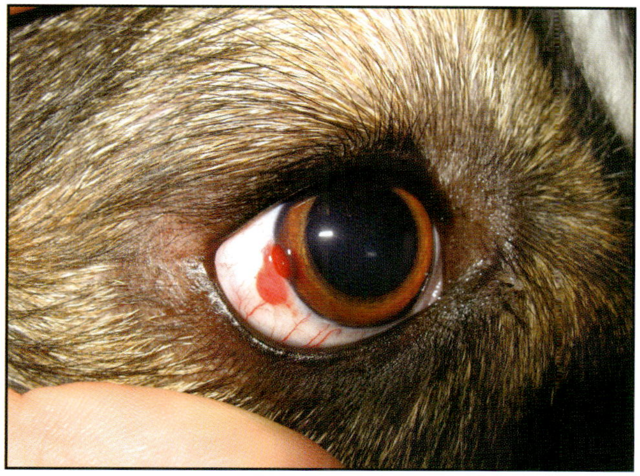

Figure 79.2 Typical presentation associated with corneoscleral hemangioma/hemangiosarcoma.

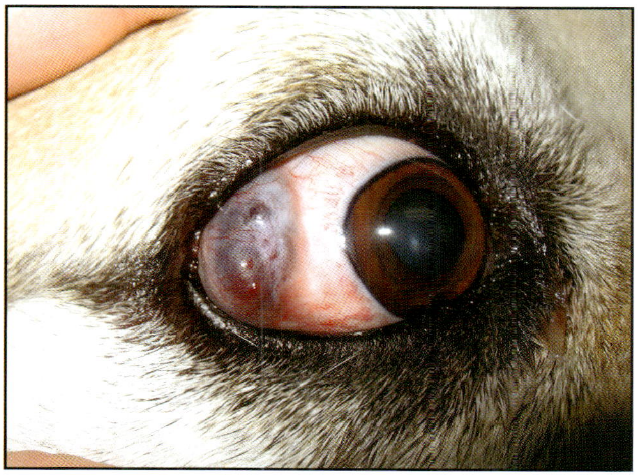

Figure 79.3 Typical presentation associated with corneoscleral hemangioma/hemangiosarcoma.

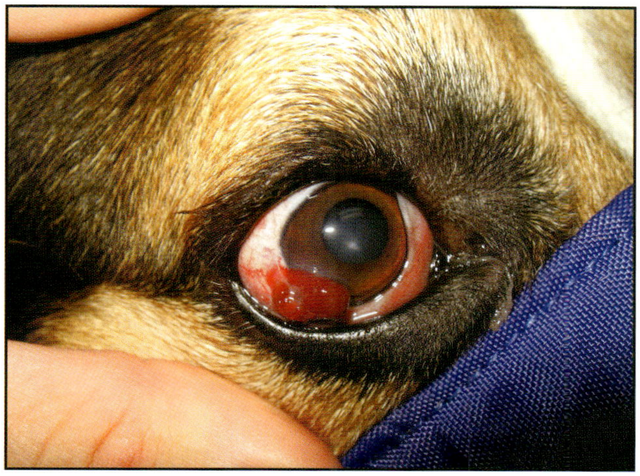

Figure 79.4 Typical presentation associated with corneoscleral hemangioma/hemangiosarcoma.

CHAPTER 80
CORNEOSCLERAL LYMPHOMA

PRESENTATION

Corneoscleral tissues are not infrequently affected by lymphoma. In some cases, ocular and/or adnexal symptoms may be the initial presentation for the disease, which may also remain localized to the adnexal region. Clinical findings may encompass a spectrum of lesions from mild peripheral infiltration around the corneoscleral limbus to localized nodular and/or diffuse cream-colored tissue infiltration. Other ocular tissues and/or more generalized involvement may also develop. Both canine and feline species as well as any breed or crossed breed may be affected (see also Cutaneous Epitheliotropic Lymphoma (CEL), Conjunctival Lymphoma, Uveal Lymphoma, Retinal/Choroidal Lymphoma, and Retrobulbar Neoplasia).

DIAGNOSIS AND TREATMENT

A definitive diagnosis of lymphoma is based on tissue biopsy and wherever lymphoma is suspected, samples should be harvested before the initiation of therapy in order to facilitate the planning of an accurate treatment protocol. Treatment comprises topical anti-inflammatory therapy (typically utilizing a corticosteroid) as well as systemic chemotherapy. Associated ophthalmic changes such as elevated intraocular pressure should be addressed as appropriate (see also Secondary (Postinflammatory) Glaucoma). Staging via local lymph node (and/or organ/bone marrow) aspiration, three-view radiography, and complete blood count (CBC)/chemistry analysis is recommended, before initiation of systemic chemotherapy. Diagnostic testing for the presence of infectious viruses including FeLV, FIV, and FIP is additionally recommended in feline patients. Individual chemotherapeutic protocols are most ideally designed by a veterinary oncologist; however, they typically include a variable combination of prednisone, vincristine, cyclophosphamide, and/or doxorubicin.

Potential Drug-Side-Effects

Potential adverse effects associated with the use of systemic corticosteroids include polyphagia, polydipsia, polyuria, hair coat changes, weight gain, pancreatitis, gastrointestinal (GI) distress, muscle damage, hepatic impairment, and diabetes. Potential adverse effects associated with the use of vincristine include stomatitis, GI distress, neuropathy, hepatopathy, and myelosuppression. Potential adverse effects associated with the use of cyclophosphamide include GI distress, pancreatitis, hepatotoxicity, and myelosuppression. Potential adverse affects associated with the use of doxorubicin include hypersensitivity, GI distress, cardiac dysfunction, and myelosuppression.

The prognosis varies depending on the extent of disease present before initiating therapy.

SELECTED REFERENCES

Nola M, Lukenda A, Bollmann M, Kalauz M, Petrovecki M, Bollmann R. Outcome and prognostic factors in ocular adnexal lymphoma. *Croat Med J*. 2004;**45**(3):328–332.

Ota-Kuroki J, Ragsdale JM, Bawa B, Wakamatsu N, Kuroki K. Intraocular and periocular lymphoma in dogs and cats: a retrospective review of 21 cases (2001–2012). *Vet Ophthalmol*. 2013. doi: 10.1111/vop.12106.

Rutley M, MacDonald V. Managing the canine lymphosarcoma patient in general practice. *Can Vet J*. 2007;**48**(9):977–979.

Clinical Atlas of Canine and Feline Ophthalmic Disease, First Edition. Douglas Esson.

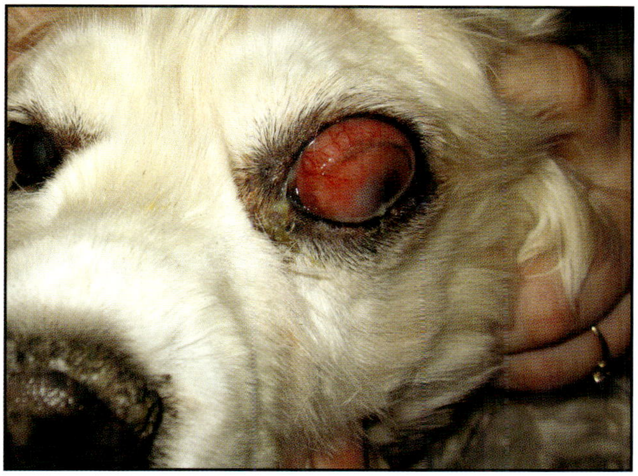

Figure 80.1 Typical presentation associated with corneoscleral lymphoma.

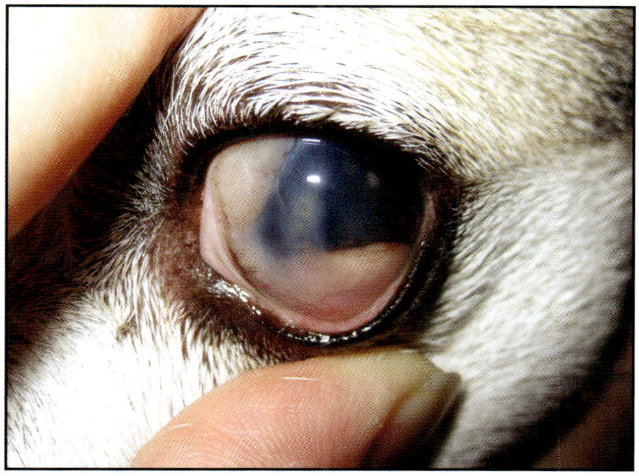

Figure 80.2 Typical presentation associated with corneoscleral lymphoma.

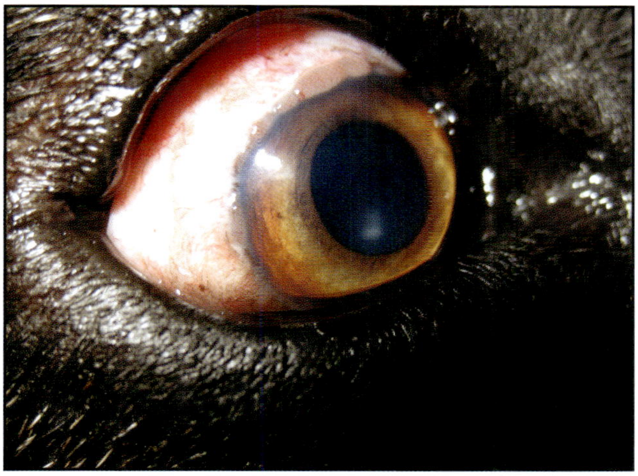

Figure 80.3 Typical presentation associated with corneoscleral lymphoma.

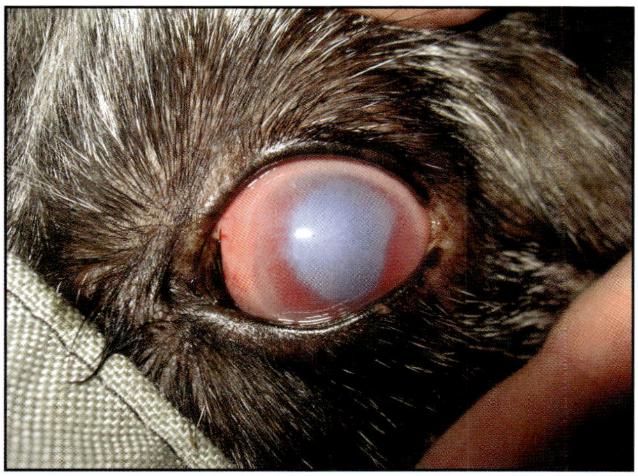

Figure 80.4 Typical presentation associated with corneoscleral lymphoma.

CHAPTER 81
CORNEAL SQUAMOUS CELL CARCINOMA

PRESENTATION

Hereditary factors, exposure to UV sunlight and/or chronic inflammation may contribute to the development of these lesions, with affected cells undergoing various degrees of anisocytosis, anisokaryosis, and/or dyskeratosis before progressing through low-grade or "carcinoma *in situ*" (which has not yet invaded the corneal stroma) to outright SCC. Clinically, SCC presents as a smooth, raised, gray- to pink-colored proliferative tissue, typically associated with a vascular supply and extending across the corneal surface in a variable pattern, ranging from focal/nodular to diffuse/lamellar. Commonly affected breeds include the Pug and the English Bulldog.

DIAGNOSIS AND TREATMENT

The diagnosis of SCC is made by histopathology following incisional or excisional biopsy, with SCC frequently appearing clinically similar to (and even encompassing) chronic corneal inflammation/granulation. Systemic health and/or involvement should be evaluated via local lymph node aspiration, three-view radiography, and complete blood count (CBC)/chemistry analysis. Treatment comprises resection of neoplastic tissue with or without the adjunctive application of cryotherapy and/or B-radiation. Cryotherapy should only be undertaken using an appropriate nitrous oxide–cooled unit. Focal swelling is common postoperatively; however, inflammation rapidly resolves. Postoperative care comprises topical and or systemic anti-inflammatory and/or antimicrobial therapy as appropriate and the use of an Elizabethan collar to prevent self-trauma.

SELECTED REFERENCES

Dreyfus J, Schobert CS, Dubielzig RR. Superficial corneal squamous cell carcinoma occurring in dogs with chronic keratitis. *Vet Ophthalmol.* 2011;**14**(3):161–168. doi: 10.1111/j.1463-5224.2010.00858.x.

Montiani-Ferreira F, Kiupel M, Muzolon P, Truppel J. Corneal squamous cell carcinoma in a dog: a case report. *Vet Ophthalmol.* 2008;**11**(4):269–272. doi: 10.1111/j.1463-5224.2008.00622.x.

Takiyama N, Terasaki E, Uechi M. Corneal squamous cell carcinoma in two dogs. *Vet Ophthalmol.* 2010;**13**(4):266–269. doi: 10.1111/j.1463-5224.2010.00792.x.

Clinical Atlas of Canine and Feline Ophthalmic Disease, First Edition. Douglas Esson.

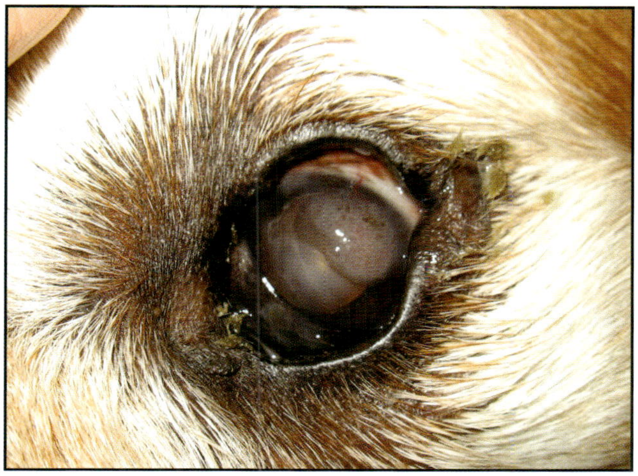

Figure 81.1 Typical presentation associated with the presence of corneal squamous cell carcinoma.

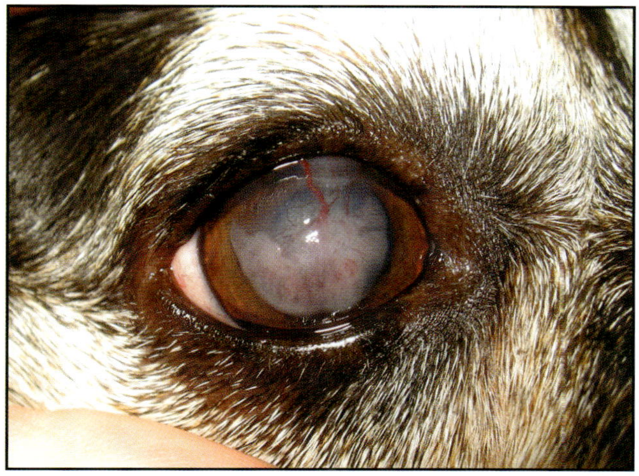

Figure 81.2 Typical presentation associated with the presence of corneal squamous cell carcinoma.

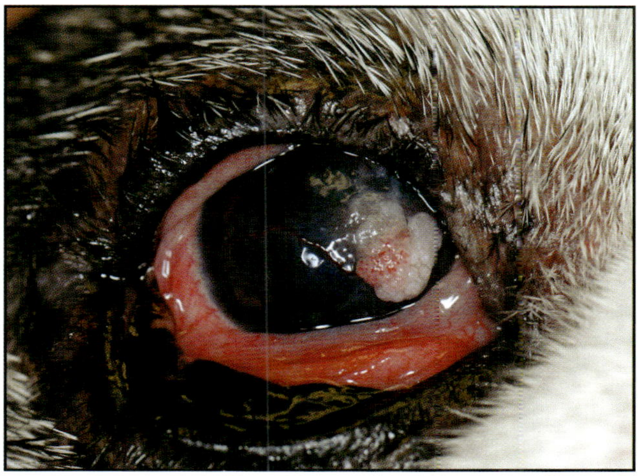

Figure 81.3 Typical presentation associated with the presence of corneal squamous cell carcinoma.

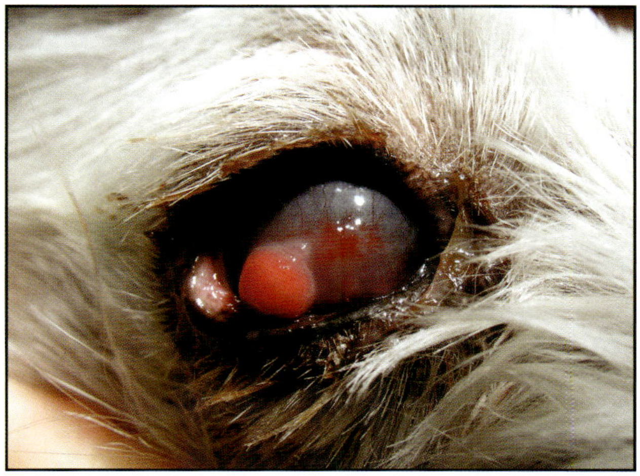

Figure 81.4 Typical presentation associated with the presence of corneal squamous cell carcinoma.

Section 5

Diseases of the Uvea

CHAPTER 82
PERSISTENT PUPILLARY MEMBRANES (PPMs)

PRESENTATION

Persistent pupillary membranes (PPMs) occur secondary to the incomplete resorption of embryonic lenticular vasculature, a process which is usually complete by several weeks after birth but which may continue for several months in some dogs. Occasionally, the remnants of this process may be recognized as a collection of fine, punctate, tan to brown spots on the axial anterior lens capsule. PPMs may extend from iris to iris, iris to lens, iris to corneal endothelium, and/or extend to float freely into the anterior chamber. The condition may be unilateral but is more commonly bilateral. Large or multiple PPMs may result in corneal opacification (due to endothelial damage, traction, and fibrosis) and/or secondary cataract formation. Commonly affected dog breeds include the Basenji, Pembroke Welsh Corgi, Mastiff, and Chow Chow.

DIAGNOSIS AND TREATMENT

The diagnosis of PPMs is made on the basis of characteristic clinical findings. It may occasionally be challenging to differentiate hereditary PPMs from postinflammatory synechiae, the latter potentially being associated with other signs of prior ocular inflammation or trauma including adjacent corneal fibrosis, iridal synechiation, pigment deposition, and/or cataract formation. Treatment is not typically necessary, although in rare cases the surgical or laser-mediated resection of PPMs and treatment of associated inflammation may be indicated. Similarly, significant cataracts, if present, may be surgically removed.

SELECTED REFERENCES

Collins BK, Collier LL, Johnson GS, Shibuya H, Moore CP, da Silva Curiel JM. Familial cataracts and concurrent ocular anomalies in chow chows. *J Am Vet Med Assoc*. 1992;**200**(10):1485–1491.

James RW. Persistent pupillary membrane in basenji dogs. *Vet Rec*. 1991;**128**(12):287–288.

Glaze MB. Congenital and hereditary ocular abnormalities in cats. *Clin Tech Small Anim Pract*. 2005;**20**(2):74–82.

Clinical Atlas of Canine and Feline Ophthalmic Disease, First Edition. Douglas Esson.

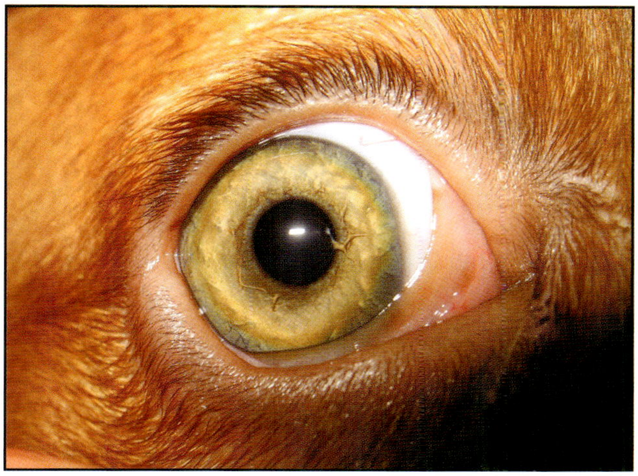

Figure 82.1 Typical presentation associated with persistent pupillary membranes. Iris to lens adhesions are present.

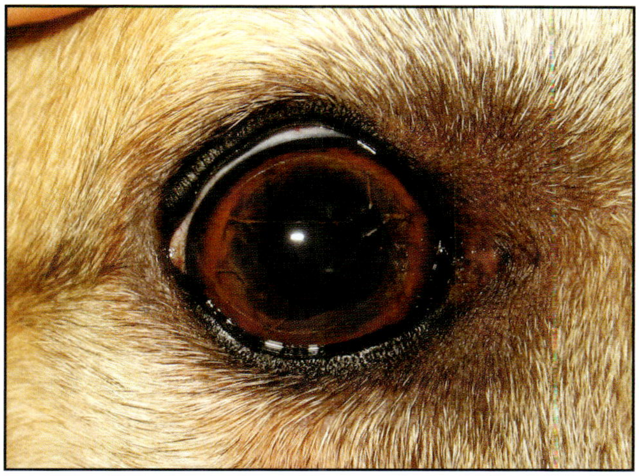

Figure 82.2 Typical presentation associated with persistent pupillary membranes. Iris to cornea adhesions are present.

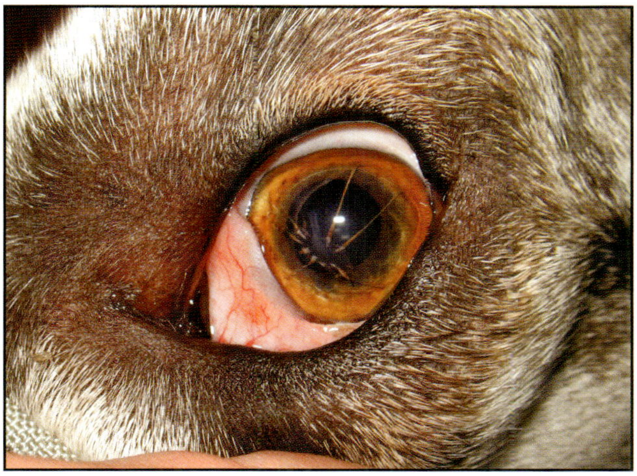

Figure 82.3 Typical presentation associated with persistent pupillary membranes. Iris to cornea adhesions are present.

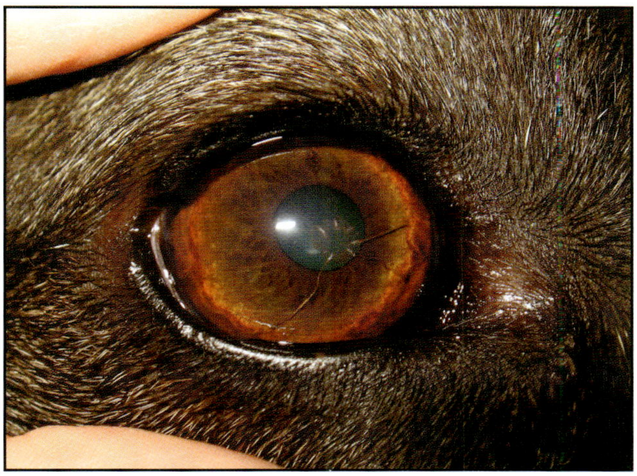

Figure 82.4 Typical presentation associated with persistent pupillary membranes. Iris to cornea adhesions are present.

CHAPTER 83
IRIS COLOBOMAS

PRESENTATION

Iris colobomas are defects occurring in any/all layers of developing iridal tissue, as a result of inappropriate embryonic differentiation. Coloboma(s) located within the iridal body may result in the false appearance of multiple pupillary openings or "pseudopolycoria." The complete absence of iris tissue (termed "aniridia") is rare. Clinically, most iris colobomas typically appear as "notch" defects within the iris. Commonly affected breeds include the Australian Shepherd and Collie breeds.

DIAGNOSIS AND TREATMENT

The diagnosis of iris coloboma is made on the basis of characteristic clinical findings. Treatment of iridal colobomas is not typically indicated.

SELECTED REFERENCES

Barnett KC, Knight GC. Persistent pupillary membrane and associated defects in the Basenji. *Vet Rec*. 1969;**85**(9):242–248.
Cook CS. Embryogenesis of congenital eye malformations. *Vet Comp Ophthalmol*. 1995;**5**:109–123.
Startup FG. Congenital abnormalities of the iris of the dog. *J Small Anim Pract*. 1966;**7**(1):99–100.

Clinical Atlas of Canine and Feline Ophthalmic Disease, First Edition. Douglas Esson.

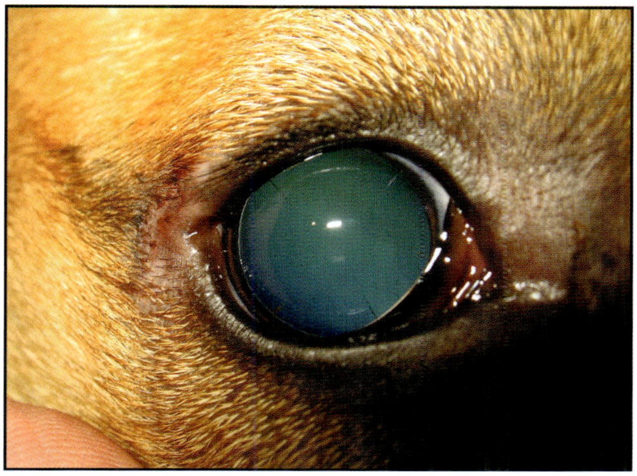

Figure 83.1 Rare complete aniridia.

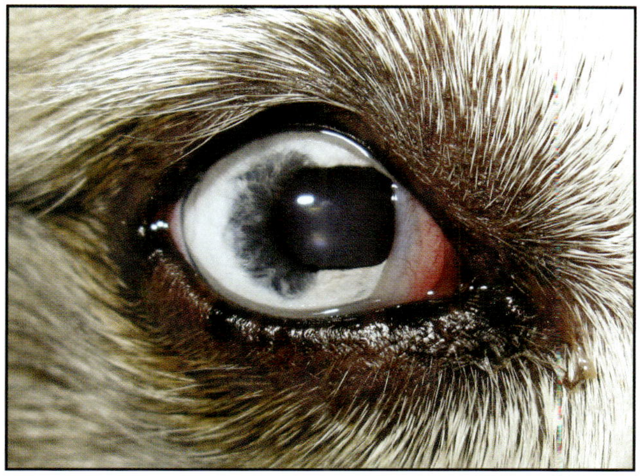

Figure 83.2 Colobomatous "notch" defect within iris tissue.

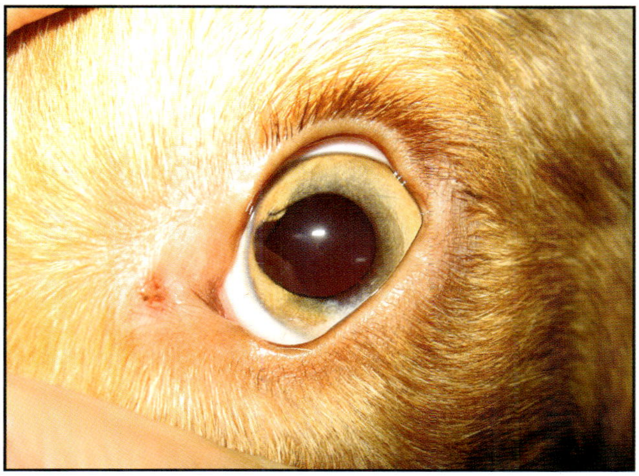

Figure 83.3 Colobomatous "notch" defect within iris tissue.

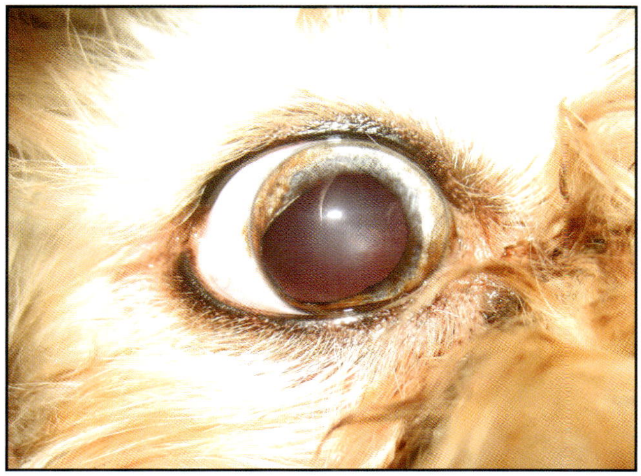

Figure 83.4 Colobomatous "notch" defect within iris tissue.

CHAPTER 84
SENILE IRIS ATROPHY

PRESENTATION

Senile iris atrophy results from the progressive loss of iridal tissue, which may occur with advanced age. Clinical findings may include thinning/translucency of iridal tissue (notably at the pupillary margin), resultant irregularities of the pupillary opening, outright pupillary dyscoria, the optical illusion of an apparently mydriatic (and poorly responsive) pupil and/or the presence of full-thickness iris defects resulting in the appearance of multiple apparent pupillary openings or "pseudopolycoria." Senile iris atrophy is typically bilateral, although not always symmetrical. Senile atrophy of iridal tissues is common in small-breed dogs.

DIAGNOSIS AND TREATMENT

The diagnosis of senile iris atrophy is made on the basis of clinical findings. It may be challenging to differentiate iridal atrophy from congenital pupillary abnormalities (notably iridal colobomas) and/or neurological disease (notably pathology resulting in mydriasis) (see also Iris Colobomas). Pharmacologic testing using topical pilocarpine will differentiate mechanical from neurologic mydriasis. No specific treatment is indicated; however, significant iridal atrophy and the resultant enlargement of the pupillary orifice may increase the relative risk of degenerate vitreous herniation and/or lenticular (sub)luxation in predisposed breeds, so that the long-term administration of miotic agents may occasionally be indicated.

SELECTED REFERENCES

Grahn BH, Cullen CL. Diagnostic ophthalmology. Iris atrophy. *Can Vet J* 2004;**45**(1):77–78.
Petrick SW. The incidence of eye disease in dogs in a veterinary academic hospital: 1772 cases. *J S Afr Vet Assoc* 1996;**67**(3):108–110.
Whiting RE, Yao G, Narfström K, Pearce JW, Coates JR, Dodam JR, Castaner LJ, Katz ML. Quantitative assessment of the canine pupillary light reflex. *Invest Ophthalmol Vis Sci* 2013;**54**(8):5432–5440. DOI: 10.1167/iovs.13-12012.

Clinical Atlas of Canine and Feline Ophthalmic Disease, First Edition. Douglas Esson.

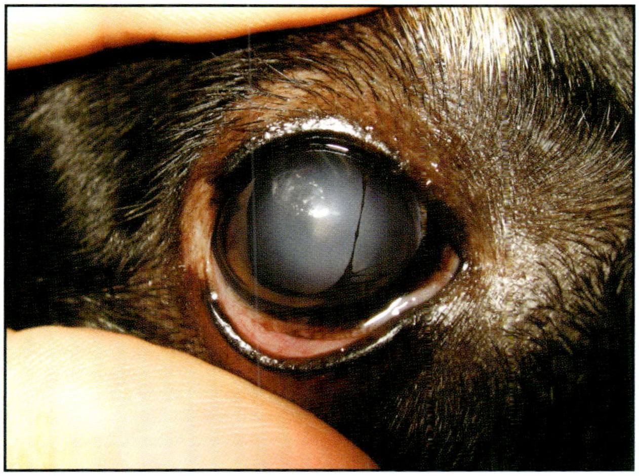

Figure 84.1 Typical presentation associated with senile iris atrophy.

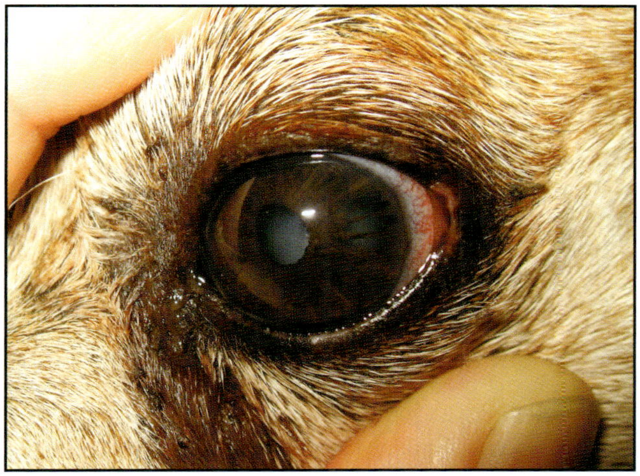

Figure 84.2 Typical presentation associated with senile iris atrophy.

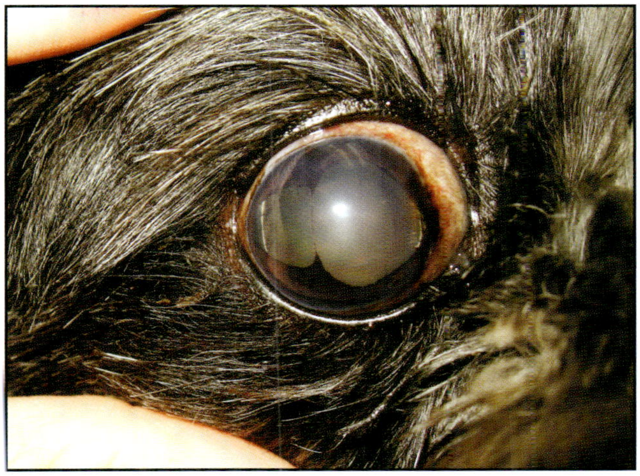

Figure 84.3 Typical presentation associated with senile iris atrophy.

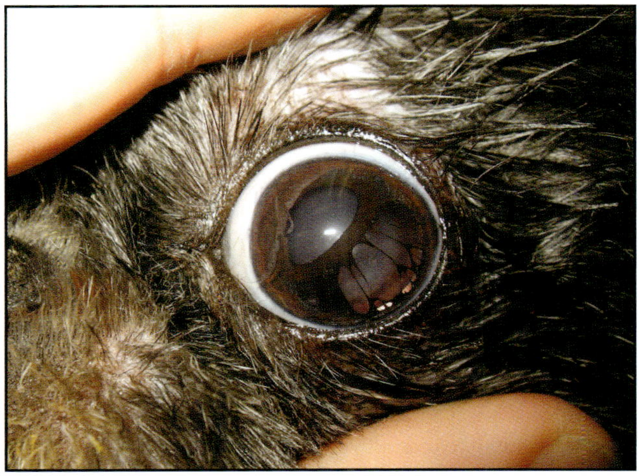

Figure 84.4 Typical presentation associated with senile iris atrophy.

CHAPTER 85
UVEAL CYSTS

PRESENTATION

Uveal cysts (sometimes also referred to as *iris cysts*) may arise from the posterior iridal or ciliary body epithelium as a result of hereditary factors, cystic hyperplasia, and/or chronic inflammation. Clinically, uveal cysts comprise oval to round, thin-walled, translucent to dark brown structures that may be attached to the ciliary tissue, float freely within the anterior or posterior chambers (or rarely within degenerate vitreous), and/or rupture and adhere against intracameral surfaces including the lens capsule and/or corneal endothelium. Uveal cysts may occur unilaterally or bilaterally and may vary significantly in both size and number. Commonly affected breeds include the Labrador Retriever, Golden Retriever, Boston Terrier, Great Dane, and American Bulldog.

DIAGNOSIS AND TREATMENT

The diagnosis of uveal cyst(s) is made on the basis of clinical findings, supported if necessary by B-mode ultrasonography. Occasionally, intracameral neoplasia (particularly melanocytoma/melanoma) may represent challenging differentials (see also Uveal Melanoma). Most uveal cysts are benign and do not require treatment. The presence of uveal cysts in Golden Retrievers should raise concern for the presence of additional ocular findings, which may suggest the development of more serious breed-associated pigmentary and cystic uveitis/glaucoma (see Golden Retriever-Associated Pigmentary Uveitis and Glaucoma). In addition, the presence of uveal cysts has been associated with other ocular changes and elevated intraocular pressure in some breeds including the American Bulldog and Great Dane. The administration of systemic topical and/or anti-inflammatory agents (either steroidal or nonsteroidal) may be indicated in cases affected by chronic intracameral inflammation. Surgical intervention may be indicated in cases where cystic proliferation results in visual impairment and/or compromised aqueous outflow. Where indicated, cysts may be removed by surgical extraction, surgical aspiration, and/or diode laser photoablation.

Potential Drug-Side-Effects

Potential adverse effects associated with the use of topical corticosteroids include impaired wound healing and corneal degeneration.

SELECTED REFERENCES

Delgado E, Pissarra H, Sales-Luís J, Peleteiro MC. Amelanotic uveal cyst in a Yorkshire terrier dog. *Vet Ophthalmol* 2010;**13**(5):343–347. DOI: 10.1111/j.1463-5224.2010.00825.x.

Gemensky-Metzler AJ, Wilkie DA, Cook CS. The use of semiconductor diode laser for deflation and coagulation of anterior uveal cysts in dogs, cats and horses: a report of 20 cases. *Vet Ophthalmol* 2004;**7**(5):360–368.

Townsend WM, Gornik KR. Prevalence of uveal cysts and pigmentary uveitis in Golden Retrievers in three Midwestern states. *J Am Vet Med Assoc* 2013;**243**(9):1298–1301. DOI: 10.2460/javma.243.9.1298.

Clinical Atlas of Canine and Feline Ophthalmic Disease, First Edition. Douglas Esson.

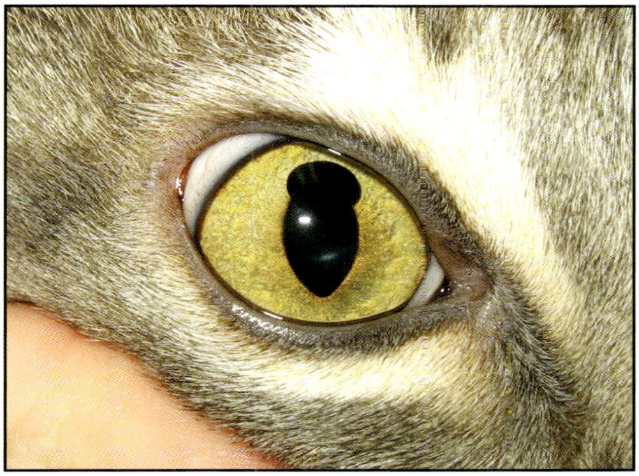

Figure 85.1 Single, heavily pigmented uveal cyst.

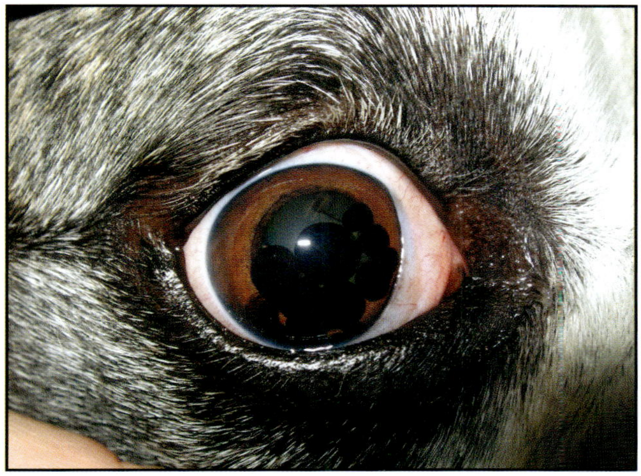

Figure 85.2 Multiple uveal cysts.

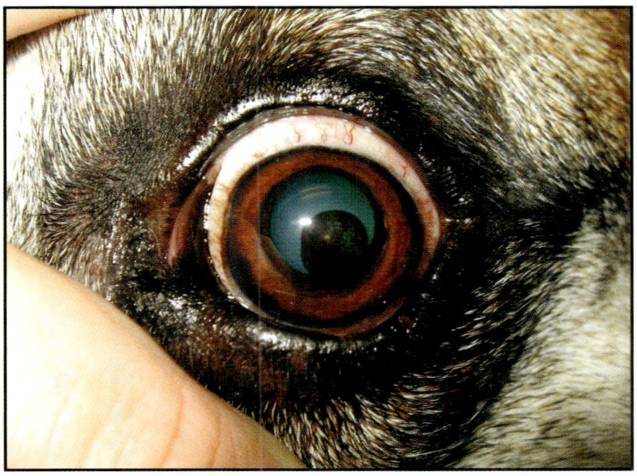

Figure 85.3 Single translucent uveal cyst.

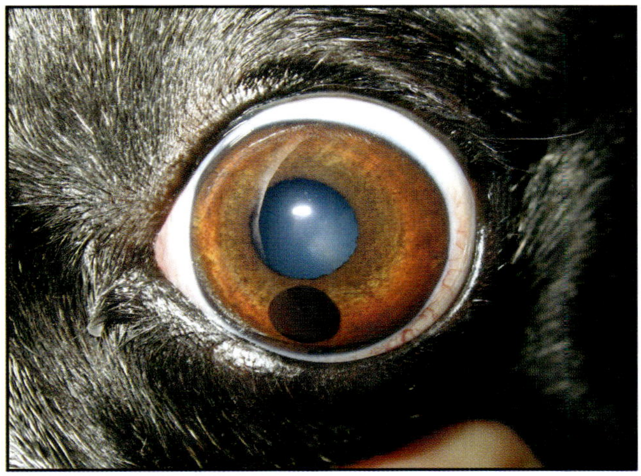

Figure 85.4 Single pigmented uveal cyst.

CHAPTER 86
MERLE OCULAR DYSGENESIS (MOD)

PRESENTATION

Merle ocular dysgenesis (MOD) is a hereditary, congenital condition, which may affect animals displaying merled coat coloration. MOD results from abnormal embryonic differentiation of tissues and may lead to multiple ocular abnormalities, including any combination of microphthalmos, microcornea, scleral staphyloma, persistent pupillary membranes (PPMs), heterochromia iris, iridal hypoplasia/coloboma (with resultant dyscoria/corectopia), pseudopolycoria, iridocorneal angle dysplasia, lenticular coloboma/cataract/subluxation, choroidal hypoplasia, optic nerve coloboma, retinal dysplasia, and/or retinal detachment (with or without hyphema). Changes are bilateral but not always symmetrical. Affected dogs (notably homozygous "white" merles) may also be congenitally deaf. Commonly affected breeds include the Australian Shepherd, (merled) Collies, Shetland Sheepdog, Harlequin Great Dane and (merled) Long-Haired Dachshund.

DIAGNOSIS AND TREATMENT

The diagnosis of MOD is made on the basis of a combination of signalment and clinical findings. Primary treatment of this disorder is not possible; however, secondary complications, such as hyphema or cataract development, may be treated symptomatically. Surgical intervention in order to address scleral, lenticular, and/or retinal pathology may also be indicated in select cases. Selective breeding reduces the incidence and severity of disease.

SELECTED REFERENCES

Gelatt KN, McGill LD. Clinical characteristics of microphthalmia with colobomas of the Australian Shepherd Dog. *J Am Vet Med Assoc* 1973;**162**(5):393–396.

Gelatt KN, Powell NG, Huston K. Inheritance of microphthalmia with coloboma in the Australian shepherd dog. *Am J Vet Res* 1981;**42**(10):1686–1690.

Strain GM, Clark LA, Wahl JM, Turner AE, Murphy KE. Prevalence of deafness in dogs heterozygous or homozygous for the merle allele. *J Vet Intern Med* 2009;**23**(2):282–286. DOI: 10.1111/j.1939-1676.2008.0257.x. Epub 2009 Feb 3.

Clinical Atlas of Canine and Feline Ophthalmic Disease, First Edition. Douglas Esson.

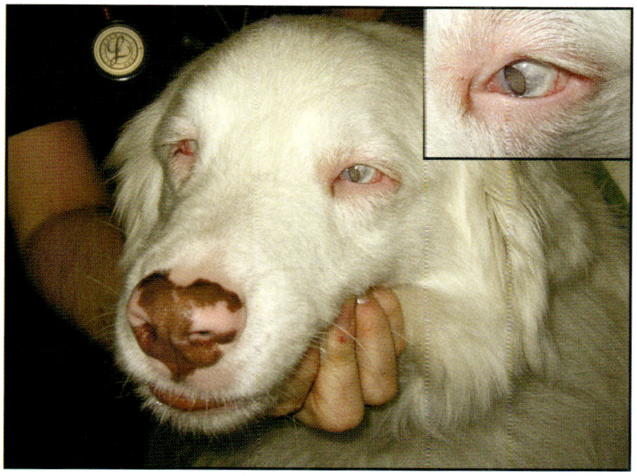

Figure 86.1 Typical presentation associated with merle ocular dysgenesis (MOD). Inset demonstrates the presence of a cataract.

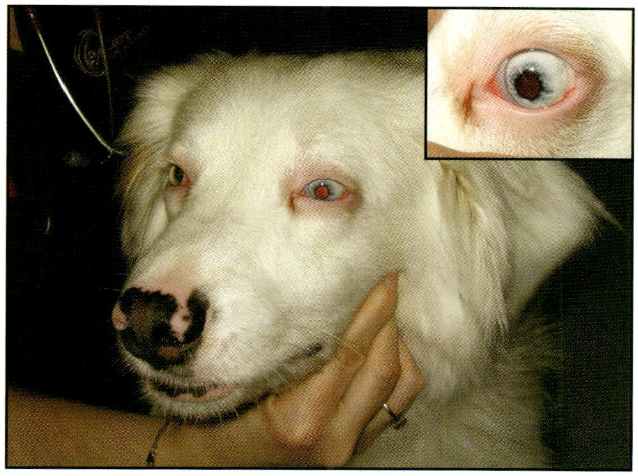

Figure 86.2 Typical presentation associated with merle ocular dysgenesis (MOD). Inset demonstrates the presence of a cataract.

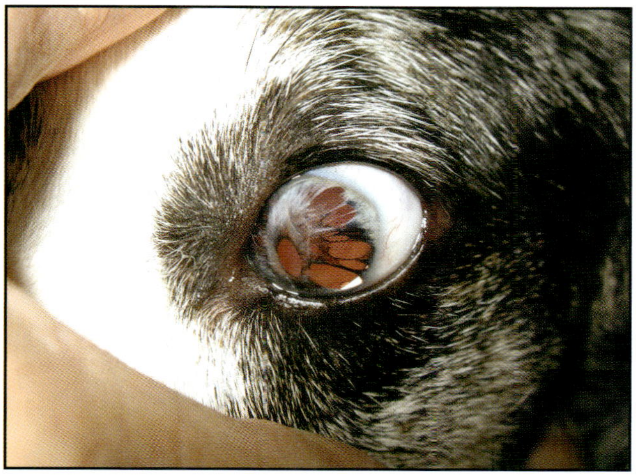

Figure 86.3 Typical presentation associated with merle ocular dysgenesis (MOD).

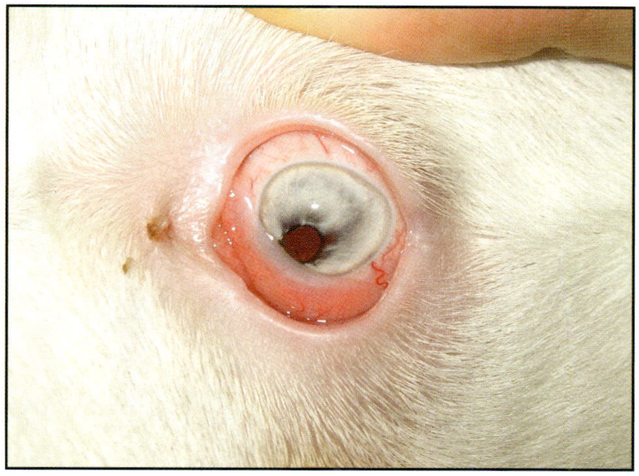

Figure 86.4 Typical presentation associated with merle ocular dysgenesis (MOD).

CHAPTER 87
FELINE ANTERIOR UVEITIS

PRESENTATION

The uveal tract is composed of anterior (iris and ciliary body) and posterior (choroidal) tissues. These tissues contain components of the "blood–ocular barrier" which regulates the passage of protein into the aqueous humor. The term uveitis describes inflammation of any of these tissues and is typically associated with variable breakdown of the blood–ocular barrier. Inflammation of the anterior uveal tissues may occur with or without significant clinical involvement of posterior uveal tissue (see also Feline Chorioretinitis). The spectrum of clinical symptoms potentially associated with feline anterior uveitis may include vascular keratitis, corneal edema, and/or the accumulation of proteinaceous keratic precipitates, aqueous proteinaceous flare, iridal thickening/hyperemia/infiltration (diffuse or nodular) or hemorrhage, iridal adhesions (anterior or posterior), outright iris bombe', secondary cataract formation, vitritis, and variable degrees of chorioretinitis (with or without retinal detachment). Initially, intraocular pressures are typically decreased in cases of uveitis; however, secondary glaucoma may occur as a later complication (see also Secondary (Postinflammatory) Glaucoma). One or both eyes may be affected. Bilateral uveitis should prompt concern for the presence of systemic disease.

DIAGNOSIS AND TREATMENT

The diagnosis of anterior uveitis is made on the basis of clinical findings. Potential etiologies include hereditary factors, lens-associated inflammation (see also Phacolytic Uveitis and Phacoclastic Uveitis), trauma, systemic disease, exposure to infectious organisms, and/or the presence of (local or systemic) neoplasia. Infectious etiologies that may be associated with the development of anterior uveitis in cats include viral (notably FeLV, FIV, FIP, FHV), protozoal (notably *Toxoplasma gondii*), bacterial (notably *Bartonella* spp.), and fungal (notably *cryptococcus*, *coccidioidomycosis*, *aspergillus*, *blastomyces*, and *histoplasmosis*) organisms. Frustratingly, the etiology of uveitis remains unclear in a significant proportion of cases. In addition, clinical uveitis may be chronic and/or recurrent in its behavior. Treatment encompasses addressing underlying systemic, infectious, or neoplastic disease. In addition, topical and/or systemic anti-inflammatory therapy (nonsteroidal or steroidal) is typically warranted. Long-term treatment may be indicated in order to minimize the risk of secondary glaucoma. Mydriatic agents (atropine/tropicamide) should be used with caution and only where specifically indicated (i.e., in the presence painful ciliary spasm and/or significant blood–aqueous barrier (BAB) breakdown). Clindamycin generally represents a suitable initial, empirical antimicrobial choice when treating feline patients.

Potential Drug-Side-Effects
Potential side effects associated with the use of clindamycin include gastrointestinal (GI) distress.

SELECTED REFERENCES

Colitz CM. Feline uveitis: diagnosis and treatment. *Clin Tech Small Anim Pract* 2005;**20**(2):117–120.

Townsend WM. Canine and feline uveitis. *Vet Clin North Am Small Anim Pract* 2008;**38**(2):323–346, vii. DOI: 10.1016/j.cvsm.2007.12.004.

van der Woerdt A. Management of intraocular inflammatory disease. *Clin Tech Small Anim Pract* 2001;**16**(1):58–61.

Clinical Atlas of Canine and Feline Ophthalmic Disease, First Edition. Douglas Esson.

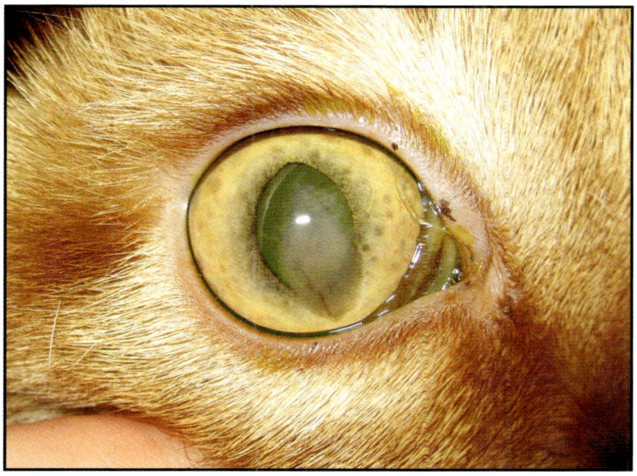

Figure 87.1 Changes associated with feline anterior uveitis including nodular iridal proliferation, iritis and the accumulation of fibrin within the anterior chamber.

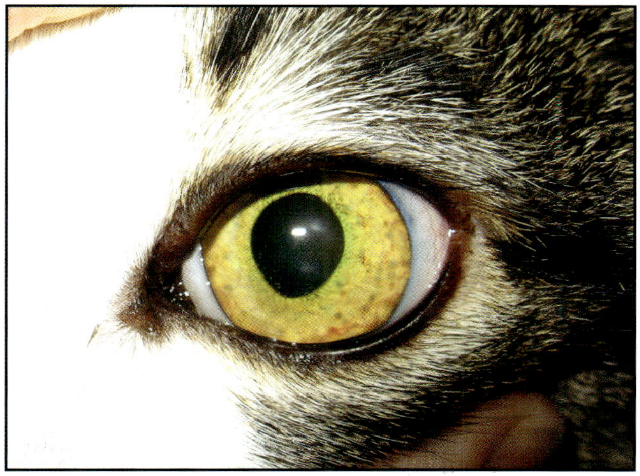

Figure 87.2 Changes associated with feline anterior uveitis including nodular iridal proliferation, iritis and endothelial keratic precipitate formation.

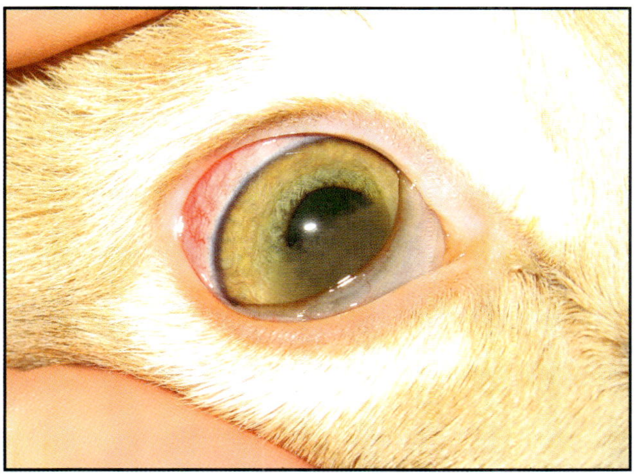

Figure 87.3 Changes associated with feline anterior uveitis including iritis and the accumulation of fibrin within the anterior chamber.

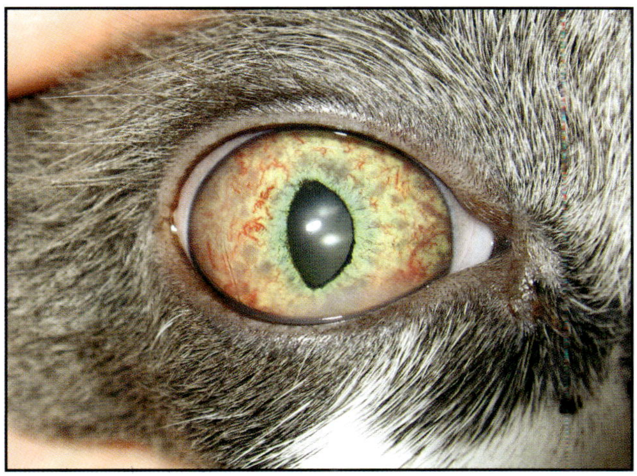

Figure 87.4 Changes associated with feline anterior uveitis including nodular iridal proliferation and iritis.

CHAPTER 88
CANINE ANTERIOR UVEITIS

PRESENTATION

The uveal tract is composed of the anterior (iris and ciliary body) and posterior (choroidal) tissues. These tissues contain components of the "blood–ocular barrier," which regulates the passage of protein into the aqueous humor. The term uveitis describes inflammation of any of these tissues and is typically associated with variable breakdown of the blood–ocular barrier. Inflammation of the anterior uveal tissues may occur with or without significant clinical involvement of posterior uveal tissue (see also Canine Chorioretinitis). The spectrum of clinical symptoms potentially associated with canine anterior uveitis may include vascular keratitis, corneal edema, and/or the accumulation of proteinaceous keratic precipitates, aqueous proteinaceous flare, iridal thickening/hyperemia/infiltration (diffuse or nodular) or hemorrhage, iridal adhesions (anterior or posterior), outright iris bombe', secondary cataract formation, vitritis, and variable degrees of chorioretinitis (with or without retinal detachment). Initially, intraocular pressures are typically decreased in cases of uveitis; however, secondary glaucoma may occur as a later complication (see also Secondary (Postinflammatory) Glaucoma). One or both eyes may be affected. Bilateral uveitis should prompt concern for the presence of systemic disease.

DIAGNOSIS AND TREATMENT

The diagnosis of anterior uveitis is made on the basis of clinical findings. Potential etiologies include hereditary factors, trauma, lens-associated inflammation (see also Phacolytic Uveitis and Phacoclastic Uveitis), systemic disease, exposure to infectious organisms, and/or the presence of (local or systemic) neoplasia. Infectious etiologies that may be associated with the development of anterior uveitis in dogs include viral (notably canine adenovirus-1 and canine parvovirus), protozoal (notably *Toxoplasma gondii*), bacterial (notably *Ehrlichia canis*, *Rickettsia rickettsii*, *Leptospira* spp., and *Borrelia* spp.) and fungal (notably *coccidioidomycosis, aspergillus, blastomyces, and histoplasmosis*) organisms. Frustratingly, the precise etiology of uveitis remains unclear in a significant proportion of cases. In addition, clinical uveitis may be chronic and/or recurrent in its behavior. Treatment encompasses addressing underlying systemic, infectious, or neoplastic disease. In addition, topical and/or systemic anti-inflammatory therapy (nonsteroidal or steroidal) is typically warranted. Long-term treatment may be indicated in order to minimize the risk of secondary glaucoma. Mydriatic agents (atropine/tropicamide) should be used with caution and only where specifically indicated (i.e., in the presence of painful ciliary spasm and/or significant blood–aqueous barrier (BAB) breakdown). Doxycycline generally represents a suitable initial, empirical antimicrobial choice when treating canine patients.

Potential Drug-Side-Effects
Potential side effects associated with the use of doxycycline, include gastrointestinal (GI) distress.

SELECTED REFERENCES

Massa KL, Gilger BC, Miller TL, Davidson MG. Causes of uveitis in dogs: 102 cases (1989–2000). *Vet Ophthalmol* 2002;**5**(2):93–98.
Townsend WM. Canine and feline uveitis. *Vet Clin North Am Small Anim Pract* 2008;**38**(2):323–346, vii. DOI: 10.1016/j.cvsm.2007.12.004.
Wasik B, Adkins E. Canine anterior uveitis. *Compend Contin Educ Vet* 2010;**32**(11):E1.

Clinical Atlas of Canine and Feline Ophthalmic Disease, First Edition. Douglas Esson.

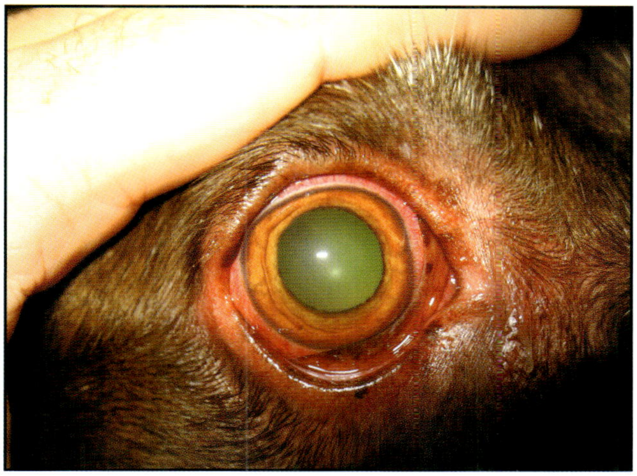

Figure 88.1 Changes associated with canine anterior uveitis including iritis.

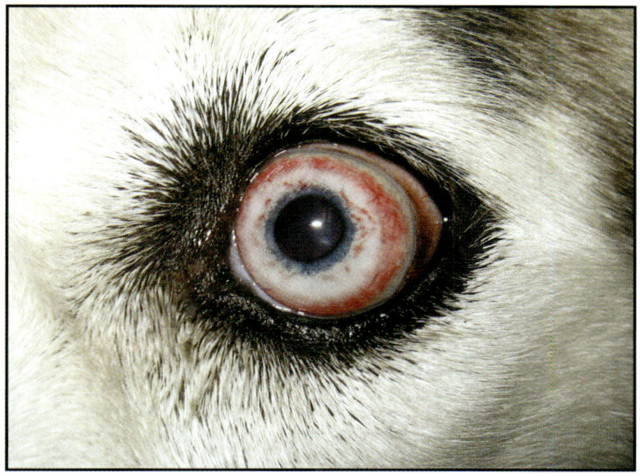

Figure 88.2 Changes associated with canine anterior uveitis including iritis.

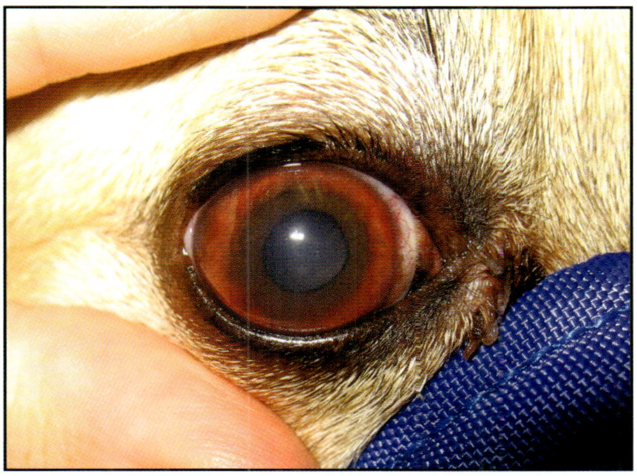

Figure 88.3 Changes associated with canine anterior uveitis including iritis and hemorrhage.

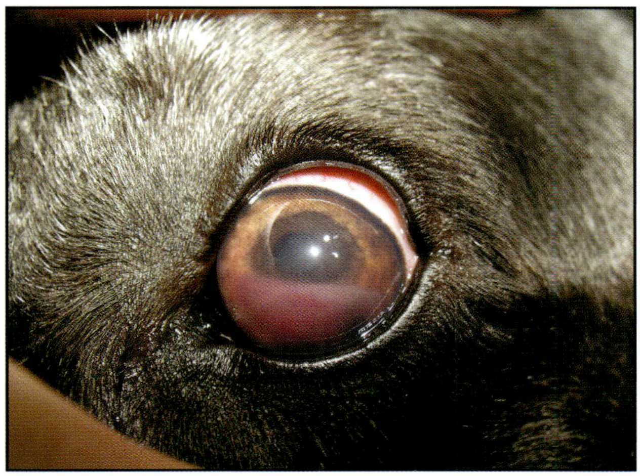

Figure 88.4 Changes associated with canine anterior uveitis including iritis and hypopyon.

CHAPTER 89
GOLDEN RETRIEVER–ASSOCIATED UVEITIS AND GLAUCOMA

PRESENTATION

A syndrome comprising slowly progressive intraocular changes, typically culminating in secondary glaucoma, is well recognized within the Golden Retriever breed. This syndrome has been variably described as "pigmentary uveitis," "Golden Retriever uveitis," and "pigmentary and cystic glaucoma of Golden Retrievers." Findings may include any combination of conjunctival and/or episcleral hyperemia, corneal decompensation, thin-walled uveal cysts within the anterior or posterior chambers, proteinaceous exudation within the anterior chamber, anterior and/or posterior iridal adhesions, pigment dispersion within the anterior chamber and/or onto the anterior lens capsule, cataract formation, hyphema and/or secondary glaucoma. Uveal cysts may detach and move into the anterior chamber where they may rupture against corneal endothelial and/or iridal surfaces or collapse and rupture within the iridocorneal angle. The hallmark of this syndrome has been described as the appearance of pigment on the anterior lens capsule, typically distributed in a radial orientation. Initial symptoms are frequently noted around middle age and are usually bilateral, although not necessarily symmetrical. The etiology of this syndrome is poorly understood; however, genetic factors have been proposed on the basis of breed predilection as well as the absence of demonstrable infectious or neoplastic causes.

DIAGNOSIS AND TREATMENT

The diagnosis of Golden Retriever–associated uveitis is made on the basis of a combination of signalment and clinical findings. Treatment is generally empirical, frequently comprising topical and/or systemic anti-inflammatory (either steroidal or nonsteroidal), immune-modulating (azathioprine or cyclosporine) as well as antiglaucoma agents; however, secondary glaucoma is frequently the endpoint of this disease.

Potential Drug-Side-Effects

Potential adverse effects associated with the use of systemic corticosteroids include polyphagia, polydipsia, polyuria, hair coat changes, weight gain, pancreatitis, enteritis, muscular damage, hepatic impairment, and diabetes. Potential adverse effects associated with the use of azathioprine include gastrointestinal (GI) distress, pancreatitis, hepatotoxicity, and myelosuppression. Potential adverse affects associated with the use of cyclosporine include hypersensitivity and GI distress.

Patients affected by advanced disease represent high-risk candidates for either cataract or glaucoma surgery based on the frequency and severity of complications encountered. Ultimately, a procedure of comfort (enucleation, cryosurgery, intrascleral prosthesis placement, or chemical ciliary body ablation) may be necessary in order to address blind and/or painful eyes.

SELECTED REFERENCES

Deehr AJ, Dubielzig RR. A histopathological study of iridociliary cysts and glaucoma in Golden Retrievers. *Vet Ophthalmol* 1998;**1**(2–3):153–158.

Esson D, Armour M, Mundy P, Schobert CS, Dubielzig RR. The histopathological and immunohistochemical characteristics of pigmentary and cystic glaucoma in the Golden Retriever. *Vet Ophthalmol* 2009;**12**(6):361–368.

Sapienza JS, Simó FJ, Prades-Sapienza A. Golden Retriever uveitis: 75 cases (1994–1999). *Vet Ophthalmol* 2000;**3**(4):241–246.

Townsend WM, Gornik KR. Prevalence of uveal cysts and pigmentary uveitis in Golden Retrievers in three Midwestern states. *J Am Vet Med Assoc* 2013;**243**(9):1298–1301. DOI: 10.2460/javma.243.9.1298.

Clinical Atlas of Canine and Feline Ophthalmic Disease, First Edition. Douglas Esson.

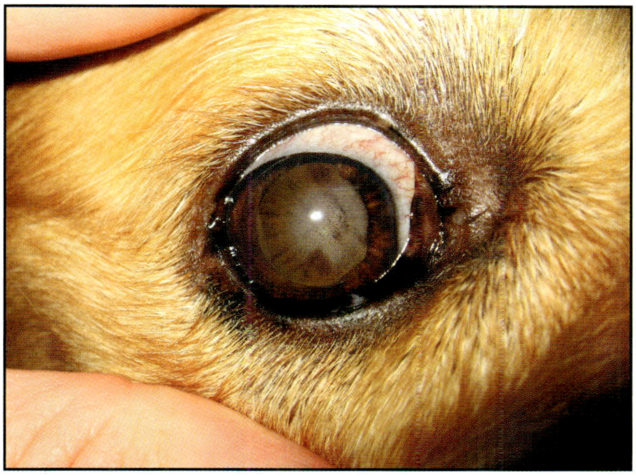

Figure 89.1 Typical clinical presentation associated with the presence of Golden Retriever-associated uveitis. Increased iridal pigmentation and radial pigment deposition on the anterior lens capsule are notable.

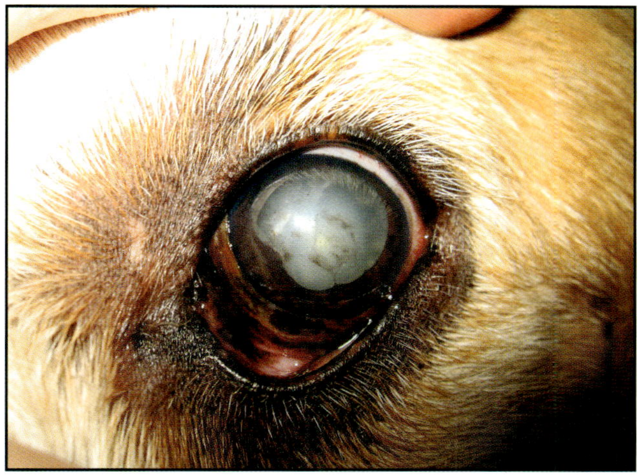

Figure 89.2 Typical clinical presentation associated with the presence of Golden Retriever–associated uveitis. Increased iridal pigmentation, posterior synechiation and secondary cataract are notable.

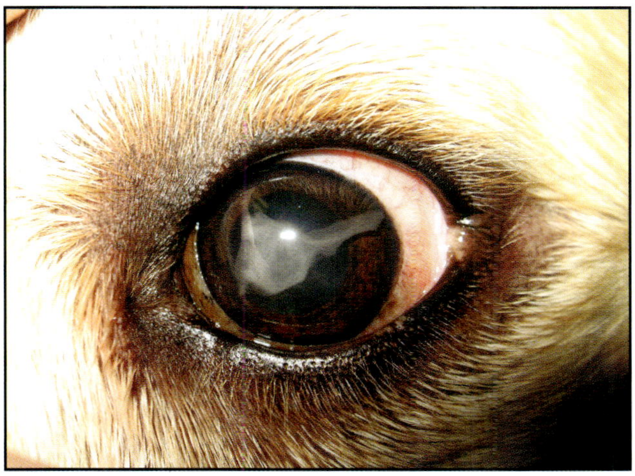

Figure 89.3 Typical clinical presentation associated with the presence of Golden Retriever–associated uveitis. Increased iridal pigmentation and anterior chamber protein exudation are notable.

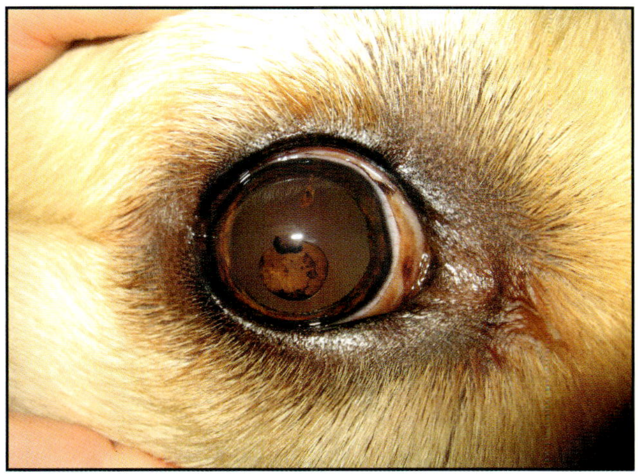

Figure 89.4 Typical clinical presentation associated with the presence of Golden Retriever–associated uveitis. Increased iridal pigmentation and thin-walled uveal cysts are notable.

CHAPTER 90
VACCINE-ASSOCIATED UVEITIS

PRESENTATION

Infection with canine adenovirus type-1 (CAV-1) and/or vaccination with modified live CAV-1 strains may be associated with anterior uveitis and/or endotheliitis (see also Endotheliitis). Ocular symptoms may include the presence of aqueous flare, pupillary miosis, and/or corneal edema secondary to endothelial cell dysfunction. Potential ocular sequela include bullous keratopathy, ulcerative keratitis, and/or secondary glaucoma. The Afghan hound has been described as being at increased risk.

DIAGNOSIS AND TREATMENT

The diagnosis of vaccine-associated uveitis is made on the basis of history (including that of recent vaccination), clinical examination, routine complete blood count (CBC)/chemistry analysis, and/or testing for the presence of infectious organisms. Treatment typically encompasses the administration of topical and systemic (steroidal) anti-inflammatory therapy, unless contraindicated. In many cases, symptoms will resolve if appropriately treated early in the course of the disease. Secondary pathologies including corneal ulceration and/or glaucoma should be managed as appropriate, if present.

Potential Drug-Side-Effects

Potential adverse effects associated with the use of topical corticosteroids include impaired wound healing and corneal degeneration. Potential adverse effects associated with the use of systemic corticosteroids include polyphagia, polydipsia, polyuria, hair coat changes, weight gain, pancreatitis, gastrointestinal (GI) distress, muscle damage, hepatic impairment, and diabetes.

SELECTED REFERENCES

Aguirre G, Carmichael L, Bistner S. Corneal endothelium in viral induced anterior uveitis. Ultrastructural changes following canine adenovirus type 1 infection. *Arch Ophthalmol* 1975;**93**(3):219–224.

Curtis R, Barnett KC. Canine adenovirus-induced ocular lesions in the Afghan hound. *Cornell Vet* 1981;**71**(1):85–95.

Curtis R, Barnett KC. The 'blue eye' phenomenon. *Vet Rec* 1983;**112**(15):347–353.

Clinical Atlas of Canine and Feline Ophthalmic Disease, First Edition. Douglas Esson.

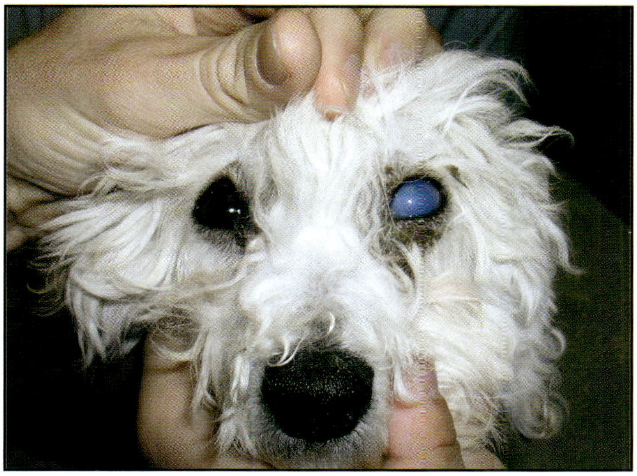

Figure 90.1 Changes as a result of vaccine-associated uveitis. Corneal edema is notable.

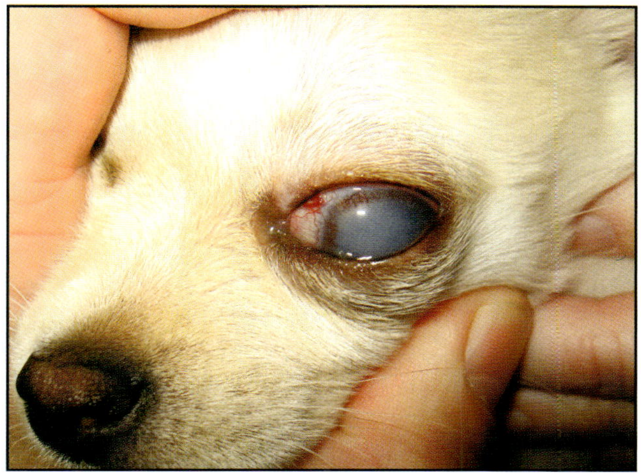

Figure 90.2 Changes as a result of vaccine-associated uveitis. Corneal edema is notable.

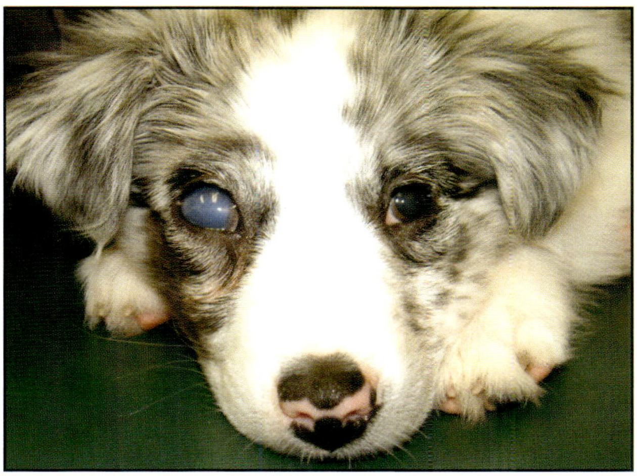

Figure 90.3 Changes as a result of vaccine-associated uveitis. Buphthalmos has developed as a result of secondary glaucoma.

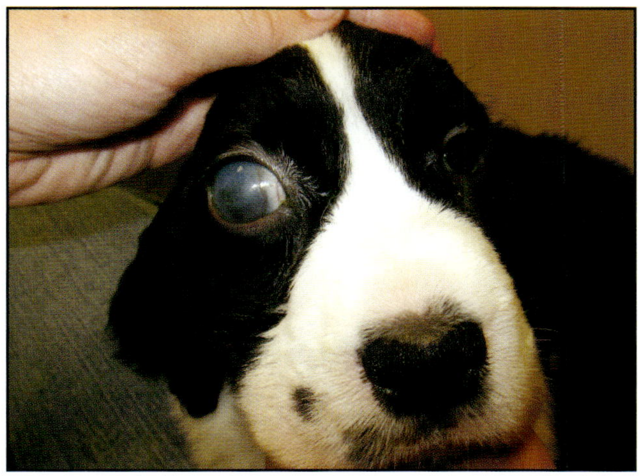

Figure 90.4 Changes as a result of vaccine-associated uveitis. Buphthalmos has developed as a result of secondary glaucoma.

CHAPTER 91
UVEODERMATOLOGIC SYNDROME (UDS)-ASSOCIATED UVEITIS

PRESENTATION

Canine uveodermatologic syndrome (UDS) represents an immune-mediated disease affecting melanocytic tissue, which likely has a hereditary etiology and which exhibits many similarities to Vogt-Koyanagi-Harada (VKH) disease in humans. Ocular symptoms associated with UDS may include inflammation marked by any combination of anterior uveitis, chorioretinitis, or panuveitis. Secondary changes may include any combination of cataract formation, retinal detachment, hyphema and/or glaucoma. Typically, both eyes are affected to a variable degree. Additional symptoms may include any combination of periocular, mucocutaneous oral and/or nasal vitiligo (loss of pigment), poliosis (whitening of hair), and/or ulcerative dermatitis. Typically, these symptoms are relatively bilaterally symmetrical in appearance (see also Autoimmune Blepharitis and Uveodermatologic Syndrome (UDS)-Associated Chorioretinitis). Commonly affected breeds include the Akita, Siberian Husky, Samoyed, Chow Chow, German Shepherd, and Shetland Sheepdog.

DIAGNOSIS AND TREATMENT

The diagnosis of UDS is made on the basis of a combination of signalment and clinical findings. Where representative adnexal or dermal changes are present, the harvesting of a small incisional skin biopsy for histopathological interpretation may support the diagnosis. Treatment usually comprises aggressive, long-term anti-inflammatory, and/or immune-modulating therapy. Typically, this involves the topical administration of corticosteroids and the systemic administration of corticosteroids with or without the adjunctive use of additional agents including cyclosporine and/or azathioprine.

Potential Drug-Side-Effects

Potential adverse effects associated with the use of topical corticosteroids include impaired wound healing and corneal degeneration. Potential adverse effects associated with the use of systemic corticosteroids include polyphagia, polydipsia, polyuria, hair coat changes, weight gain, pancreatitis, enteritis, muscular damage, hepatic impairment, and diabetes. Potential adverse effects associated with the use of azathioprine include gastrointestinal (GI) distress, pancreatitis, hepatotoxicity, and myelosuppression. Potential adverse affects associated with the use of cyclosporine include hypersensitivity and GI distress.

SELECTED REFERENCES

Angles JM, Famula TR, Pedersen NC. Uveodermatologic (VKH-like) syndrome in American Akita dogs is associated with an increased frequency of DQA1*00201. *Tissue Antigens* 2005;**66**(6):656–665.

Carter WJ, Crispin SM, Gould DJ, Day MJ. An immunohistochemical study of uveodermatologic syndrome in two Japanese Akita dogs. *Vet Ophthalmol* 2005;**8**(1):17–24.

Horikawa T, Vaughan RK, Sargent SJ, Toops EE, Locke EP. Pathology in practice. Uveodermatologic syndrome. *J Am Vet Med Assoc* 2013;**242**(6):759–761. DOI: 10.2460/javma.242.6.759.

Clinical Atlas of Canine and Feline Ophthalmic Disease, First Edition. Douglas Esson.

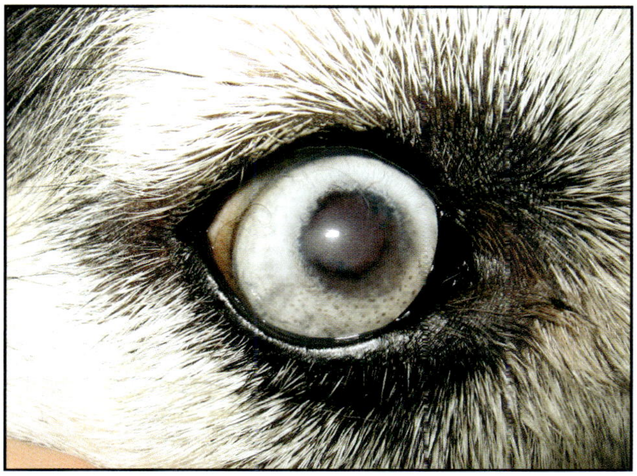

Figure 91.1 Changes associated with uveodermatologic syndrome–associated uveitis. Endothelial keratic precipitates are notable.

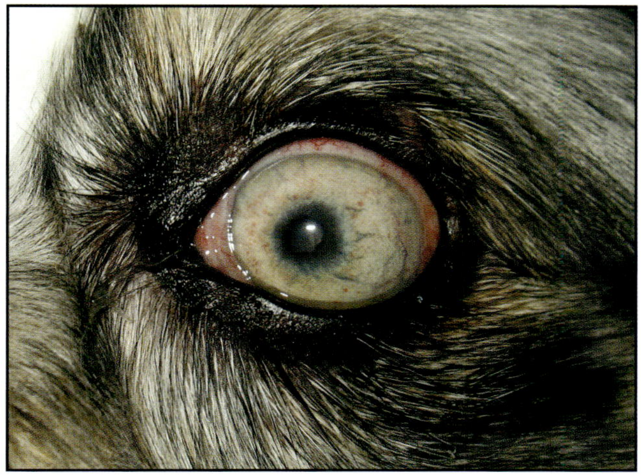

Figure 91.2 Changes associated with uveodermatologic syndrome–associated uveitis. Iritis is notable.

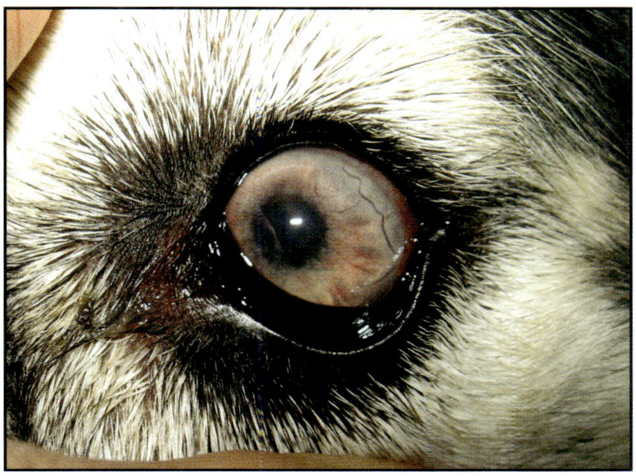

Figure 91.3 Changes associated with uveodermatologic syndrome–associated uveitis. Iritis is notable.

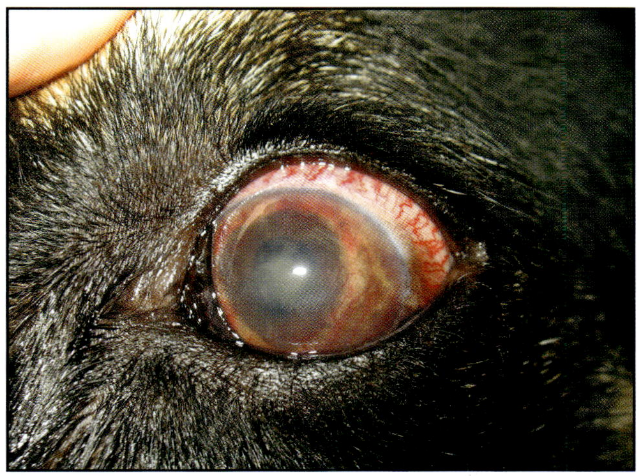

Figure 91.4 Changes associated with uveodermatologic syndrome–associated uveitis. Iritis and hyphema are notable.

CHAPTER 92
HYPHEMA

PRESENTATION

Hyphema describes the presence of free blood within the anterior chamber (AC). Clinically, the appearance of affected eyes may include varying degrees of tan to red discoloration of the AC (or in the case of longstanding hemorrhage, purple to black discoloration—sometimes referred to as "8-ball" hemorrhage). Hyphema presents a significant diagnostic challenge, potential causes including;

- Congenital anomalies (including collie eye anomaly, retinal dysplasia, merle ocular dysgenesis and persistent hyaloid vasculature)
- Trauma
- Coagulopathies (including hereditary, immune-mediated, and toxic)
- Vasculopathies
- Severe uveitis
- Systemic disease (including infectious disease and/or hypertension)
- Neoplasia (particularly lymphoma)
- Retinal detachment

DIAGNOSIS AND TREATMENT

The diagnosis of hyphema is made based on clinical findings. Potentially life-threatening injuries/disease should be addressed and the patient stabilized prior to further ophthalmic investigation/treatment. B-mode ultrasonography permits assessment of intraocular structures and scleral integrity in the presence of severe hyphema. Routine CBC, chemistry infectious-titer testing, coagulation times, and blood-pressure measurement are generally indicated when pursuing the diagnostic algorithm for hyphema. Radiography will rule out the presence of penetrating metallic foreign bodies such as air gun pellets and/or the presence of orbital fractures. Bilateral hyphema should raise suspicion of systemic disease/toxicity and/or neoplasia. Medical treatment largely comprises topical and/or systemic anti-inflammatory therapy (typically steroidal, unless contra indicated) as well as addressing underlying pathology. The administration of mydriatic agents when treating severe hyphema is controversial, shorter-acting agents such as tropicamide, potentially being safer than longer acting agents like atropine. The intracameral injection of a fibrinolytic agent (tissue plasminogen activator) may be indicated in some cases, generally being administered within 72 h of fibrin organization. Although, mild to moderate hyphema typically responds well to medical therapy, secondary glaucoma remains a persistent danger in cases of significant hyphema. Even if vision cannot be salvaged, the appropriate management of hemorrhage will minimize the risk of secondary glaucoma and globe loss (see also Secondary (Post-inflammatory) Glaucoma).

SELECTED REFERENCES

Bayón A, Tovar MC, Fernández del Palacio MJ, Agut A. Ocular complications of persistent hyperplastic primary vitreous in three dogs. *Vet Ophthalmol* 2001;**4**(1):35–40.

Mandell DC. Ophthalmic emergencies. *Clin Tech Small Anim Pract* 2000;**15**(2):94–100.

Nelms SR, Nasisse MP, Davidson MG, Kirschner SE. Hyphema associated with retinal disease in dogs: 17 cases (1986–1991). *J Am Vet Med Assoc* 1993;**202**(8):1289–1292.

Clinical Atlas of Canine and Feline Ophthalmic Disease, First Edition. Douglas Esson.

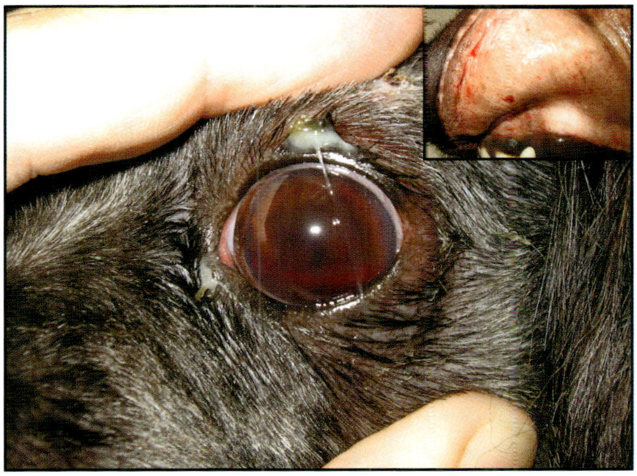

Figure 92.1 Hyphema as a result of warfarin-toxicity. Inset demonstrates multiple mucous membrane-associated petechial hemorrhages.

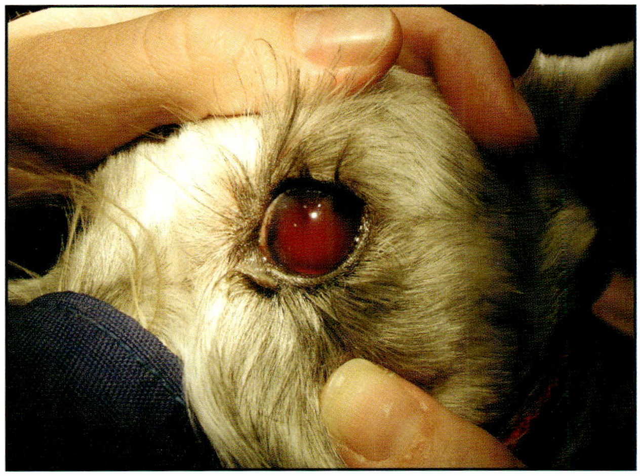

Figure 92.2 Hyphema as a result of retinal detachment secondary to chronic lens-induced uveitis in a diabetic patient.

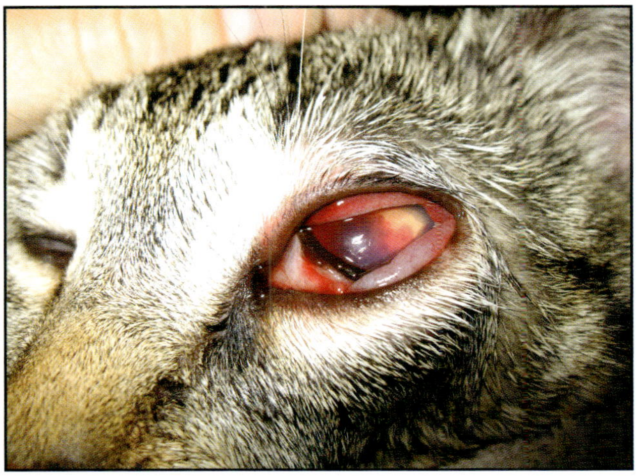

Figure 92.3 Hyphema due to a penetrating foreign body (air gun pellet).

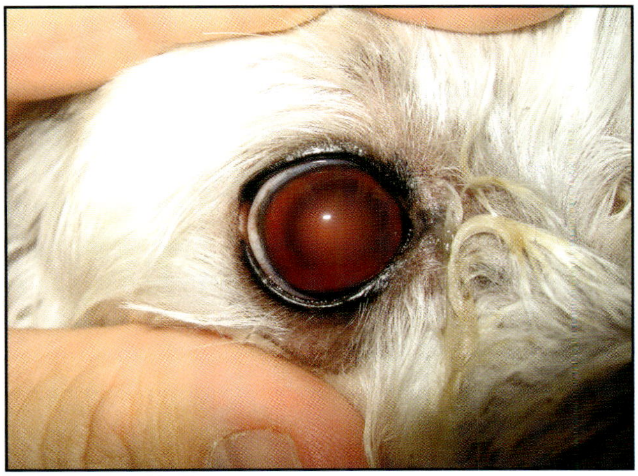

Figure 92.4 Hyphema in association with systemic hypertension.

CHAPTER 93
AQUEOUS LIPIDOSIS

PRESENTATION

Aqueous lipidosis describes a condition in which elevated levels of lipoproteins move across an incompetent and/or overloaded blood-ocular-barrier (BAB) into the anterior chamber. Changes may occur spontaneously as a result of primary hyperlipoproteinemia, following significant dietary indiscretion, in association with underlying metabolic disease and/or as a result of anterior uveitis. The condition may be either unilateral or bilateral and typically develops acutely. Commonly affected breeds include the Beagle, Miniature Schnauzer, and Shetland Sheepdog.

DIAGNOSIS AND TREATMENT

The diagnosis of aqueous lipidosis is made on the basis of clinical findings, with affected anterior chambers appearing cloudy/white. Focal, illuminated examination may reveal the presence of "rivulets" of clear aqueous within the anterior chamber. In some cases, lipid accumulation within the corneal tissue and/or lipemia of the retinal vasculature may also be noted. Complete blood count (CBC)/chemistry analysis is typically supportive of the clinical diagnosis, frequently reflecting elevated serum cholesterol and/or triglyceride levels. More specific "lipid panels" as well as further evaluation of hepatic, renal, pancreatic, and/or thyroid function may provide additional diagnostic information. Addressing underlying metabolic and/or dietary imbalances as well as concurrent uveitis, if present, typically results in rapid resolution of symptoms. In selected cases, treatment using fibrates (such as gemfibrozil) and/or statins (such as atorvastatin) may be indicated; however, the use of these products in canine patients has not been approved. Treatment typically encompasses the topical administration of (steroidal or nonsteroidal) anti-inflammatory agents as well as the judicious use of a short-term mydriatic agent such as tropicamide in order to stabilize the blood–aqueous barrier (BAB) and minimize the risk of secondary glaucoma.

Potential Drug-Side-Effects

Potential adverse effects associated with the use of topical corticosteroids include impaired wound healing and corneal degeneration.

SELECTED REFERENCES

Bauer JE. Lipoprotein-mediated transport of dietary and synthesized lipids and lipid abnormalities of dogs and cats. *J Am Vet Med Assoc* 2004;**224**(5):668–675.

Crispin S. Ocular lipid deposition and hyperlipoproteinaemia. *Prog Retin Eye Res* 2002;**21**(2):169–224.

Mori N, Lee P, Muranaka S, Sagara F, Takemitsu H, Nishiyama Y, Yamamoto I, Yagishita M, Arai T. Predisposition for primary hyperlipidemia in Miniature Schnauzers and Shetland sheepdogs as compared to other canine breeds. *Res Vet Sci* 2010;**88**(3):394–399. DOI: 10.1016/j.rvsc.2009.12.003. Epub 2010 Jan 12.

Xenoulis PG, Steiner JM. Lipid metabolism and hyperlipidemia in dogs. *Vet J* 2010;**183**(1):12–21. DOI: 10.1016/j.tvjl.2008.10.011. Epub 2009 Jan 23.

Clinical Atlas of Canine and Feline Ophthalmic Disease, First Edition. Douglas Esson.

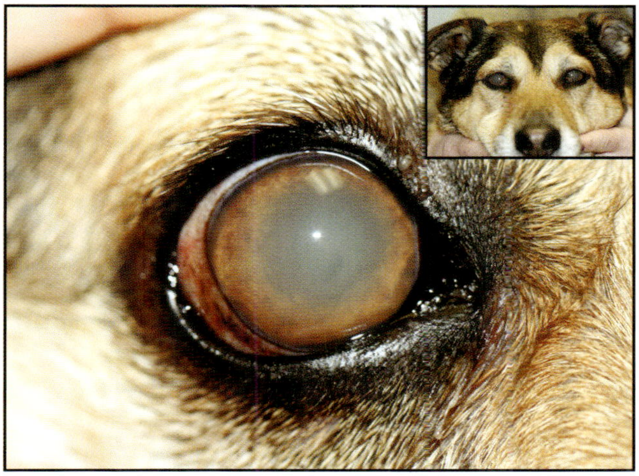

Figure 93.1 Typical clinical presentation associated with aqueous lipidosis. Inset demonstrates the frequently bilateral nature of the condition.

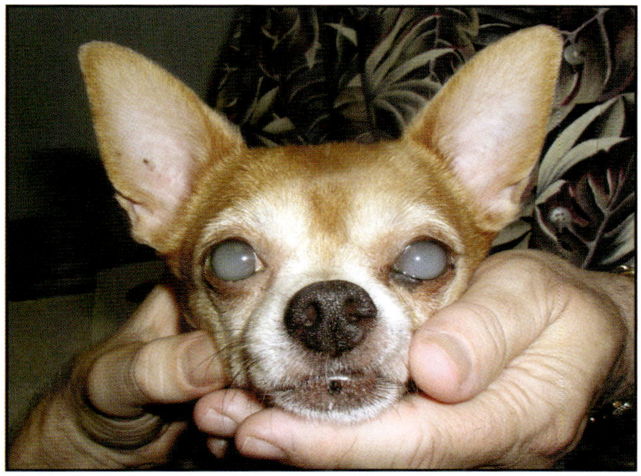

Figure 93.2 Typical clinical presentation associated with aqueous lipidosis.

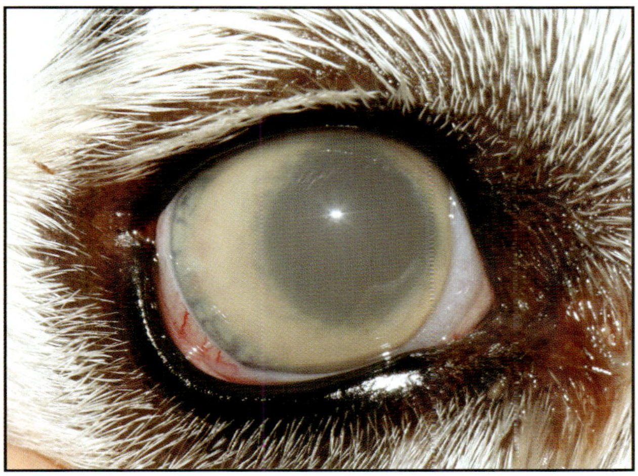

Figure 93.3 Typical clinical presentation associated with aqueous lipidosis.

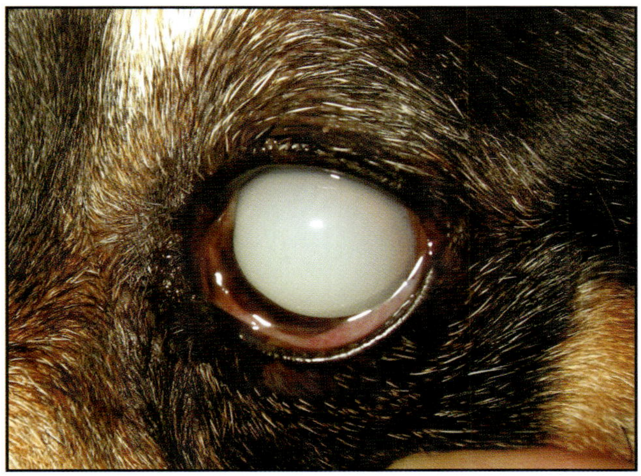

Figure 93.4 Typical clinical presentation associated with aqueous lipidosis.

CHAPTER 94
IRIS BOMBE'

PRESENTATION

Iris bombe' is not a specific disease entity, rather a manifestation of post-inflammatory changes. Presentation comprises 360 synechiation around the pupillary opening, between the posterior iris and anterior lens capsule. As a result of impaired aqueous flow, iridal tissue "balloons" forward. Associated findings may include varying degrees of uveitis, hypopyon, fibrin, hyphema, pigment deposition, cataract formation, and/or glaucoma. Both canine and feline species of any breed or crossed breed may be affected by iris bombe'.

DIAGNOSIS AND TREATMENT

The diagnosis of iris bombe' is made on the basis of clinical findings. Active uveitis should be managed if present (see also Feline Anterior Uveitis and Canine Anterior Uveitis), Similarly, elevated intraocular pressure (IOP) should be managed if present (see feline and canine secondary glaucoma). Surgical resection of iridal adhesions, laser iridotomy, and/or lenticular removal may be attempted in selected cases; however, the likelihood of recurrent iridal adhesion and/or secondary postoperative glaucoma is high. The presence of iris bombe' reflects chronic preexisting intraocular inflammation and, as a consequence, the prognosis for affected eyes is considered guarded.

SELECTED REFERENCES

Deehr AJ, Dubielzig RR. A histopathological study of iridociliary cysts and glaucoma in Golden Retrievers. *Vet Ophthalmol* 1998;**1**(2–3):153–158.

Sigle KJ, McLellan GJ, Haynes JS, Myers RK, Betts DM. Unilateral uveitis in a dog with uveodermatologic syndrome. *J Am Vet Med Assoc* 2006;**228**(4):543–548.

Strubbe T. Uveitis and pupillary block glaucoma in an aphakic dog. *Vet Ophthalmol* 2002;**5**(1):3–7.

Clinical Atlas of Canine and Feline Ophthalmic Disease, First Edition. Douglas Esson.

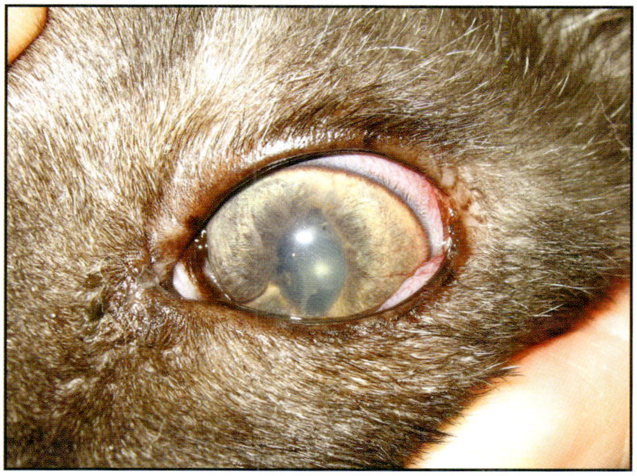

Figure 94.1 Typical clinical presentation associated with iris bombe'.

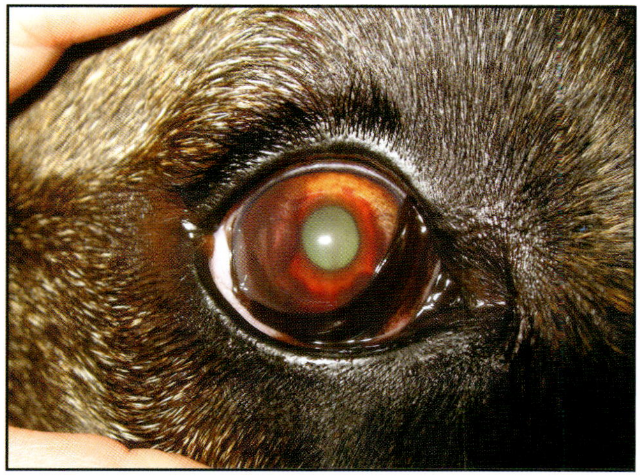

Figure 94.2 Typical clinical presentation associated with iris bombe'.

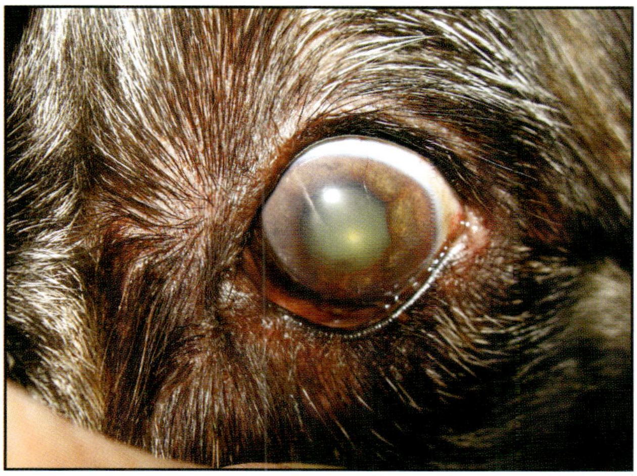

Figure 94.3 Typical clinical presentation associated with iris bombe'.

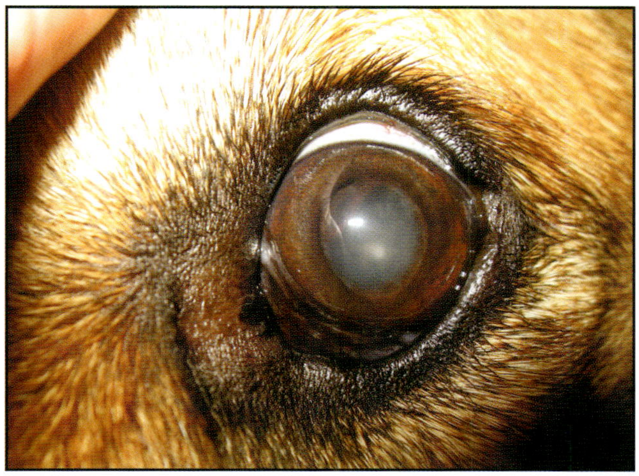

Figure 94.4 Typical clinical presentation associated with iris bombe'.

CHAPTER 95
FELINE IRIS MELANOSIS (FIM)

PRESENTATION

Clinically, feline iris melanosis (FIM) presents as one or more tan to brown, focal to coalescing iris nevi (areas of iridal pigmentation). Generally, the extent and density of these lesions increases slowly over time (typically over months to years). One or both eyes may be affected. Associated clinical uveitis is not usually present. Histologically, this process comprises the accumulation of pigmented melanocytes within the anterior iridal tissue. With time, some cases display deeper iris invasion and may additionally develop histologic characteristics of malignancy, representing true feline (diffuse) iris melanoma (FDIM), harboring the potential for metastatic spread of neoplastic cells to other regions of the body. In addition, melanomas may result in progressive effacement of normal iridal tissue and/or invasion into iridocorneal drainage structures and or adjacent uveal tissues and may result in severe secondary pathology, most commonly glaucoma.

DIAGNOSIS AND TREATMENT

The management of FIM (and its differentiation from iris melanoma) represents a challenge to the practitioner. Options include

- benign neglect/clinical monitoring only (particularly relevant in cases displaying only minimally progressive focal nevi which are not elevated above the level of the iris)
- transcorneal diode laser photoablation of affected tissues (particularly relevant in cases showing relatively rapid progression or beginning to invade ICA structures)
- enucleation (particularly relevant in cases displaying changes suggestive of outright uveal neoplastic progression and/or secondary glaucoma). Clinical changes suggestive of neoplastic proliferation may include the development of a "velvety" appearance to focal lesions and/or obvious elevation of lesions above the iridal surface and resultant pupillary dyscoria.

In cases where neoplastic progression is suspected, the evaluation of systemic health and/or involvement via local lymph node aspiration, three-view radiography, and complete blood count (CBC)/chemistry analysis, is encouraged before enucleation.

SELECTED REFERENCES

Grahn BH, Peiffer RL, Cullen CL, Haines DM. Classification of feline intraocular neoplasms based on morphology, histochemical staining, and immunohistochemical labeling. *Vet Ophthalmol* 2006;**9**(6):395–403.

Kalishman JB, Chappell R, Flood LA, Dubielzig RR. A matched observational study of survival in cats with enucleation due to diffuse iris melanoma. *Vet Ophthalmol* 1998;**1**(1):25–29.

Planellas M, Pastor J, Torres MD, Peña T, Leiva M. Unusual presentation of a metastatic uveal melanoma in a cat. *Vet Ophthalmol* 2010;**13**(6):391–4. DOI: 10.1111/j.1463-5224.2010.00839.x.

Clinical Atlas of Canine and Feline Ophthalmic Disease, First Edition. Douglas Esson.

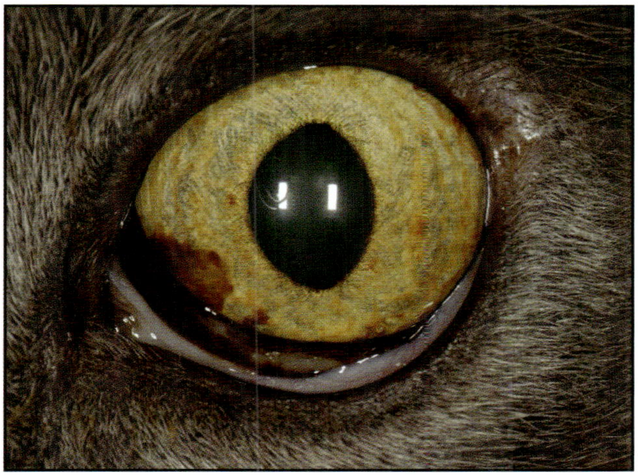

Figure 95.1 Focal iris melanosis ("iris nevus").

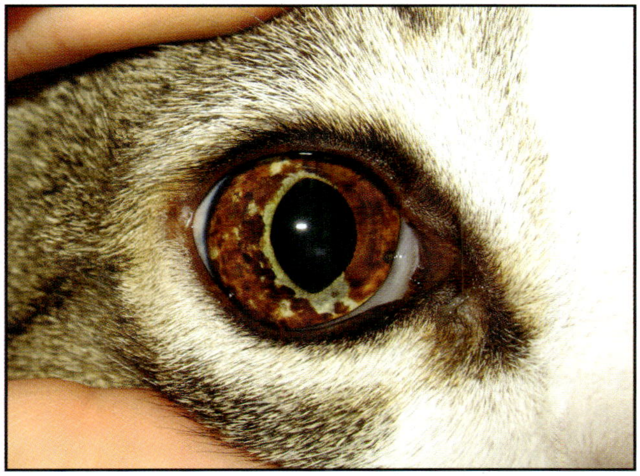

Figure 95.2 Diffuse iris melanosis.

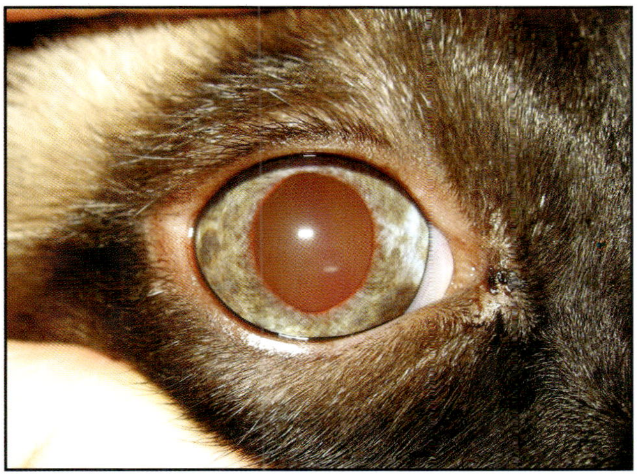

Figure 95.3 Diffuse iris melanosis displaying a 'velvety" appearance.

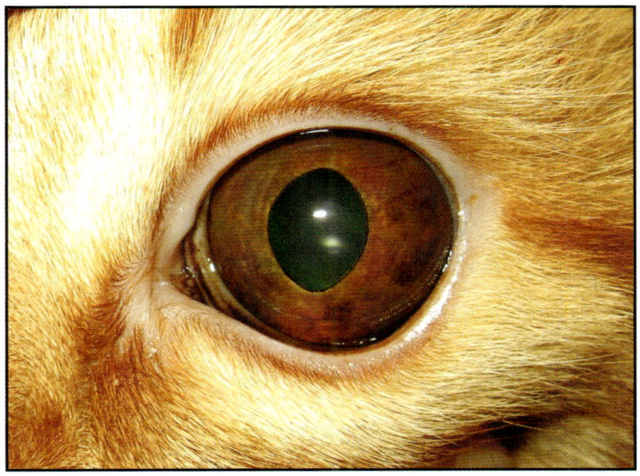

Figure 95.4 Diffuse iris melanosis displaying iridal thickening.

CHAPTER 96
UVEAL MELANOMA

PRESENTATION

Melanocytic neoplasia of the uveal tract encompasses a spectrum extending from relatively benign melanocytoma to malignant melanoma (see also Feline Iris Melanosis (FIM)). Melanocytomas typically affect the anterior uveal tissues and only rarely extend beyond the globe or metastasize to other tissues. Malignant melanomas occur less frequently and may be more likely to metastasize or extend beyond the tissues of the globe. Less commonly, these tumors may arise from choroidal tissue. Clinically, uveal melanocytic tumors present as focal or multifocal areas of progressive iridal thickening and increased pigmentation. Rarely, amelanotic melanocytomas/melanomas may appear tan to pink in color. Secondary changes may include pupillary dyscoria, hyphema, retinal detachment, keratitis, and/or secondary glaucoma. Both feline and canine eyes may be affected by melanocytoma/melanoma. Commonly affected canine breeds include the Labrador Retriever and Golden Retriever.

DIAGNOSIS AND TREATMENT

A tentative diagnosis of uveal melanoma may be made on the basis of clinical findings. Soft tissue imaging modalities including ultrasonography, computed tomography (CT) and/or magnetic resonance imaging (MRI) may also contribute to the clinical diagnosis; however, definitive diagnosis and the assessment of biologic behavior is made on the basis of histopathological evaluation of representative tissue, often following enucleation or evisceration. Treatment options include diode laser photoablation of neoplastic tissue where indicated, surgical resection of neoplastic tissue where possible, or enucleation of the globe. The evaluation of systemic health and/or potential metastasis via complete blood count (CBC)/chemistry analysis, local lymph node aspiration, and/or three-view radiography is recommended before surgical intervention. The potential value of vaccine-mediated immunotherapy in the treatment of uveal melanomas has not been fully evaluated.

SELECTED REFERENCES

Galán A, Martín-Suárez EM, Molleda JM, Raya A, Gómez-Laguna J, Martín De Las Mulas J. Presumed primary uveal melanoma with brain extension in a dog. *J Small Anim Pract* 2009;**50**(6):306–310.

Grahn BH, Sandmeyer LS, Bauer B. Diagnostic ophthalmology. Extrascleral extension of an uveal melanoma. *Can Vet J* 2008;**49**(7):723–724.

Yi NY, Park SA, Park SW, Jeong MB, Kang MS, Jung JH, Choi MC, Kim DY, Nam TC, Seo KM. Malignant ocular melanoma in a dog. *J Vet Sci* 2006;**7**(1):89–90.

Clinical Atlas of Canine and Feline Ophthalmic Disease, First Edition. Douglas Esson.

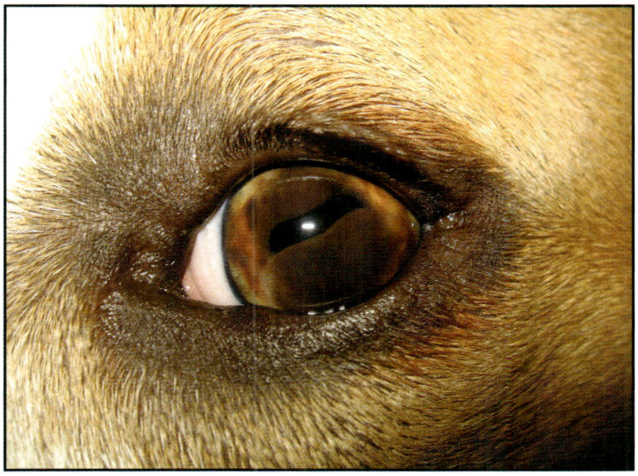

Figure 96.1 Typical clinical presentation associated with uveal melanocytoma/melanoma.

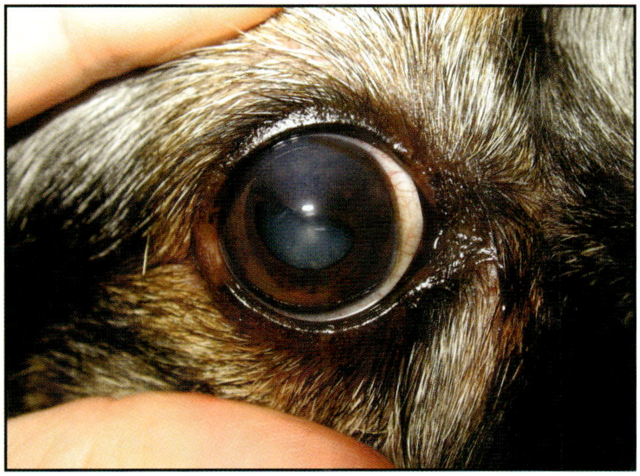

Figure 96.2 Typical clinical presentation associated with uveal melanocytoma/melanoma.

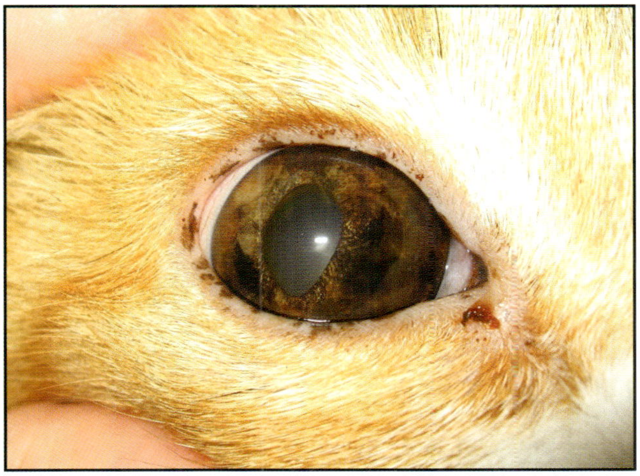

Figure 96.3 Typical clinical presentation associated with uveal melanocytoma/melanoma.

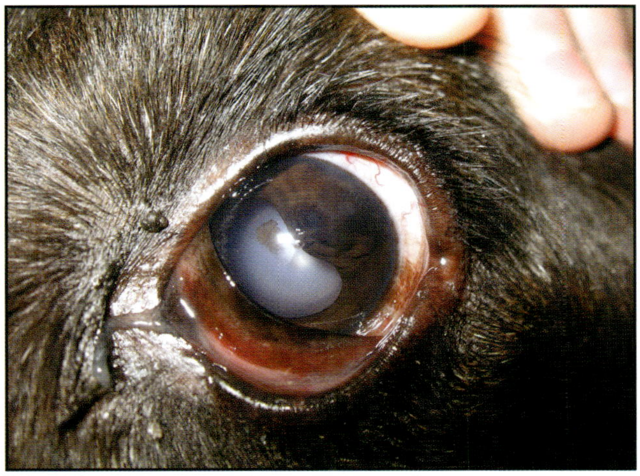

Figure 96.4 Typical clinical presentation associated with uveal melanocytoma/melanoma.

CHAPTER 97
UVEAL ADENOMA/ADENOCARCINOMA

PRESENTATION

Although not as common as uveal melanoma, iridal epithelial tumors are relatively common intraocular neoplasms. These tumors arise from the ciliary epithelium and typically present as slowly enlarging well-defined pink to tan colored masses, which may be noted to arise or to emerge behind the pupil and/or deform the iridal tissue. Secondary intraocular complications may include uveitis, retinal detachment, hyphema, and/or glaucoma. The behavior of these tumors encompasses the spectrum from relatively benign adenomas (which although unlikely to metastasize, typically result in globe loss through secondary complications) to adenocarcinomas, which behave in a more malignant manner and may be more likely to metastasize to distant tissues. Both dogs and cats may be affected. Commonly affected canine breeds include the Labrador Retriever and Golden Retriever.

DIAGNOSIS AND TREATMENT

A tentative diagnosis may be made on the basis of clinical findings. Definitive diagnosis and the assessment of biologic behavior, however, is made on the basis of histopathological evaluation of representative tissue, typically either following enucleation or evisceration. Treatment options include diode laser photoablation of neoplastic tissue where indicated, surgical resection of neoplastic tissue where possible or enucleation of the globe. The evaluation of systemic health and/or involvement via local lymph node aspiration, three-view radiography, and complete blood count (CBC)/chemistry analysis is encouraged before surgical intervention.

SELECTED REFERENCES

Dubielzig RR, Steinberg H, Garvin H, Deehr AJ, Fischer B. Iridociliary epithelial tumors in 100 dogs and 17 cats: a morphological study. *Vet Ophthalmol* 1998;**1**(4):223–231.

Duke FD, Strong TD, Bentley E, Dubielzig RR. Canine ocular tumors following ciliary body ablation with intravitreal gentamicin. *Vet Ophthalmol.* 2013;**16**(2):159–162. DOI: 10.1111/j.1463-5224.2012.01050.x. Epub 2012 Jul 19.

Zarfoss MK, Dubielzig RR. Metastatic iridociliary adenocarcinoma in a labrador retriever. *Vet Pathol* 2007;**44**(5):672–676.

Clinical Atlas of Canine and Feline Ophthalmic Disease, First Edition. Douglas Esson.

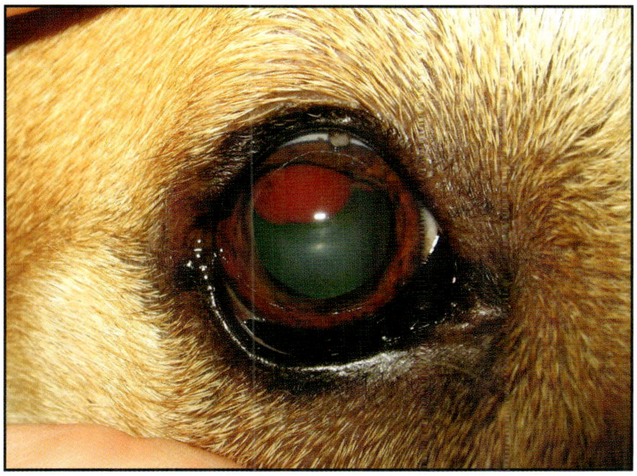

Figure 97.1 Typical clinical presentation associated with uveal adenoma/adenocarcinoma.

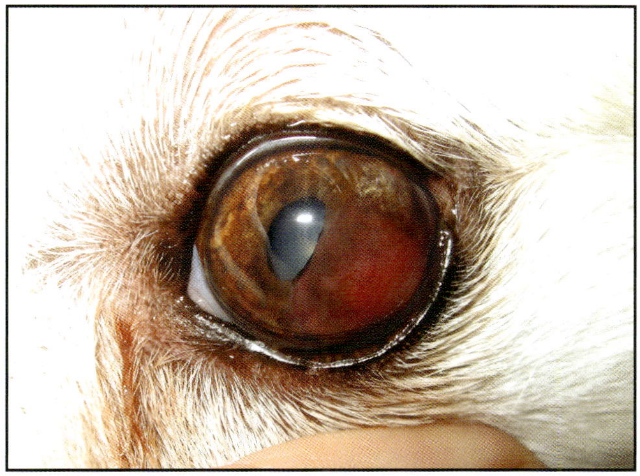

Figure 97.2 Typical clinical presentation associated with uveal adenoma/adenocarcinoma.

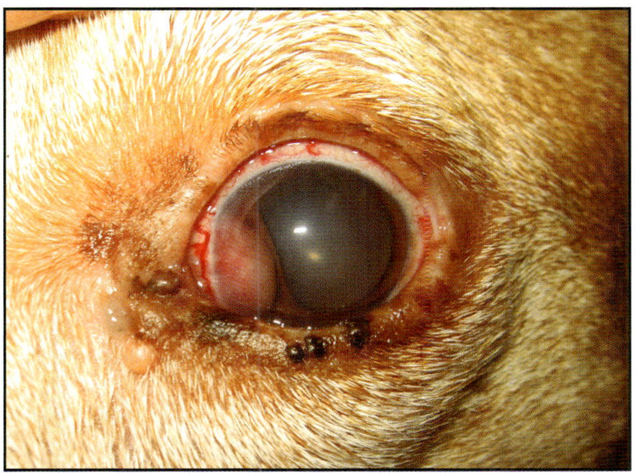

Figure 97.3 Typical clinical presentation associated with uveal adenoma/adenocarcinoma.

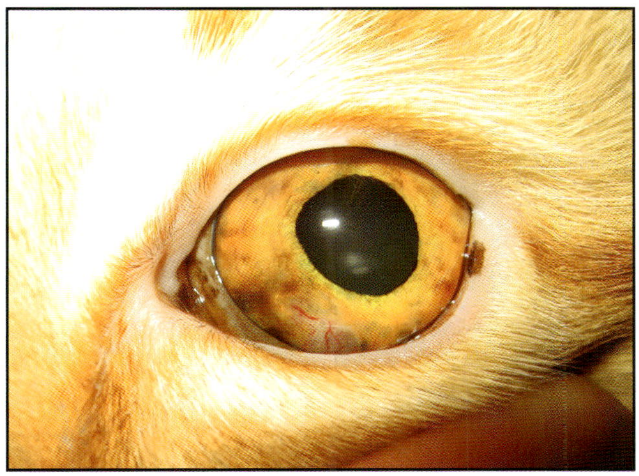

Figure 97.4 Typical clinical presentation associated with uveal adenoma/adenocarcinoma.

CHAPTER 98
UVEAL LYMPHOMA

PRESENTATION

Uveal lymphoma is a relatively common presentation, frequently occurring in combination with systemic disease, although ocular changes may precede systemic symptoms. One, or more commonly both, eye(s) may be affected and associated ocular findings may include any combination of corneal edema, anterior uveitis, chorioretinitis or panuveitis, hypopyon, hyphema, diffuse or nodular iridal thickening, retinal hemorrhage and/or detachment and/or glaucoma (see also Feline Chorioretinitis, Canine Chorioretinitis, Choroidal Lymphoma, and Retrobulbar Neoplasia). Systemic symptoms may include any combination of weight loss, lethargy, inappetence, gastrointestinal (GI) distress, pyrexia, lymphadenopathy, organomegaly, hypercalcemia, and/or anemia. Both feline and canine species of any breed or crossed breed may be affected.

DIAGNOSIS AND TREATMENT

The diagnosis of lymphoma may be made on the basis of clinical findings, ancillary imaging, cytological/histological interpretation, polymerase chain reaction (PCR) analysis of samples obtained by aqueocentesis as well as lymph node and/or affected organ aspiration/biopsy. Treatment comprises topical anti-inflammatory therapy (typically utilizing a corticosteroid) as well as systemic chemotherapy. Associated ophthalmic changes such as elevated intraocular pressure should be addressed as appropriate. Staging via local lymph node (and/or organ/bone marrow) aspiration, three-view radiography, and complete blood count (CBC)/chemistry analysis should be undertaken before initiation of systemic chemotherapy. Diagnostic testing for the presence of infectious viruses including FelV, FIV, and FIP is additionally recommended in feline patients. Individual chemotherapeutic protocols are most ideally designed by a veterinary oncologist; however, they typically include a variable combination of prednisone, vincristine, cyclophosphamide, and/or doxorubicin.

Potential Drug-Side-Effects

Potential adverse effects associated with the use of systemic corticosteroid sinclude polyphagia, polydipsia, polyuria, hair coat changes, weight gain, pancreatitis, GI distress, muscle damage, hepatic impairment, and diabetes. Potential adverse effects associated with the use of vincristine include stomatitis, GI distress, neuropathy, hepatopathy, and myelosuppression. Potential adverse effects associated with the use of cyclophosphamide include GI distress, pancreatitis, hepatotoxicity, and myelosuppression. Potential adverse affects associated with the use of doxorubicin include hypersensitivity, GI distress, cardiac dysfunction, and myelosuppression.

The prognosis varies depending on the extent of disease present before initiation of therapy.

SELECTED REFERENCES

Massa KL, Gilger BC, Miller TL, Davidson MG. Causes of uveitis in dogs: 102 cases (1989–2000). *Vet Ophthalmol* 2002;**5**(2):93–98.

Nerschbach V, Eule JC, Eberle N, Höinghaus R, Betz D. Ocular manifestation of lymphoma in newly diagnosed cats. *Vet Comp Oncol* 2013. DOI: 10.1111/vco.12061.

Ota-Kuroki J, Ragsdale JM, Bawa B, Wakamatsu N, Kuroki K. Intraocular and periocular lymphoma in dogs and cats: a retrospective review of 21 cases (2001–2012). *Vet Ophthalmol* 2013. DOI: 10.1111/vop.12106.

Rutley M, MacDonald V. Managing the canine lymphosarcoma patient in general practice. *Can Vet J* 2007;**48**(9):977–979.

Clinical Atlas of Canine and Feline Ophthalmic Disease, First Edition. Douglas Esson.

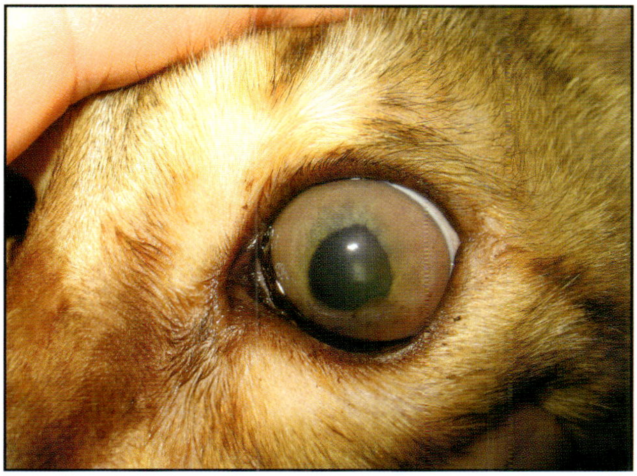

Figure 98.1 Typical clinical presentation associated with uveal lymphoma. Diffuse iridal thickening is present.

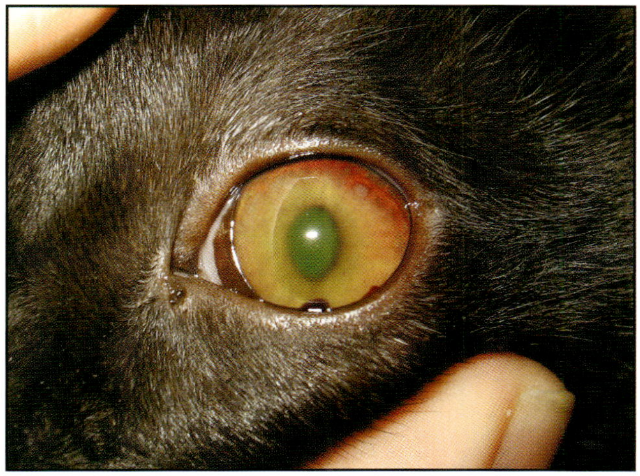

Figure 98.2 Typical clinical presentation associated with uveal lymphoma. Nodular iridal thickening is present.

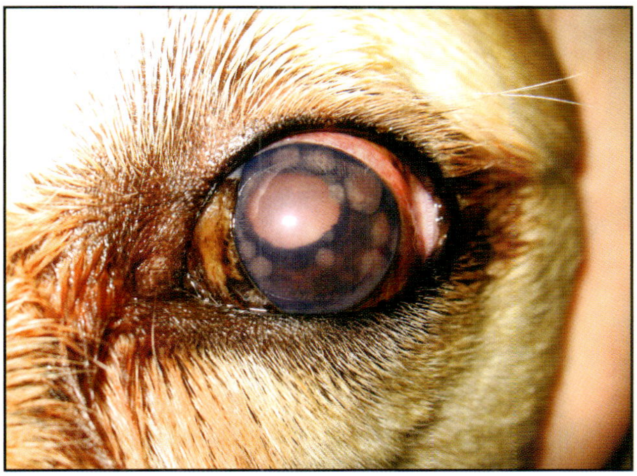

Figure 98.3 Typical clinical presentation associated with uveal lymphoma. Nodular iridal thickening is present.

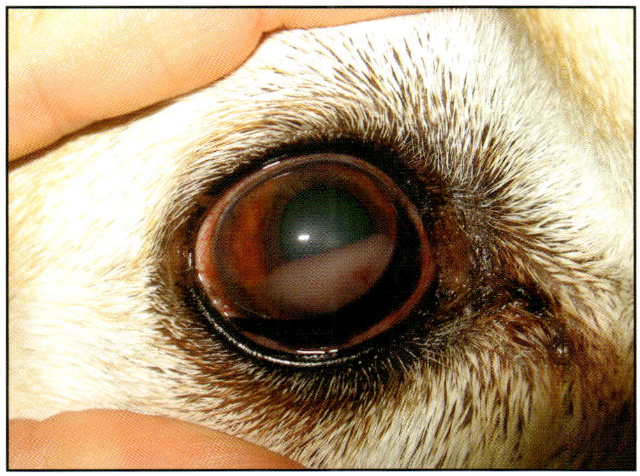

Figure 98.4 Typical clinical presentation associated with uveal lymphoma. Diffuse iridal thickening and hypopyon are present.

Section 6

Diseases of the Lens

CHAPTER 99
MICROPHAKIA/SPHEROPHAKIA

PRESENTATION

Congenital microphakia describes an abnormally small lens. This condition results from aberrant embryonic differentiation and frequently occurs in combination with spherophakia (a spherically shaped lens). Other potential abnormalities include lentiglobus (a globoid-shaped lens), lenticonus (a cone-shaped lens), lenticular subluxation, and/or cataracts. Affected animals may additionally develop glaucoma. Commonly affected canine breeds include the Beagle, Doberman Pinscher, and Miniature Schnauzer. Commonly affected feline breeds include the Burmese.

TREATMENT

The diagnosis of microphakia (and/or spherophakia) is made on the basis of clinical findings, supported if necessary by B-mode ultrasonography. Treatment may include benign neglect, medical management using a long-term miotic agent in order to minimize the risk of complete lenticular luxation, and/or surgical lens removal/replacement. Appropriate long-term miotic agents include demecarium bromide and the prostaglandin analogues (such as latanoprost).

Potential Drug-Side-Effects

Potential complications associated with the use of demecarium bromide include ocular discomfort and gastrointestinal (GI) distress.

SELECTED REFERENCES

Arnbjerg J, Jensen O. Spontaneous microphthalmia in two Doberman puppies with anterior chamber cleavage syndrome. *J Am Anim Hosp Assoc* 1982;**18**:481–484.

Binder DR, Herring IP, Gerhard T. Outcomes of nonsurgical management and efficacy of demecarium bromide treatment for primary lens instability in dogs: 34 cases (1990–2004). *J Am Vet Med Assoc* 2007;**231**(1):89–93.

Curtis R. Lens luxation in the dog and cat. *Vet Clin North Am Small Anim Pract* 1990;**20**(3):755–773.

Clinical Atlas of Canine and Feline Ophthalmic Disease, First Edition. Douglas Esson.

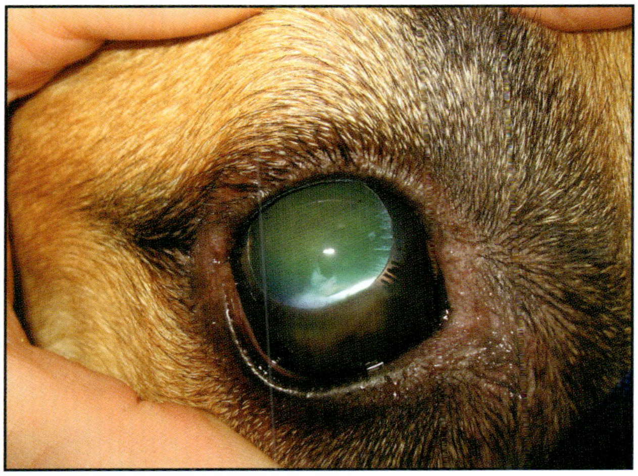

Figure 99.1 Typical presentation associated with microphakia/spherophakia. Notable are the stretched ciliary processes.

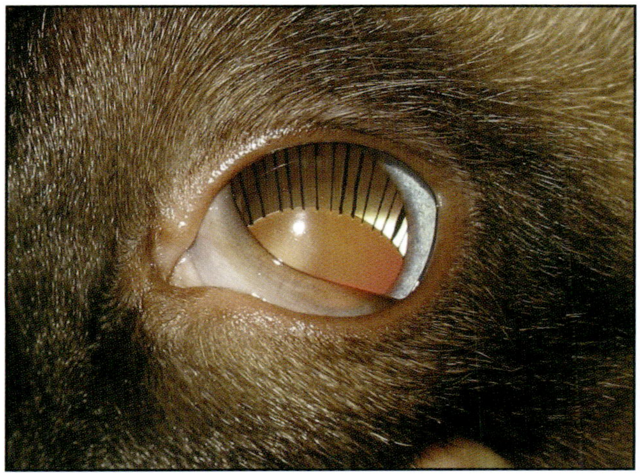

Figure 99.2 Typical presentation associated with microphakia/spherophakia. Notable are the stretched ciliary processes.

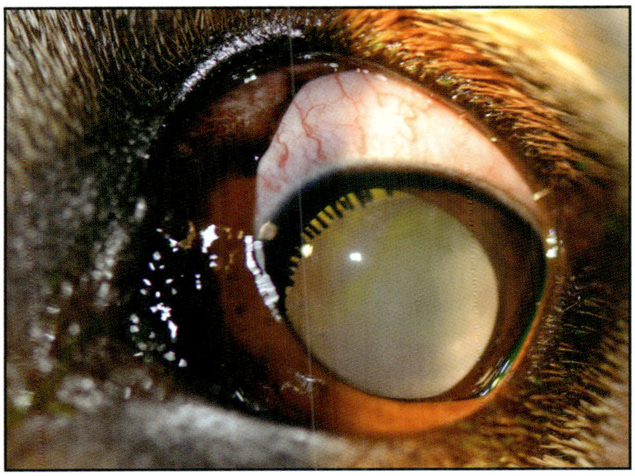

Figure 99.3 Typical presentation associated with microphakia/spherophakia. Notable are the stretched ciliary processes.

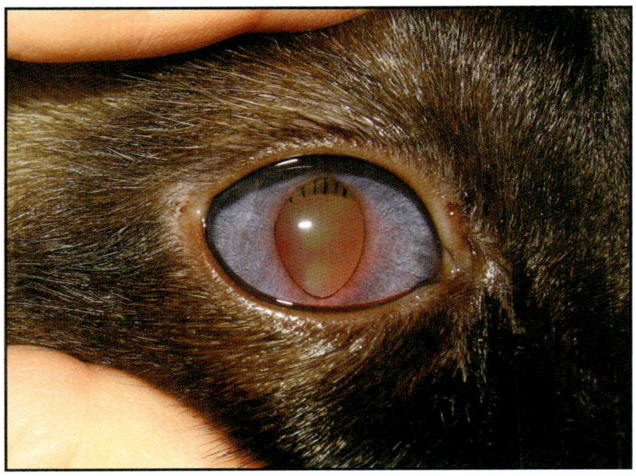

Figure 99.4 Typical presentation associated with microphakia/spherophakia. Notable are the stretched ciliary processes.

CHAPTER 100
PERSISTENT HYALOID VASCULATURE (PHV)

PRESENTATION

During embryogenesis, the vascular supply to the developing lens regresses. Failure of this process results in the presence of visible (and in some cases patent) vascular remnants, associated with the lens and/or lens capsule, typically leading to cataract formation and visual impairment. Findings associated with this condition have been described as persistent hyperplastic tunica vasculosa lentis/persistent hyperplastic primary vitreous (PHTVL/PHPV). Commonly affected breeds include the Doberman Pinscher, Greyhound, and Staffordshire Bull Terrier.

TREATMENT

The diagnosis of persistent hyaloid vasculature (PHV) is made on the basis of clinical findings (confirmed by B-mode ultrasonography where necessary). Where indicated, the lens and opacified lens capsule as well as associated vascular tissue may be surgically removed and patent vessels cauterized; however, the risk of intra- and postoperative complications associated with this procedure are significant.

SELECTED REFERENCES

Bayón A, Tovar MC, Fernández del Palacio MJ, Agut A. Ocular complications of persistent hyperplastic primary vitreous in three dogs. *Vet Ophthalmol* 2001;**4**(1):35–40.

Boevé MH, van der Linde-Sipman JS, Stades FC. Early morphogenesis of the canine lens capsule, tunica vasculosa lentis posterior, and anterior vitreous body. A transmission electron microscopic study. *Graefes Arch Clin Exp Ophthalmol* 1989;**227**(6):589–594.

Cullen CL, Grahn BH. Diagnostic ophthalmology. Persistent hyperplastic tunica vasculosa lentis and primary vitreous. *Can Vet J* 2004;**45**(5):433–434. No abstract available.

Gemensky-Metzler AJ, Wilkie DA. Surgical management and histologic and immunohistochemical features of a cataract and retrolental plaque secondary to persistent hyperplastic tunica vasculosa lentis/persistent hyperplastic primary vitreous (PHTVL/PHPV) in a Bloodhound puppy. *Vet Ophthalmol* 2004;**7**(5):369–375.

Clinical Atlas of Canine and Feline Ophthalmic Disease, First Edition. Douglas Esson.

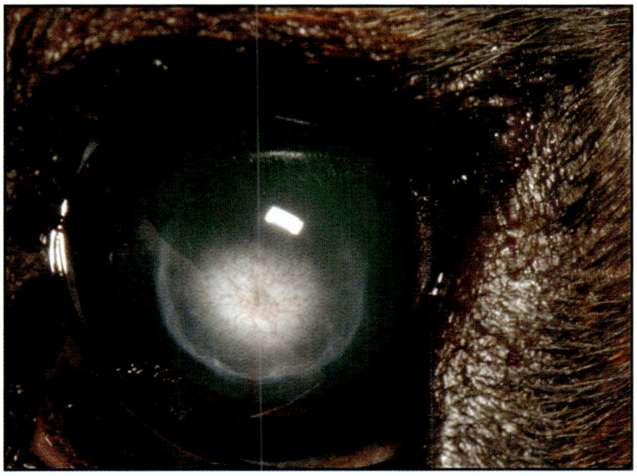

Figure 100.1 Clinical presentation associated with persistent hyaloid vasculature (PHV). Notable are fine vessels radiating across the posterior lens capsule.

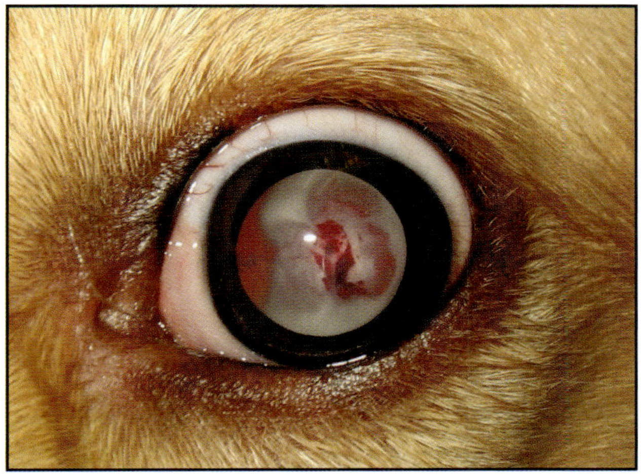

Figure 100.2 Clinical presentation associated with persistent hyaloid vasculature (PHV). Notable is free hemorrhage within the cataractous lens.

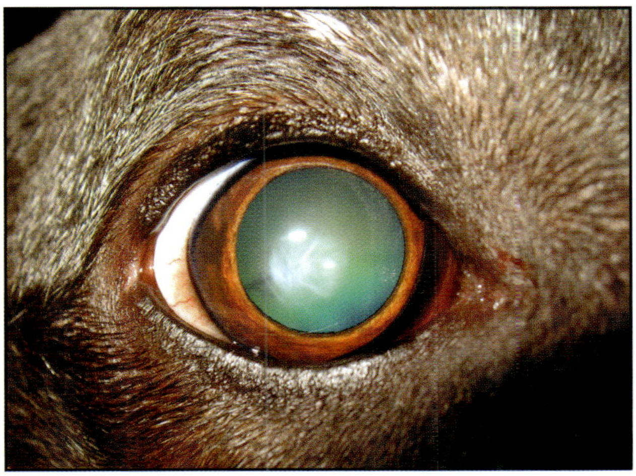

Figure 100.3 Clinical presentation associated with persistent hyaloid vasculature (PHV). Notable is the single vessel extending to the posterior lens capsule.

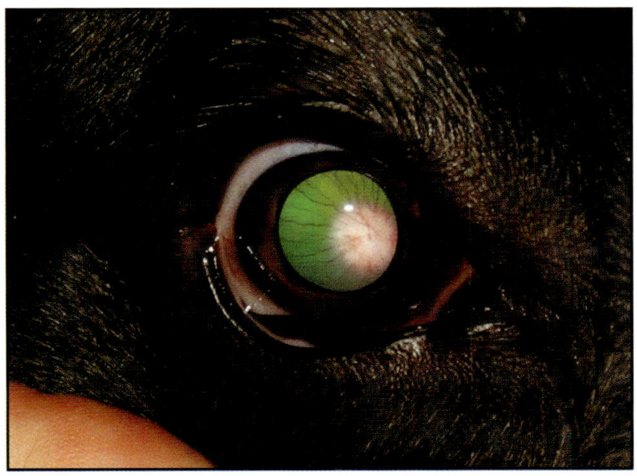

Figure 100.4 Clinical presentation associated with persistent hyaloid vasculature (PHV). Notable are fine vessels radiating across the posterior lens capsule.

CHAPTER 101
NUCLEAR SCLEROSIS

PRESENTATION

Nuclear sclerosis (or "lenticular sclerosis") describes the progressive thickening of the canine and feline lens due to ongoing (age-associated) lens-fiber deposition and resultant compression of the lenticular nucleus. Clinically, this process imparts a gray-blue appearance to the nucleus, typically becoming apparent after 7–8 years of age.

DIAGNOSIS AND TREATMENT

The diagnosis of nuclear sclerosis is made on the basis of clinical findings. The major differential is a lenticular cataract; however (unlike a cataract) nuclear sclerosis does not prevent the uninterrupted observation of a complete tapetal reflex. Although a degree of refractive error may be associated with aging changes, significant visual impairment is not generally noted clinically and neither medical nor surgical treatment of this condition is typically warranted.

SELECTED REFERENCES

Fischer CA. Geriatric ophthalmology. *Vet Clin North Am Small Anim Pract* 1989;**19**(1):103–123.

Murphy CJ, Zadnik K, Mannis MJ. Myopia and refractive error in dogs. *Invest Ophthalmol Vis Sci* 1992;**33**(8):2459–2463.

Poulos P Jr. Selenium-tocopherol treatment of senile lenticular sclerosis in dogs (four case reports). *Vet Med Small Anim Clin* 1966;**61**(10):986–988.

Clinical Atlas of Canine and Feline Ophthalmic Disease, First Edition. Douglas Esson.

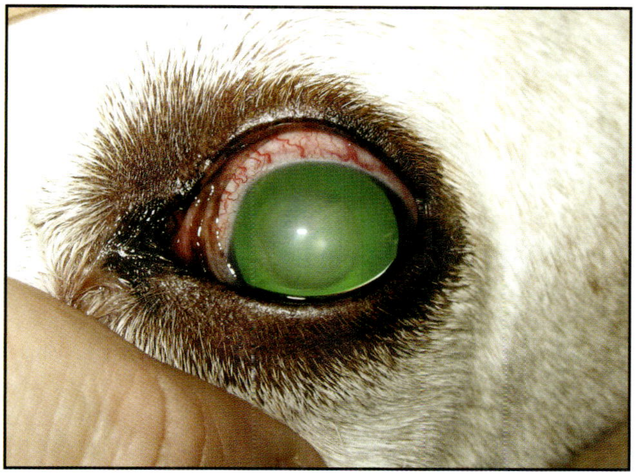

Figure 101.1 Clinical appearance of age-associated nuclear sclerosis.

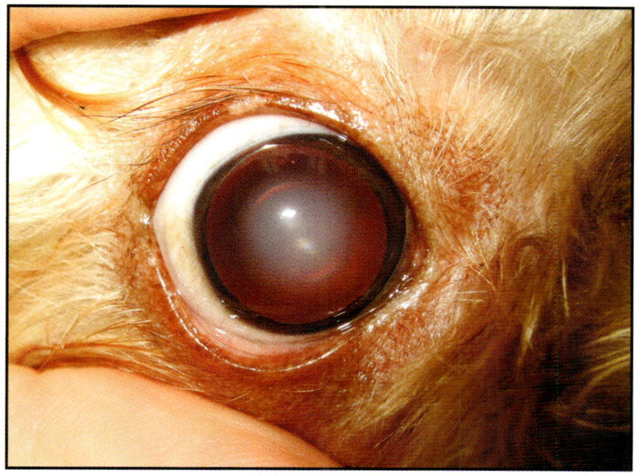

Figure 101.2 Clinical appearance of age-associated nuclear sclerosis.

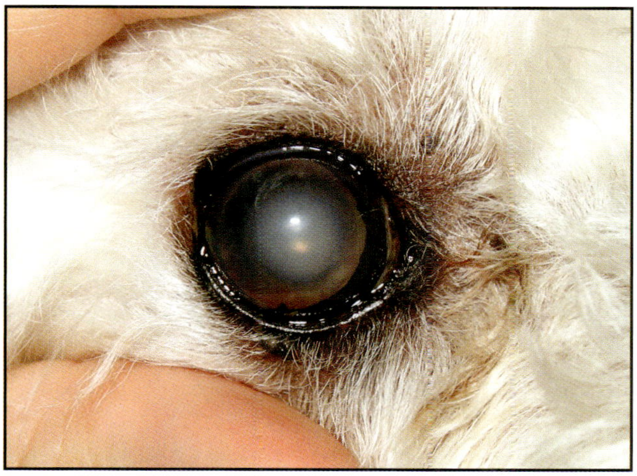

Figure 101.3 Clinical appearance of age-associated nuclear sclerosis.

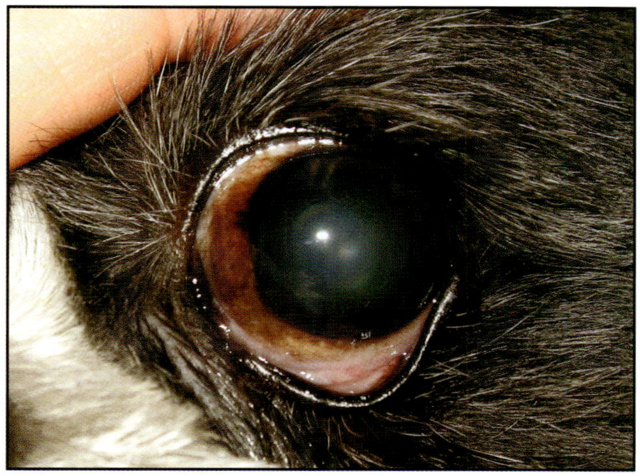

Figure 101.4 Clinical appearance of age-associated nuclear sclerosis.

CHAPTER 102
IMMATURE CATARACT

PRESENTATION

A cataract describes any opacity of the normally transparent and avascular lens. Cataractogenesis occurs most commonly as a result of hereditary factors; however, it may also result from systemic disease (notably diabetes mellitus), lenticular trauma/inflammation, dietary deficiencies (notably associated with the use of milk replacers), exposure to pharmacologic agents (notably ketoconazole), as a sequela to the retinal atrophies (RAs), and following exposure to therapeutic radiation. Changes may be unilateral or bilateral, symmetrical or asymmetrical, and may develop over varying timeframes. An "incipient" cataract describes opacification of less than 10% of the lens volume. An "immature" cataract describes a variable degree of lenticular opacification; however, the tapetal reflex remains present as does a variable degree of functional vision. Incipient/immature cataracts are not typically associated with overt uveitis. Many breeds (and mixed breeds) may be affected by hereditary cataracts, and multiple-breed-related features including age of onset and rate of progression have been described. Commonly affected breeds include the Boston Terrier, Bichon Frisé, Cocker Spaniel, Labrador Retriever, Miniature Schnauzer, Miniature Poodle, and Siberian Husky.

TREATMENT

The diagnosis is made on the basis of clinical findings. Treatment of immature cataracts is not typically necessary. Lens-associated uveitis, if present, should be treated with topical anti-inflammatory agents in order to minimize the risk of subsequent glaucoma (see also Phacolytic Uveitis). Typically, steroidal agents are avoided when treating diabetic patients. If significant visual impairment is present, cataract surgery may be indicated (pending the results of presurgical diagnostic testing including electroretinal function).

SELECTED REFERENCES

Basher AW, Roberts SM. Ocular manifestations of diabetes mellitus: diabetic cataracts in dogs. *Vet Clin North Am Small Anim Pract* 1995;**25**(3):661–676. Review.

Gelatt KN, Mackay EO. Prevalence of primary breed-related cataracts in the dog in North America. *Vet Ophthalmol* 2005;**8**(2):101–111.

Lim CC, Bakker SC, Waldner CL, Sandmeyer LS, Grahn BH. Cataracts in 44 dogs (77 eyes): a comparison of outcomes for no treatment, topical medical management, or phacoemulsification with intraocular lens implantation. *Can Vet J* 2011;**52**(3):283–288.

Clinical Atlas of Canine and Feline Ophthalmic Disease, First Edition. Douglas Esson.

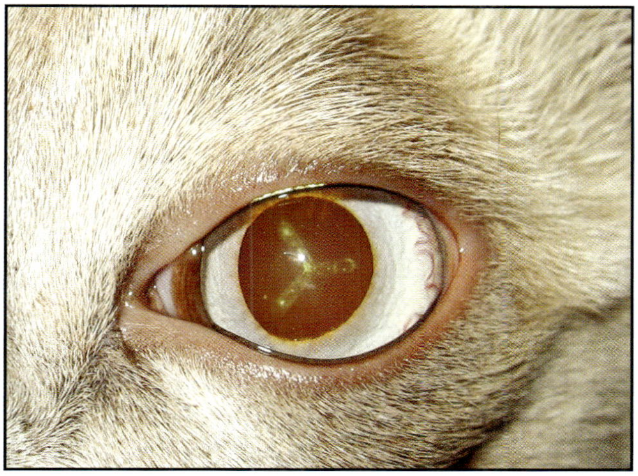

Figure 102.1 Clinical appearance of an incipient/immature cataract. The tapetal reflex remains visible.

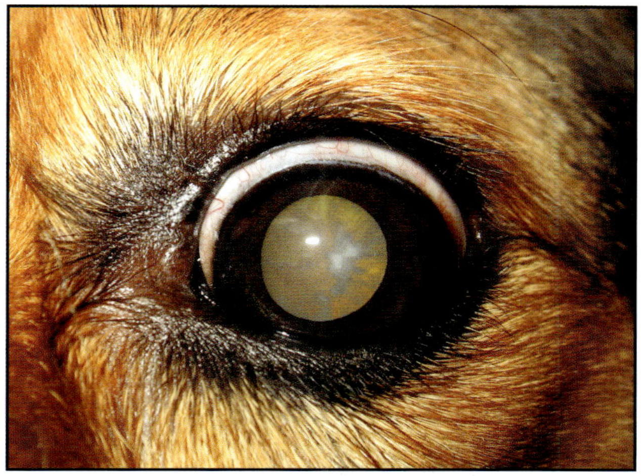

Figure 102.2 Clinical appearance of an incipient/immature cataract. The tapetal reflex remains visible.

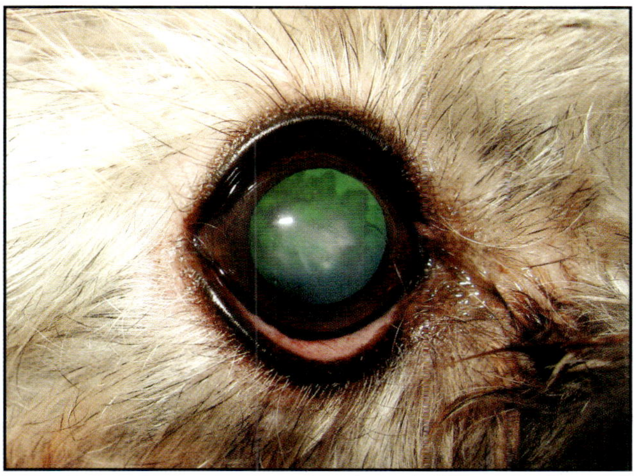

Figure 102.3 Clinical appearance of an incipient/immature cataract. The tapetal reflex remains visible.

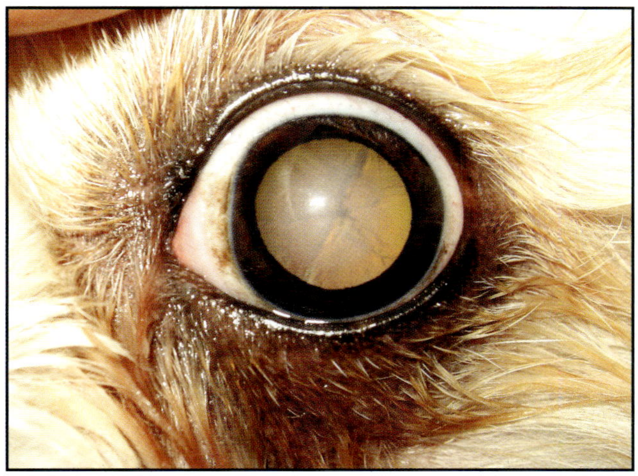

Figure 102.4 Clinical appearance of an incipient/immature cataract. The tapetal reflex remains visible.

CHAPTER 103
MATURE CATARACT

PRESENTATION

A cataract describes any opacity of the normally transparent and avascular lens. Cataractogenesis occurs most commonly as a result of hereditary factors; however, it may also result from systemic disease (notably diabetes mellitus), lenticular trauma/inflammation, dietary deficiencies (notably associated with the use of milk replacers), exposure to pharmacologic agents (notably ketoconazole), as a sequela to the retinal atrophies (RAs), and following exposure to therapeutic radiation. Changes may be unilateral or bilateral, symmetrical or asymmetrical, and may develop over varying timeframes. A "mature" cataract describes complete lenticular opacification, such that the tapetal reflex is obscured, and is associated with complete loss of functional vision. Leakage of lens proteins results in a variable degree of lens-associated inflammation (see Phacolytic Uveitis). Osmotic action may result in fluid accumulation within the lens and subsequent enlargement of overall lenticular size (described as an intumescent cataract). Rapidly forming intumescent cataracts, such as those associated with uncontrolled diabetes, may result in equatorial lens capsule rapture and severe, acute inflammation (see Phacoclastic Uveitis). Many breeds (and mixed breeds) may be affected by hereditary cataracts, and multiple breed-related features including age of onset and rate of progression are described. Commonly affected breeds include the Boston Terrier, Bichon Frisé, Cocker Spaniel, Labrador Retriever, Miniature Schnauzer, Miniature Poodle, and Siberian Husky.

TREATMENT

The diagnosis is made on the basis of clinical findings. Lens-associated uveitis, if present, should be treated with topical anti-inflammatory agents in order to minimize the risk of subsequent glaucoma (see also Phacolytic Uveitis). Typically, steroidal agents are avoided when treating diabetic patients. Chronic, uncontrolled lens-induced uveitis (LIU) may result in secondary complications including retinal detachment and/or glaucoma. Cataract surgery may be indicated (pending the results of presurgical diagnostic testing including electroretinal function).

SELECTED REFERENCES

Gelatt KN, Mackay EO. Prevalence of primary breed-related cataracts in the dog in North America. *Vet Ophthalmol* 2005;**8**(2):101–111.

Lim CC, Bakker SC, Waldner CL, Sandmeyer LS, Grahn BH. Cataracts in 44 dogs (77 eyes): a comparison of outcomes for no treatment, topical medical management, or phacoemulsification with intraocular lens implantation. *Can Vet J* 2011;**52**(3):283–288.

Wilcock BP, Peiffer RL Jr. The pathology of lens-induced uveitis in dogs. *Vet Pathol* 1987;**24**(6):549–553.

Wilkie DA, Colitz CM. Update on veterinary cataract surgery. *Curr Opin Ophthalmol* 2009;**20**(1):61–68. DOI: 10.1097/ICU.0b013e32831a98aa.

Clinical Atlas of Canine and Feline Ophthalmic Disease, First Edition. Douglas Esson.

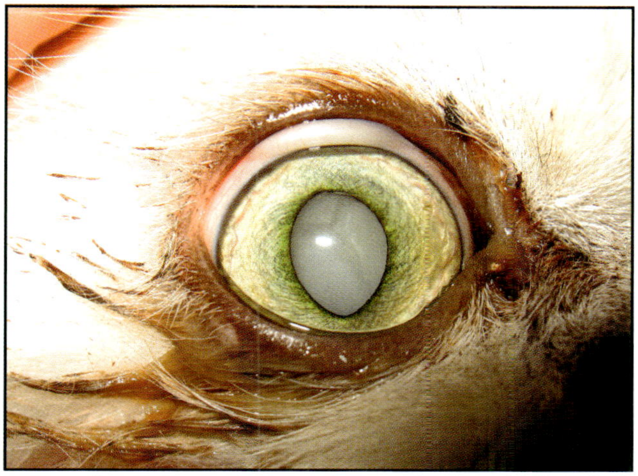

Figure 103.1 Clinical appearance of a mature cataract. The tapetal reflex is obscured.

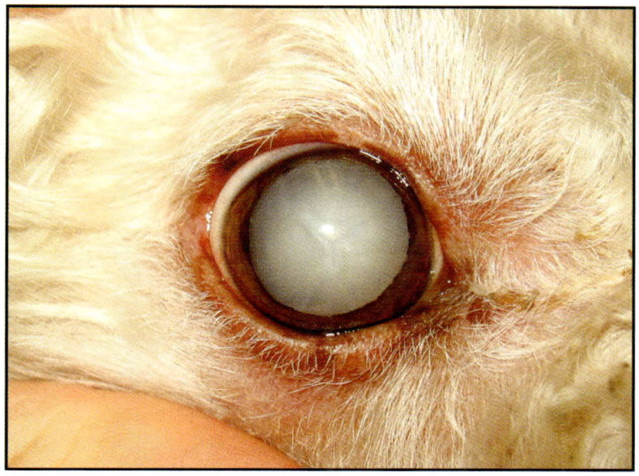

Figure 103.2 Clinical appearance of a mature cataract. The tapetal reflex is obscured.

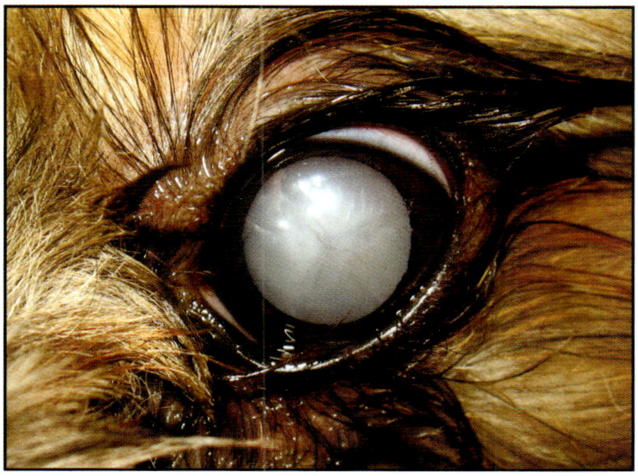

Figure 103.3 Clinical appearance of a mature cataract. The tapetal reflex is obscured.

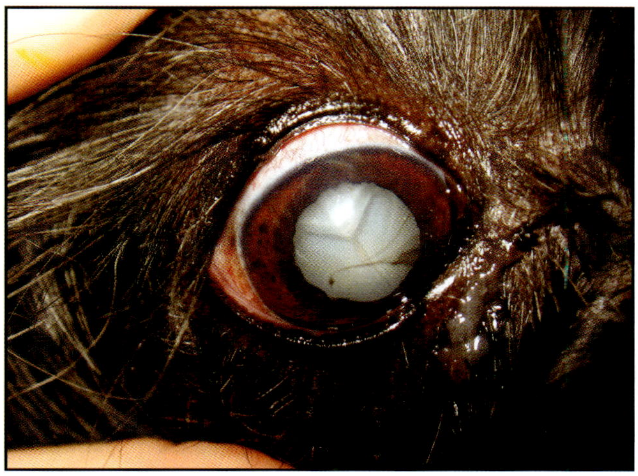

Figure 103.4 Clinical appearance of a mature cataract. The tapetal reflex is obscured. Significant "clefting" of lens material in association with intumescence is notable.

CHAPTER 104
HYPERMATURE CATARACT

PRESENTATION

A cataract describes any opacity of the normally transparent and avascular lens. Cataractogenesis occurs most commonly as a result of hereditary factors; however, it may also result from systemic disease (notably diabetes mellitus), lenticular trauma/inflammation, dietary deficiencies (notably associated with the use of milk replacers), exposure to pharmacologic agents (notably ketoconazole), as a sequela to the retinal atrophies (RAs), and following exposure to therapeutic radiation. Changes may be unilateral or bilateral, symmetrical or asymmetrical. A "hypermature" (or "Morgagnian") cataract describes a cataract in which the lens cortex has begun to liquefy and resorb. The lens nucleus may sink and the capsule shrink, fibrose, and calcify. Hypermature cataracts typically have a crystalline appearance and are frequently associated with symptoms of chronic uveitis. Variable degrees of tapetal reflectivity and/or visual impairment may be present. Many breeds (and mixed breeds) may be affected by hereditary cataracts and many breed-related features including age of onset and rate of progression are described. Commonly affected breeds include the Boston Terrier, Bichon Frisé, Cocker Spaniel, Labrador Retriever, Miniature Schnauzer, Miniature Poodle, and Siberian Husky.

TREATMENT

The diagnosis is made on the basis of clinical findings. Lens-associated uveitis should be treated with topical anti-inflammatory agents (see also Phacolytic Uveitis). Typically, steroidal agents are avoided when treating diabetic patients. Cataract surgery may be indicated (pending the results of presurgical diagnostic testing including electroretinal function). The potential for complications associated with the removal of hypermature cataracts is considered significant.

SELECTED REFERENCES

Gelatt KN, Mackay EO. Prevalence of primary breed-related cataracts in the dog in North America. *Vet Ophthalmol* 2005;**8**(2):101–111.

Gonzalez-Alonso-Alegre E, Rodriguez-Alvaro A. Spontaneous resorption of a diabetic cataract in a geriatric dog. *J Small Anim Pract* 2005;**46**(8):406–408.

Lim CC, Bakker SC, Waldner CL, Sandmeyer LS, Grahn BH. Cataracts in 44 dogs (77 eyes): A comparison of outcomes for no treatment, topical medical management, or phacoemulsification with intraocular lens implantation. *Can Vet J* 2011;**52**(3):283–288.

Wilcock BP, Peiffer RL Jr. The pathology of lens-induced uveitis in dogs. *Vet Pathol* 1987;**24**(6):549–553.

Clinical Atlas of Canine and Feline Ophthalmic Disease, First Edition. Douglas Esson.

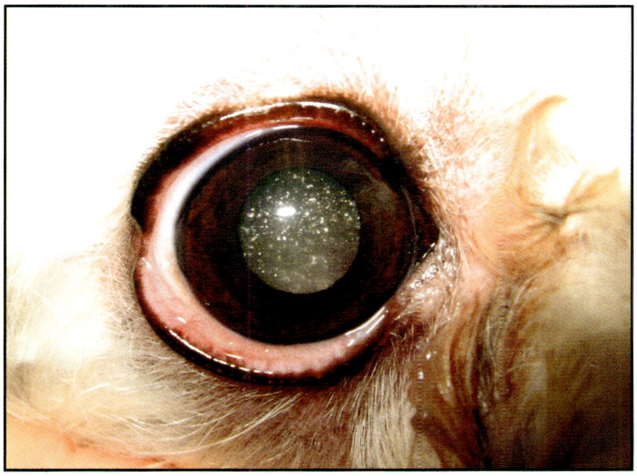

Figure 104.1 Clinical appearance of a hypermature cataract. Crystalline lens material is visible.

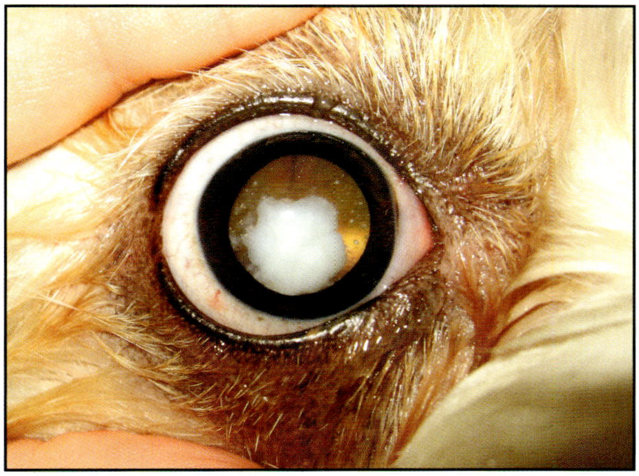

Figure 104.2 Clinical appearance of a hypermature cataract. The nucleus is visible within liquefied cortical lens material.

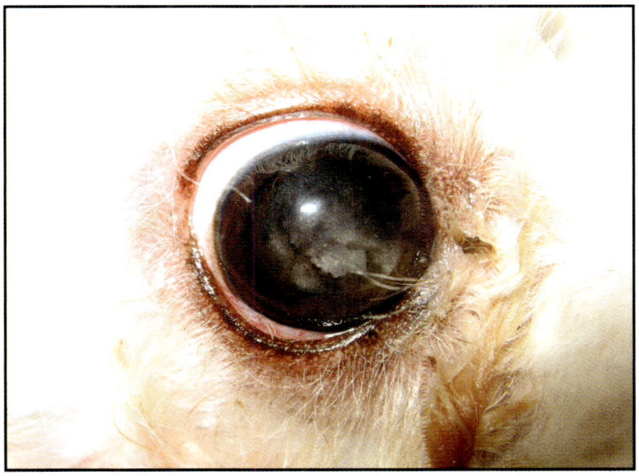

Figure 104.3 Clinical appearance of a hypermature cataract. Notable are multiple areas of iridal adhesion secondary to lens-associated inflammation.

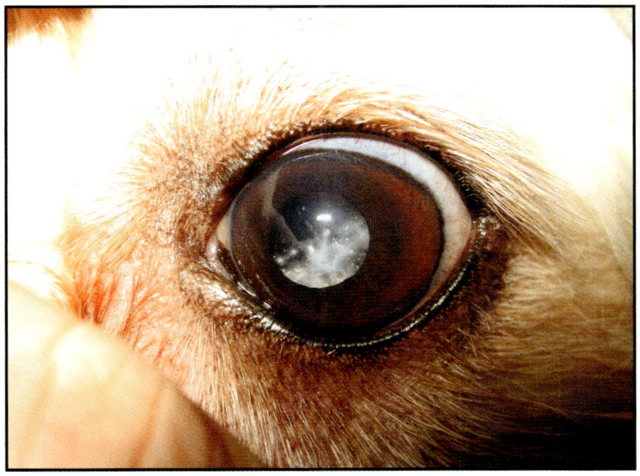

Figure 104.4 Clinical appearance of a hypermature cataract. Notable is the shrunken lens capsule.

CHAPTER 105
PHACOLYTIC UVEITIS

PRESENTATION

Phacolytic (or "lens-induced") uveitis describes inflammation of the uveal tract as a result of the leakage of lens-associated proteins across an intact lens capsule (notably in the case of rapidly forming cataracts such as those associated with diabetes mellitus). Clinically, phacolytic uveitis may manifest as any combination of conjunctival/episcleral hyperemia, corneal edema, endothelial keratic precipitates, aqueous flare, iritis, iridal adhesions, pupillary miosis, uveal cyst formation, ectropion uvea, and/or decreased intraocular pressure (IOP). Any breed or crossbreed may be affected

TREATMENT

The diagnosis of phacolytic uveitis is made on the basis of clinical findings, in conjunction with the presence of a cataract. Treatment of phacolytic uveitis should be undertaken in order to minimize the risk of secondary complications associated with chronic intraocular inflammation (notably retinal detachment and/or glaucoma). Treatment typically encompasses topical (and where necessary systemic) (steroidal or nonsteroidal) anti-inflammatory therapy. Where possible, the long-term use of steroidal agents is avoided in the management of diabetic patients.

Potential Drug-Side-Effects

Potential adverse effects associated with the use of topical corticosteroids include impaired wound healing and corneal degeneration. Potential adverse effects associated with the use of systemic cortiocosteroids include polyphagia, polydipsia, polyuria, hair coat changes, weight gain, pancreatitis, gastrointestinal (GI) distress, muscle damage, hepatic impairment, and diabetes.

SELECTED REFERENCES

Massa KL, Gilger BC, Miller TL, Davidson MG. Causes of uveitis in dogs: 102 cases (1989–2000). *Vet Ophthalmol* 2002;**5**(2):93–98.

van der Woerdt A, Nasisse MP, Davidson MG. Lens-induced uveitis in dogs: 151 cases (1985–1990). *J Am Vet Med Assoc* 1992; **201**(6):921–926.

Wilcock BP, Peiffer RL Jr. The pathology of lens-induced uveitis in dogs. *Vet Pathol* 1987;**24**(6):549–553.

Clinical Atlas of Canine and Feline Ophthalmic Disease, First Edition. Douglas Esson.

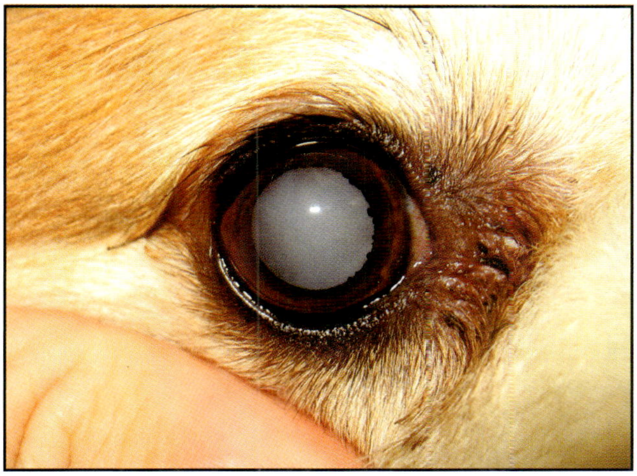

Figure 105.1 Clinical changes associated with phacolytic uveitis. "Ectropion uvea" is visible as a "crenelated" pupillary opening.

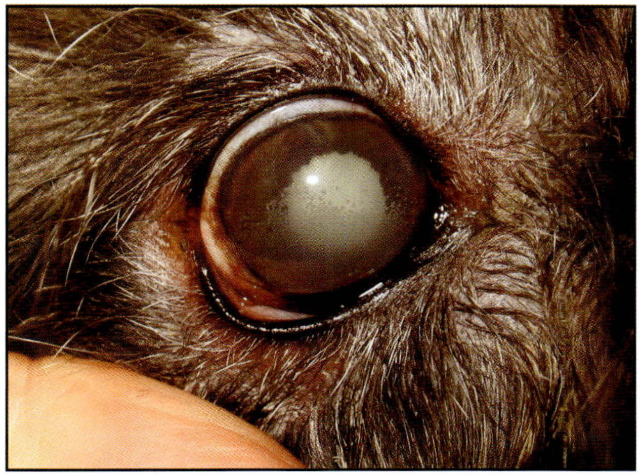

Figure 105.2 Clinical changes associated with phacolytic uveitis. Endothelial keratic precipitates are present.

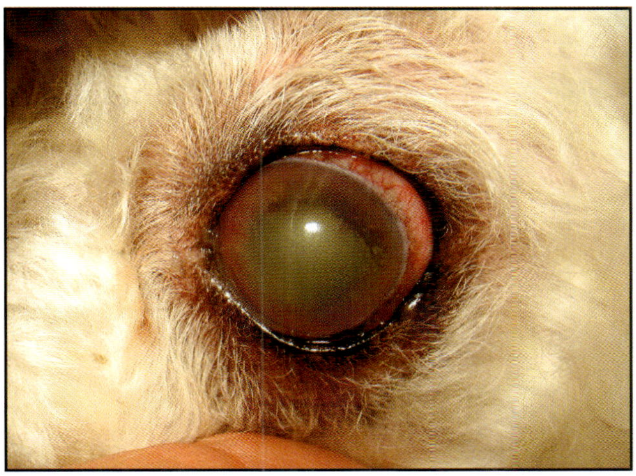

Figure 105.3 Clinical changes associated with phacolytic uveitis. Endothelial keratic precipitates are present.

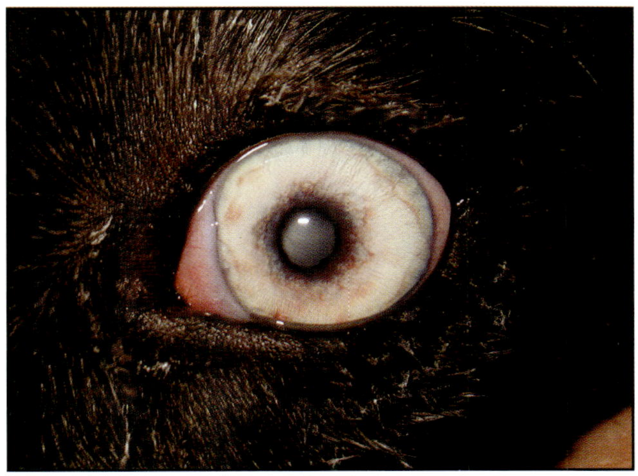

Figure 105.4 Clinical changes associated with phacolytic uveitis. "Ectropion uvea" and iritis are present.

CHAPTER 106
PHACOCLASTIC UVEITIS

PRESENTATION

Phacoclastic uveitis describes severe, acute intraocular inflammation as a result of the sudden exposure to lens-associated proteins following lens capsule laceration or rupture. Rapidly forming "intumescent" cataracts are particularly predisposed to equatorial lens-capsule rupture. Clinically, phacoclastic uveitis may manifest as any combination of conjunctival/episcelral hyperemia, corneal edema, endothelial keratic precipitates, aqueous flare, hypopyon, hyphema, iritis, iridal adhesions, pupillary miosis, dyscoria, ectropion uvea, and decreased or elevated intraocular pressure (IOP). Any breed or crossed breed may be affected.

TREATMENT

The diagnosis of phacoclastic uveitis is made on the basis of history, clinical findings, and the presence of severe intraocular inflammation. Evaluation of lens capsular integrity may be challenging as a result of difficulties associated with examining a painful patient, corneal opacity (notably as a result of corneal edema), intracameral hemorrhage/hypopyon/fibrin and/or pupillary miosis. B-mode ultrasonography may contribute to the diagnosis. Treatment typically encompasses aggressive topical and systemic (typically steroidal) anti-inflammatory therapy. Lens removal by phacoemulsification is frequently necessary in order to control severe uveitis. A unique response to lenticular trauma in the feline species is the potential for subsequent sarcoma development (also see Feline Post Traumatic Sarcoma).

Potential Drug Side-Effects

Potential adverse effects associated with the use of topical corticosteroids include impaired wound healing and corneal degeneration. Potential adverse effects associated with the use of systemic cortiocosteroids include polyphagia, polydipsia, polyuria, hair coat changes, weight gain, pancreatitis, gastrointestinal (GI) distress, muscle damage, hepatic impairment, and diabetes.

SELECTED REFERENCES

Bell CM, Pot SA, Dubielzig RR. Septic implantation syndrome in dogs and cats: a distinct pattern of endophthalmitis with lenticular abscess. *Vet Ophthalmol* 2013;**16**(3):180–185. DOI: 10.1111/j.1463-5224.2012.01046.x. Epub 2012 Jul 19.

Paulsen ME, Kass PH. Traumatic corneal laceration with associated lens capsule disruption: a retrospective study of 77 clinical cases from 1999 to 2009. *Vet Ophthalmol* 2012;**15**(6):355–368. DOI: 10.1111/j.1463-5224.2011.00990.x. Epub 2012 Feb 20.

Wilkie DA, Gemensky-Metzler AJ, Colitz CM, Bras ID, Kuonen VJ, Norris KN, Basham CR. Canine cataracts, diabetes mellitus and spontaneous lens capsule rupture: a retrospective study of 18 dogs. *Vet Ophthalmol* 2006;**9**(5):328–334.

Clinical Atlas of Canine and Feline Ophthalmic Disease, First Edition. Douglas Esson.

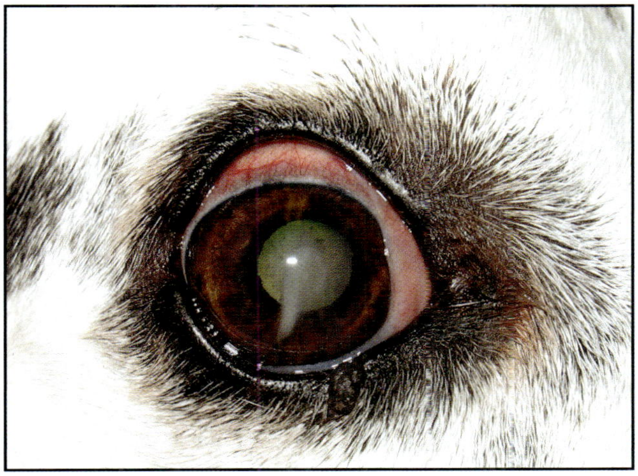

Figure 106.1 Clinical changes associated with phacoclastic uveitis secondary to lens-capsule rupture.

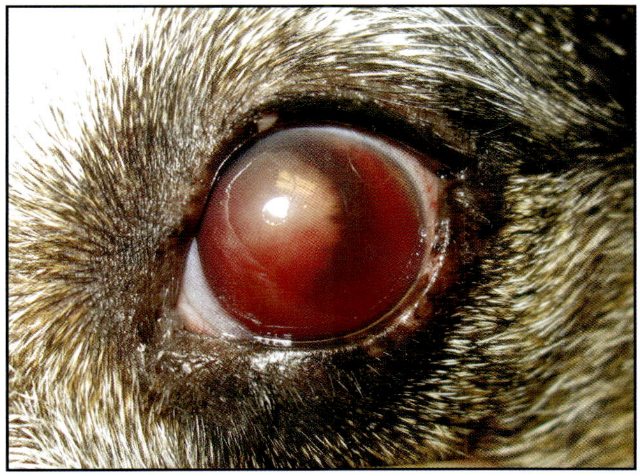

Figure 106.2 Clinical changes associated with phacoclastic uveitis secondary to lens-capsule rupture.

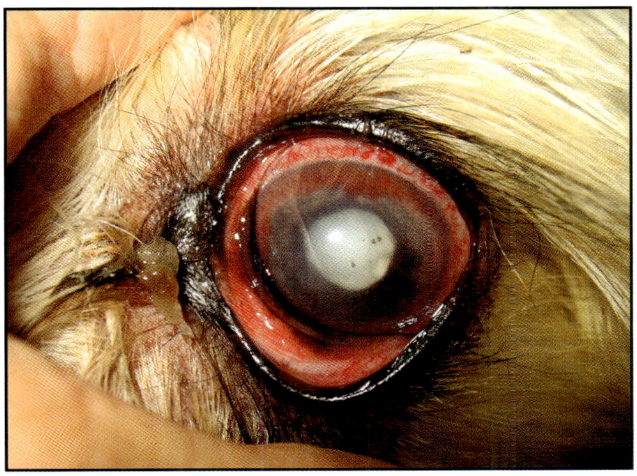

Figure 106.3 Clinical changes associated with phacoclastic uveitis secondary to lens-capsule rupture.

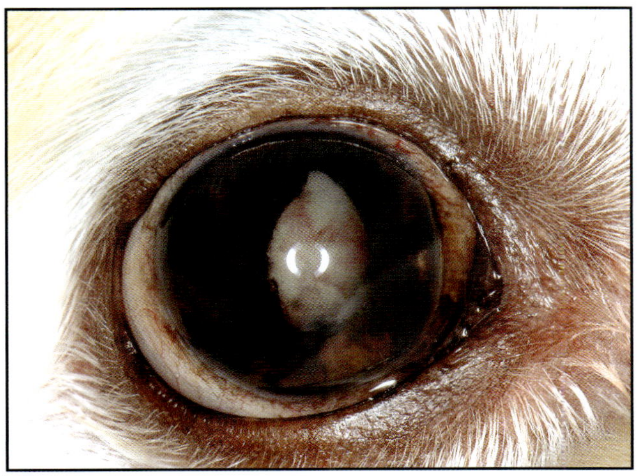

Figure 106.4 Clinical changes associated with phacoclastic uveitis secondary to lens-capsule rupture.

CHAPTER 107
ANTERIOR LENS LUXATION

PRESENTATION

The canine or feline lens may become dislocated from its normal position within the patellar fossa posterior to the iris. This may be the result of hereditary factors (predominantly abnormalities of the suspensory lens zonules and/or vitreous body), chronic intraocular inflammation, vitreous syneresis, glaucoma, and/or trauma. Anterior lenticular luxation may be partial (termed subluxation) or complete such that the lens becomes displaced into the anterior chamber. Associated changes may include corneal edema, uveitis, varying degrees of cataract formation, the presence of degenerate vitreous material within the pupillary opening and/or anterior chamber, and decreased or elevated intraocular pressure (IOP). Changes may be chronic or acute. Commonly affected breeds include multiple terrier breeds (Sealyham, Jack Russell, Wire Haired Fox, and Miniature Bull Terrier) the Australian Cattle Dog, German Shepherd and Shar Pei.

TREATMENT

The diagnosis of anterior (sub)luxation is made on the basis of clinical examination. Corneal edema and/or significant patient discomfort may render clinical diagnosis challenging, particularly in the case of non-cataractous lenses. Where indicated, diagnostic aids include sedation, anesthesia (topical or general), and/or B-mode ultrasonography. Subluxated lenses may be managed either medically (using anti-inflammatory therapy) or, more commonly, by surgical removal. The long-term use of a miotic agent in the contralateral eye may be indicated in an effort to prevent similar pathology from developing. Appropriate long-term miotic agents include demecarium bromide and the prostaglandin analogues (such as latanoprost). Miotic agents are however generally contraindicated when treating eyes affected by anterior (sub)luxation. Complete anterior lens luxation is most appropriately addressed via surgical intracapsular lens extraction (ICLE) and limited automated vitrectomy. Long-term postoperative anti-inflammatory therapy is typically indicated. Potential complications associated with lenticular (sub)luxation include chronic uveitis, retinal detachment, and/or glaucoma.

Potential Drug-Side-Effects

Potential complications associated with the use of demecarium bromide include ocular discomfort and gastrointestinal (GI) distress.

SELECTED REFERENCES

Binder DR, Herring IP, Gerhard T. Outcomes of nonsurgical management and efficacy of demecarium bromide treatment for primary lens instability in dogs: 34 cases (1990–2004). *J Am Vet Med Assoc* 2007;**231**(1):89–93.

Curtis R. Lens luxation in the dog and cat. *Vet Clin North Am Small Anim Pract* 1990;**20**(3):755–773. Review.

Glover TL, Davidson MG, Nasisse MP, Olivero DK. The intracapsular extraction of displaced lenses in dogs: a retrospective study of 57 cases (1984–1990). *J Am Anim Hosp Assoc* 1995;**31**(1):77–81.

Nasisse MP, Glover TL. Surgery for lens instability. *Vet Clin North Am Small Anim Pract* 1997;**27**(5):1175–1192. Review.

Oberbauer AM, Hollingsworth SR, Belanger JM, Regan KR, Famula TR. Inheritance of cataracts and primary lens luxation in Jack Russell Terriers. *Am J Vet Res* 2008;**69**(2):222–227. DOI: 10.2460/ajvr.69.2.222.

Clinical Atlas of Canine and Feline Ophthalmic Disease, First Edition. Douglas Esson.

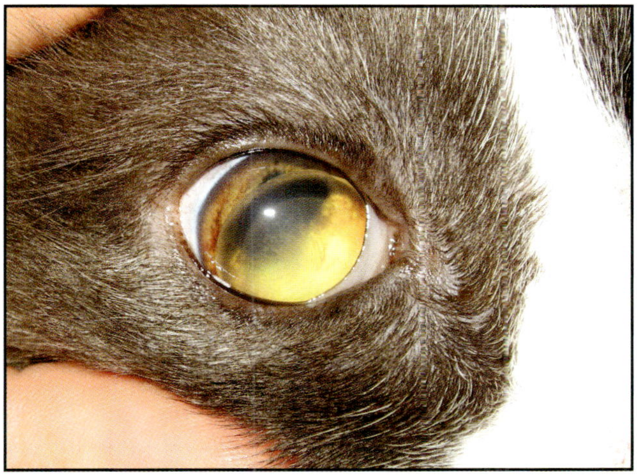

Figure 107.1 Clinical presentation associated with anterior lens luxation.

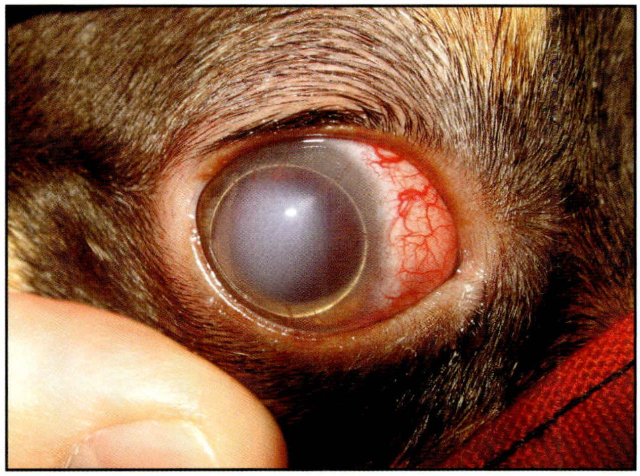

Figure 107.2 Clinical presentation associated with anterior lens luxation.

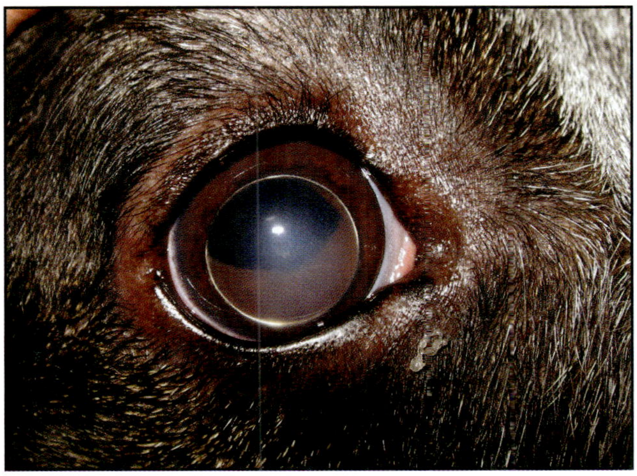

Figure 107.3 Clinical presentation associated with anterior lens luxation.

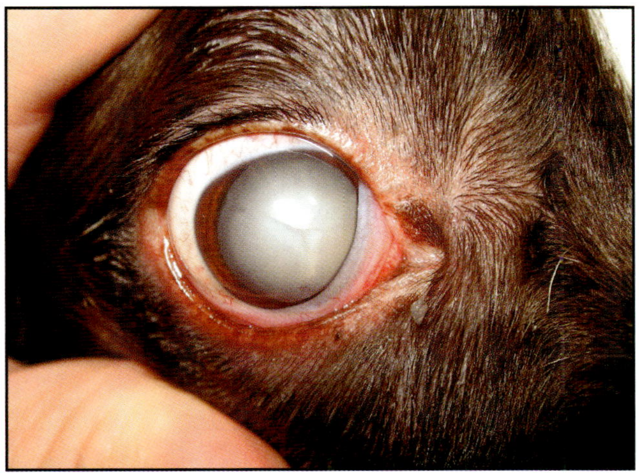

Figure 107.4 Clinical presentation associated with anterior lens luxation. A significant secondary cataract has formed.

CHAPTER 108
POSTERIOR LENS LUXATION

PRESENTATION

The canine or feline lens may become dislocated from its normal position within the patellar fossa posterior to the iris. This may be the result of hereditary factors (predominantly abnormalities of the suspensory lens zonules and/or vitreous body), chronic intraocular inflammation, vitreous syneresis, glaucoma, and/or trauma. Posterior lenticular luxation may be partial (termed subluxation) or complete. Associated changes may include uveitis, varying degrees of cataract formation, the presence of degenerate vitreous material within the pupillary opening and/or anterior chamber and decreased or elevated intraocular pressure (IOP). Changes may be chronic or acute. Commonly affected breeds include multiple terrier breeds (Sealyham, Jack Russell, Wire Haired Fox and Miniature Bull Terrier) the Australian Cattle Dog, the Chihuahua, Miniature Pinscher, and Springer Spaniel.

TREATMENT

The diagnosis of posterior (sub)luxation is made on the basis of clinical examination. Pathological shifting of the lens away from the central visual axis may result in the visualization of a semicircular region of increased tapetal reflectivity (termed an aphakic crescent). B-mode ultrasonography may be used to further define lenticular position if necessary. Subluxated lenses may be managed either medically (using a combination of miotic and/or anti-inflammatory therapy) or, where indicated, by surgical removal. Appropriate long-term miotic agents include demecarium bromide and the prostaglandin analogues (such as latanoprost). Long-term postoperative anti-inflammatory therapy is typically indicated. Potential complications associated with lenticular (sub)luxation include chronic uveitis, retinal detachment, and/or glaucoma.

Potential Drug-Side-Effects

Potential complications associated with the use of demecarium bromide include ocular discomfort and gastrointestinal (GI) distress.

SELECTED REFERENCES

Binder DR, Herring IP, Gerhard T. Outcomes of nonsurgical management and efficacy of demecarium bromide treatment for primary lens instability in dogs: 34 cases (1990–2004). *J Am Vet Med Assoc* 2007;**231**(1):89–93.

Curtis R. Lens luxation in the dog and cat. *Vet Clin North Am Small Anim Pract* 1990;**20**(3):755–773. Review.

Glover TL, Davidson MG, Nasisse MP, Olivero DK. The intracapsular extraction of displaced lenses in dogs: a retrospective study of 57 cases (1984–1990). *J Am Anim Hosp Assoc* 1995;**31**(1):77–81.

Nasisse MP, Glover TL. Surgery for lens instability. *Vet Clin North Am Small Anim Pract* 1997;**27**(5):1175–1192. Review.

Clinical Atlas of Canine and Feline Ophthalmic Disease, First Edition. Douglas Esson.

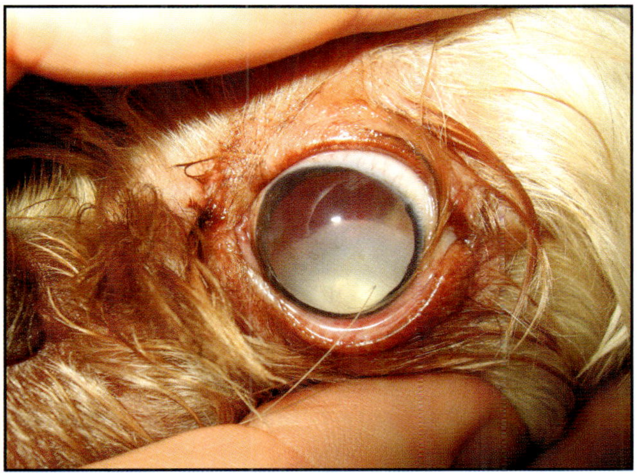

Figure 108.1 Clinical presentation associated with posterior lens luxation. An "aphakic crescent" is visible.

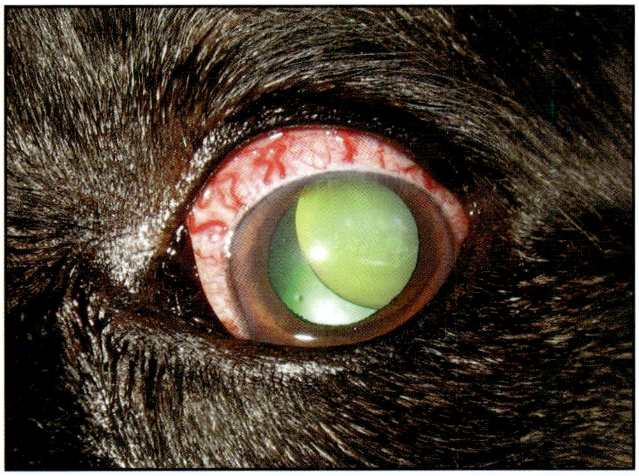

Figure 108.2 Clinical presentation associated with posterior lens luxation. An "aphakic crescent" is visible.

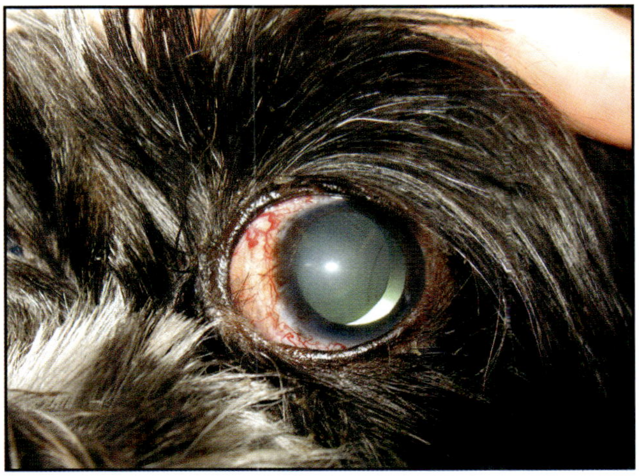

Figure 108.3 Clinical presentation associated with posterior lens luxation. An "aphakic crescent" is visible.

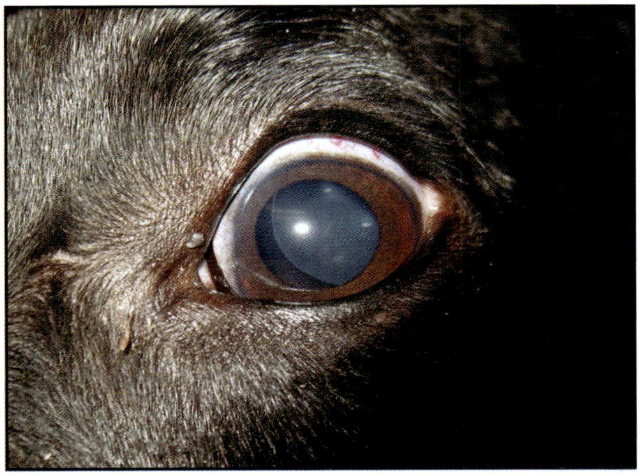

Figure 108.4 Clinical presentation associated with posterior lens luxation. An "aphakic crescent" is visible.

CHAPTER 109
FELINE POST-TRAUMATIC OCULAR SARCOMA

PRESENTATION

Feline post-traumatic ocular sarcoma (FPTOS) represents a malignant intraocular neoplasm, which may develop following severe inflammation and/or traumatic injury to the ocular structures (particularly the lens). Neoplastic changes typically take several years to develop. FPTOS encompasses several morphological variants, all of which are associated with the significant potential for extraocular extension and/or distant metastasis. Clinically, changes are typically unilateral and may include corneal edema, keratitis, corneal ulceration, uveitis, iridal thickening, and/or dyscoria, the presence of an intraocular mass, hyphema, retinal detachment, glaucoma, and/or exophthalmos.

TREATMENT

The diagnosis of FPTOS is made on the basis of clinical findings in conjunction with history. Soft tissue imaging modalities including B-mode ultrasonography, computed tomography (CT), and/or magnetic resonance imaging (MRI) may contribute to the clinical diagnosis, which is confirmed histologically either by biopsy or following enucleation/exenteration. The treatment of choice is enucleation (or exenteration where extraocular tumor extension is suspected/demonstrated). The evaluation of systemic health and/or potential metastasis via complete blood count (CBC)/chemistry analysis, local lymph node aspiration, and/or three-view radiography is indicated before surgical intervention. In general, chemical ciliary body ablation (CBA), in order to manage glaucoma, is discouraged in cats owing to the potential risk for the development of FPTOS.

SELECTED REFERENCES

Dubielzig RR, Everitt J, Shadduck JA, Albert DM. Clinical and morphologic features of post-traumatic ocular sarcomas in cats. *Vet Pathol* 1990;**27**(1):62–65.

Duke FD, Strong TD, Bentley E, Dubielzig RR. Feline ocular tumors following ciliary body ablation with intravitreal gentamicin. *Vet Ophthalmol.* 2013;**16**(Suppl 1):188–190. DOI: 10.1111/vop.12066. Epub 2013.

Zeiss CJ, Johnson EM, Dubielzig RR. Feline intraocular tumors may arise from transformation of lens epithelium. *Vet Pathol* 2003;**40**(4):355–362.

Clinical Atlas of Canine and Feline Ophthalmic Disease, First Edition. Douglas Esson.

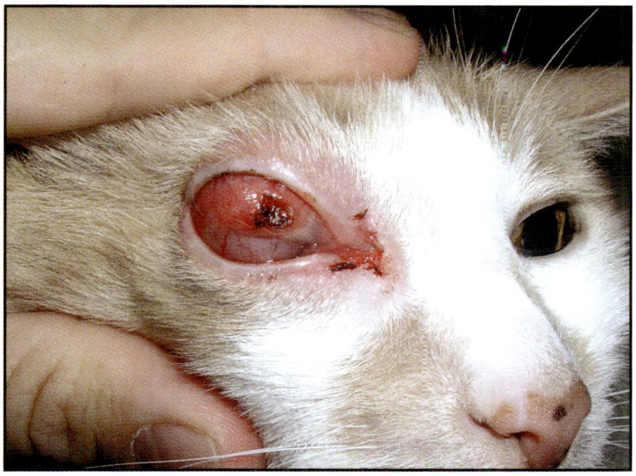

Figure 109.1 Clinical presentation associated with feline post-traumatic ocular sarcoma.

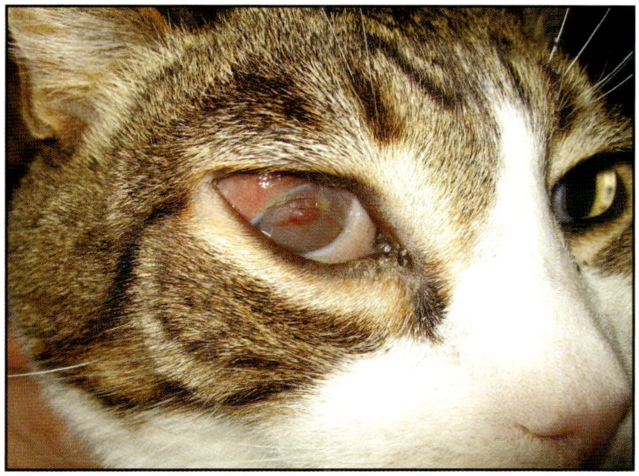

Figure 109.2 Clinical presentation associated with feline post-traumatic ocular sarcoma.

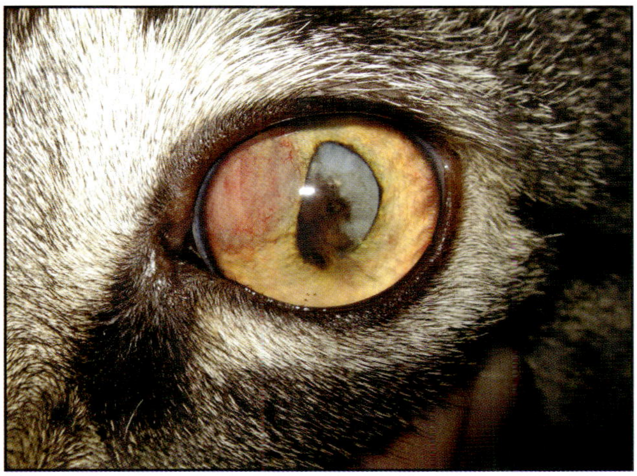

Figure 109.3 Clinical presentation associated with feline post-traumatic ocular sarcoma.

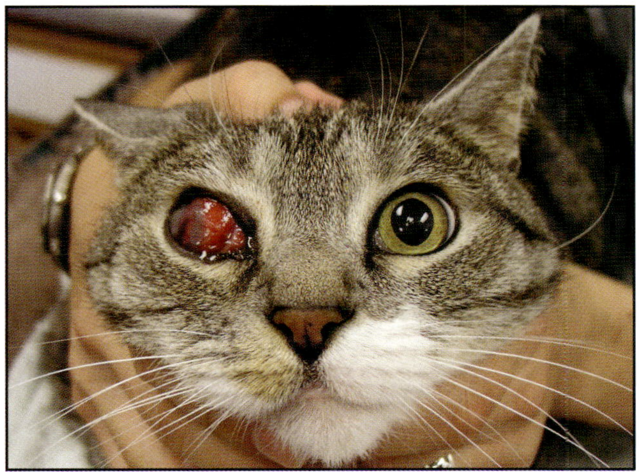

Figure 109.4 Clinical presentation associated with feline post-traumatic ocular sarcoma.

Section 7

Vitreoretinal Disease

CHAPTER 110
THE RETINAL DYSPLASIAS (RDs)

PRESENTATION

The retinal dysplasias (RDs) represent a group of inherited (bilateral) retinal diseases associated with the anomalous differentiation and proliferation of one of more layers (with or without the involvement of other ocular tissues). The majority of clinical cases occur as a result of hereditary disease; however, external factors such as viral infection (including canine adenovirus, canine herpes virus, feline panleukopenia), and radiation exposure and toxicity may induce similar changes. The RDs may involve the following:

- Multifocal linear folds of tissue (notably affecting the Labrador Retriever, American Cocker Spaniel, Beagle, Rottweiler, and Yorkshire Terrier)
- Large irregular or "geographic" areas of tissue (notably affecting the Labrador Retriever, Golden Retriever, English Springer Spaniel, and Cavalier King Charles Spaniel)
- Complete dysplasia with or without retinal detachment (notably affecting the Labrador Retriever, Australian Shepherd, Samoyed, Doberman Pinscher, Akita, and Chow Chow)

DIAGNOSIS AND TREATMENT

The diagnosis of retinal dysplasia is made on the basis of funduscopic examination, typically possible from 6 to 8 weeks of age. In some cases, small lesions and folds may disappear by follow-up examination at 6 months to 1 year. Genetic testing is also available for multiple-breed-related retinal dysplasias (www.optigen.com). No medical therapy is likely to be beneficial. Surgical management of retinal detachments may be indicated in selected cases.

SELECTED REFERENCES

MacMillan A. Retinal dysplasia in the dog and cat. *Vet Clin North Am Small Anim Pract* 1980;**10**(2):411–415.

Petersen-Jones S. Advances in the molecular understanding of canine retinal diseases. *J Small Anim Pract* 2005;**46**(8):371–380.

Whiteley HE. Dysplastic canine retinal morphogenesis. *Invest Ophthalmol Vis Sci* 1991;**32**(5):1492–1498.

Clinical Atlas of Canine and Feline Ophthalmic Disease, First Edition. Douglas Esson.

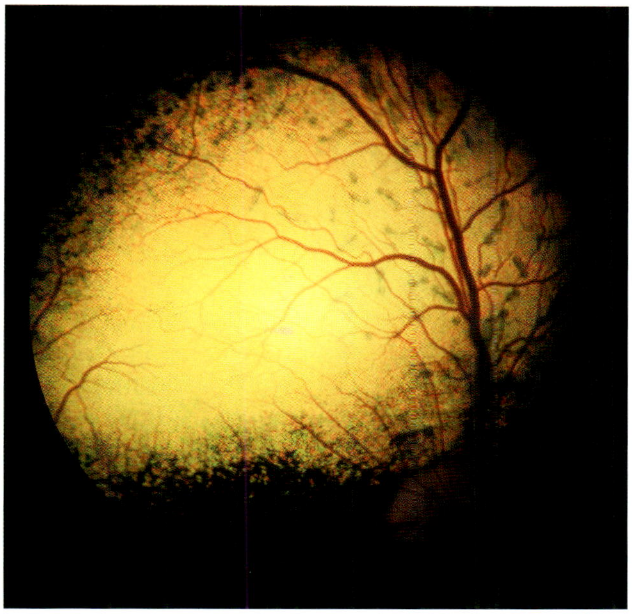

Figure 110.1 Funduscopic changes consistent with retinal dysplasia. Multiple areas of linear to vermiform dysplasia are visible.

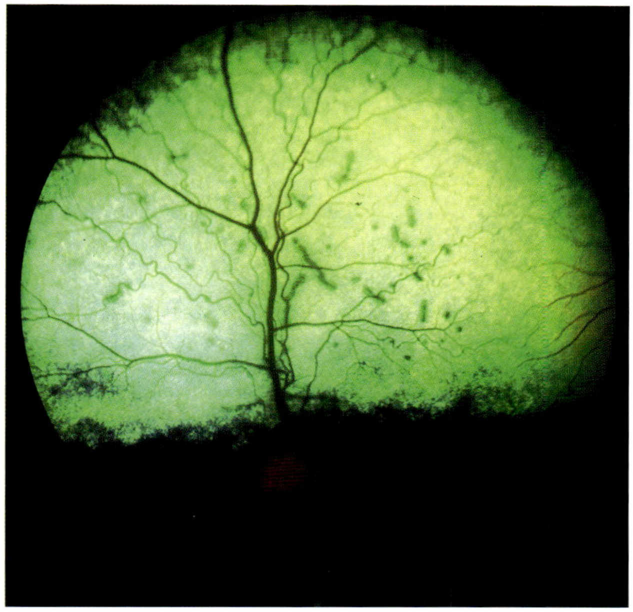

Figure 110.2 Funduscopic changes consistent with retinal dysplasia. Multiple areas of linear to vermiform dysplasia are visible.

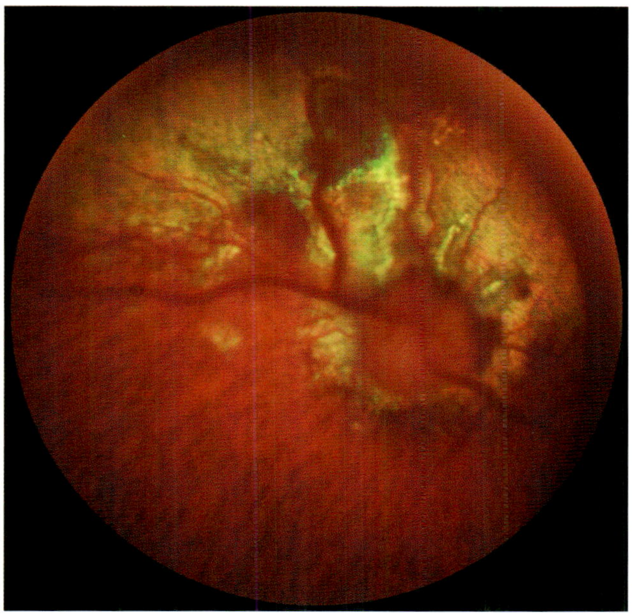

Figure 110.3 Funduscopic changes consistent with retinal dysplasia. Large irregular areas of geographic dysplasia are visible.

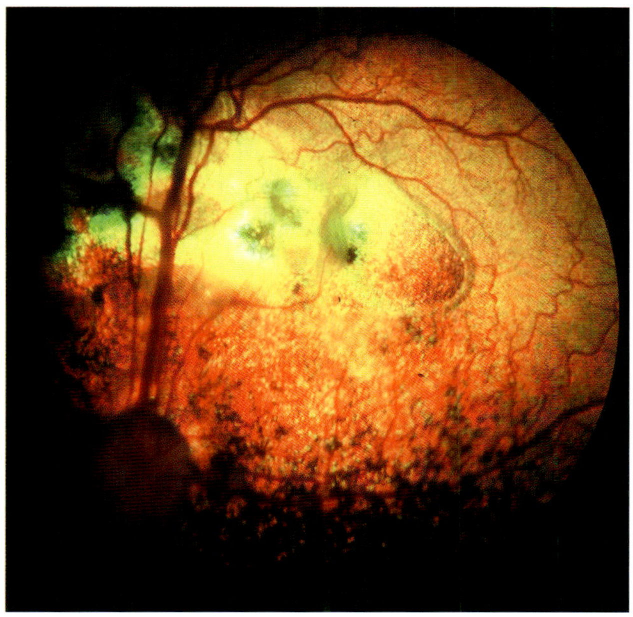

Figure 110.4 Funduscopic changes consistent with retinal dysplasia. Large irregular areas of geographic dysplasia are visible.

CHAPTER 111
OCULOSKELETAL DYSPLASIA (OSD)

PRESENTATION

Oculoskeletal dysplasia (OSD) represents a hereditary syndrome comprising varying combinations of osteochondrodysplasia and/or ocular pathology. Skeletal changes typically include shortened limbs (particularly the forelimbs), marked by varus deformities of the elbows and valgus deformities of the carpi, epiphyseal dysplasia, ununited anconeal/coronoid processes, and/or hip dysplasia. Ocular pathology may include any combination of cataracts, retinal folding/dysplasia, retinal detachment (complete or partial), hyaloid remnants, hyphema, and/or glaucoma. Affected breeds include the Labrador Retriever and Samoyed.

DIAGNOSIS AND TREATMENT

The diagnosis of OSD is made on the basis of clinical findings. Ocular ultrasonography and skeletal radiography may support the diagnosis where necessary. Genetic testing for affected breeds is also available (www.optigen.com). Specific treatment is not available; however, secondary ocular complications including cataracts, hyphema, glaucoma, and/or retinal detachment may be managed as individually appropriate.

SELECTED REFERENCES

Carrig CB, Sponenberg DP, Schmidt GM, Tvedten HW. Inheritance of associated ocular and skeletal dysplasia in Labrador retrievers. *J Am Vet Med Assoc* 1998;**193**(10):1269–1272.

Cook JL, Jordan RC. What is your diagnosis? Retinal dysplasia with concurrent developmental skeletal abnormalities in a Labrador retriever. *J Am Vet Med Assoc* 1997;**210**(3):329–330. No abstract available.

Goldstein O, Guyon R, Kukekova A, Kuznetsova TN, Pearce-Kelling SE, Johnson J, Aguirre GD, Acland GM. COL9A2 and COL9A3 mutations in canine autosomal recessive oculoskeletal dysplasia. *Mamm Genome* 2010;**21**(7–8):398–408. DOI: 10.1007/s00335-010-9276-4. Epub 2010 Aug 5.

Clinical Atlas of Canine and Feline Ophthalmic Disease, First Edition. Douglas Esson.

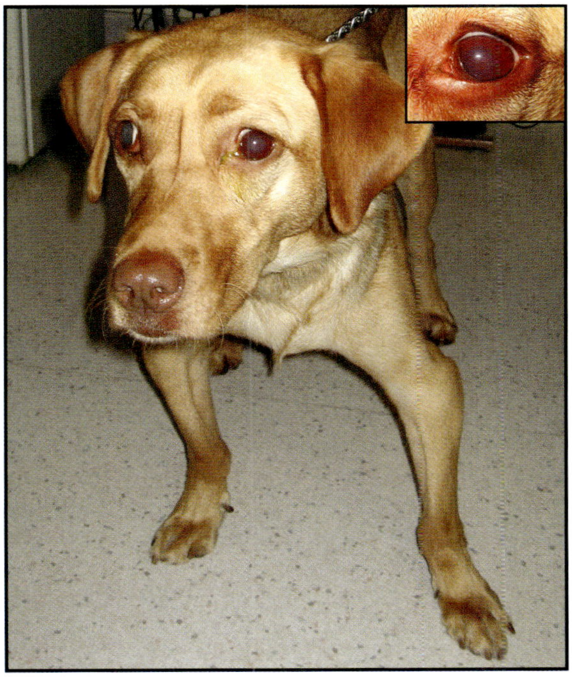

Figure 111.1 Clinical presentation associated with oculoskeletal dysplasia, including forelimb varus defects. Inset demonstrates hyphema secondary to retinal detachment.

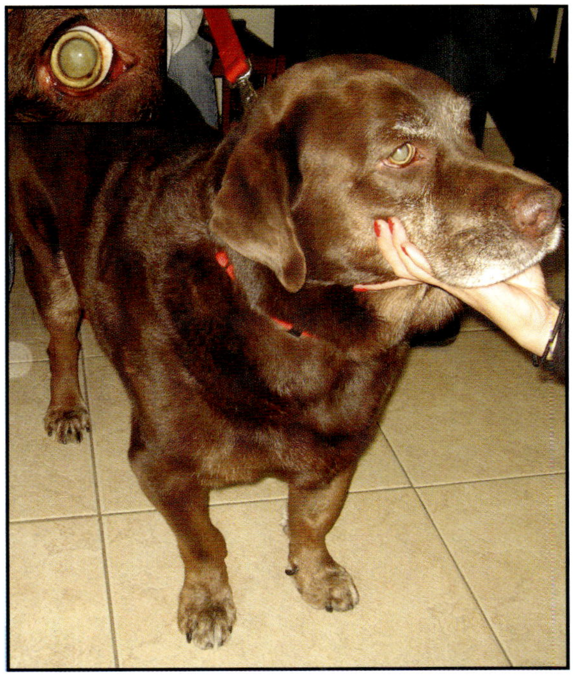

Figure 111.2 Clinical presentation associated with oculoskeletal dysplasia, including forelimb varus defects. Inset demonstrates cataractous changes.

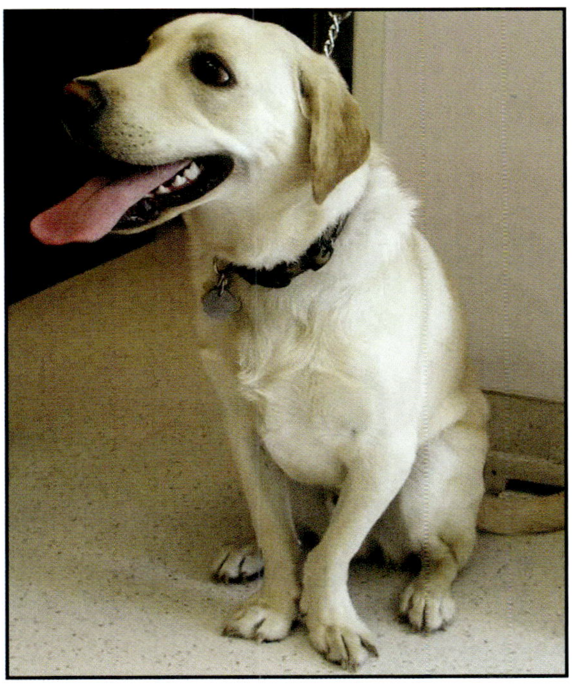

Figure 111.3 Clinical presentation associated with oculoskeletal dysplasia, including forelimb varus defects.

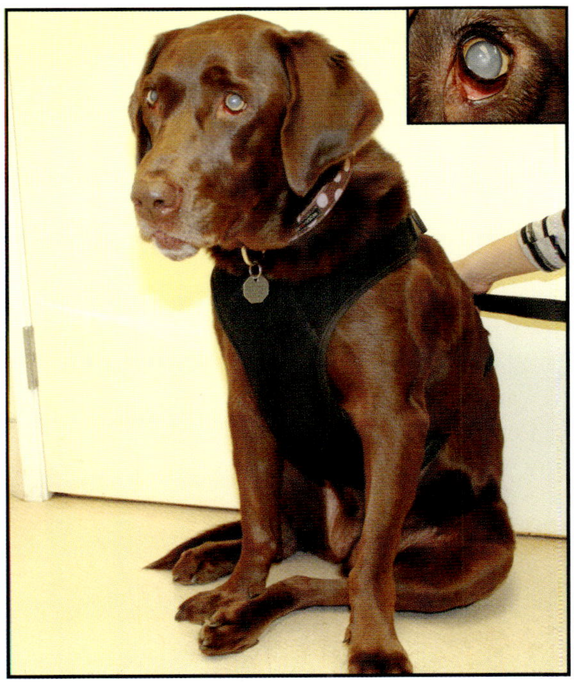

Figure 111.4 Clinical presentation associated with oculoskeletal dysplasia, including forelimb varus defects. Inset demonstrates cataractous changes.

CHAPTER 112
COLLIE EYE ANOMALY (CEA)

PRESENTATION

Collie eye anomaly (CEA) describes a congenital, hereditary disease resulting from abnormal embryonic differentiation of ocular tissues. Changes may include any combination of choroidal vascular hypoplasia, retinal pigment epithelial (RPE), and/or tapetal defects, abnormal retinal vasculature, scleral colobomas (typically involving the region surrounding the optic nerve head), retinal dysplasia, and/or retinal detachment (partial or complete). Changes are bilateral but not always symmetrical. Most affected animals are clinically asymptomatic, abnormalities only being detected upon fundic examination; however, patients may present as a result of symptoms associated with retinal detachment and/or hyphema. Commonly affected breeds include the Collie breeds, Australian Shepherd, and Shetland Sheepdog.

DIAGNOSIS AND TREATMENT

The diagnosis of CEA is made on the basis of signalment in combination with clinical findings. Genetic testing is also available for multiple-breed-related CEAs (www.optigen.com). Primary treatment of this disorder is not possible; however, secondary complications, such as hyphema, may be treated symptomatically. Surgical intervention in order to address scleral or retinal pathology may be indicated in select cases. Selective breeding reduces the incidence and severity of disease.

SELECTED REFERENCES

Lowe JK, Kukekova AV, Kirkness EF, Langlois MC, Aguirre GD, Acland GM, Ostrander EA. Linkage mapping of the primary disease locus for collie eye anomaly. *Genomics* 2003;**82**(1):86–95.

Munyard KA, Sherry CR, Sherry L. A retrospective evaluation of congenital ocular defects in Australian Shepherd dogs in Australia. *Vet Ophthalmol* 2007;**10**(1):19–22.

Parker HG, Kukekova AV, Akey DT, Goldstein O, Kirkness EF, Baysac KC, Mosher DS, Aguirre GD, Acland GM, Ostrander EA. Breed relationships facilitate fine-mapping studies: a 7.8-kb deletion cosegregates with Collie eye anomaly across multiple dog breeds. *Genome Res* 2007;**17**(11):1562–1571. Epub 2007 Oct 4.

Wallin-Håkanson B, Wallin-Håkanson N, Hedhammar A. Influence of selective breeding on the prevalence of chorioretinal dysplasia and coloboma in the rough collie in Sweden. *J Small Anim Pract* 2000;**41**(2):56–59.

Clinical Atlas of Canine and Feline Ophthalmic Disease, First Edition. Douglas Esson.

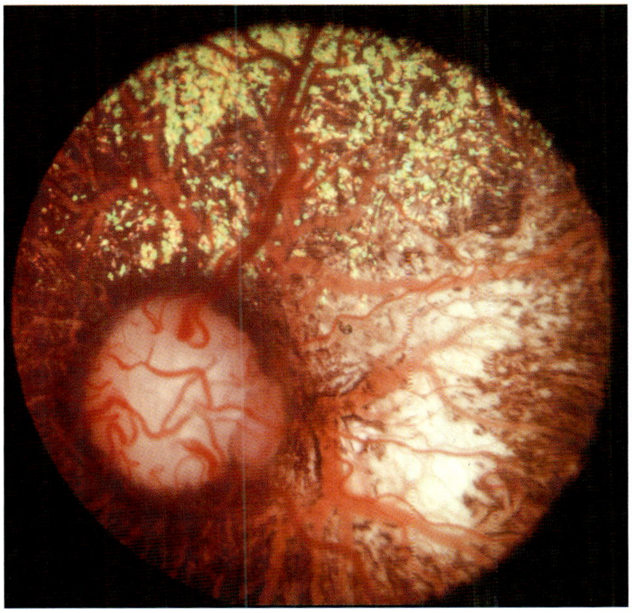

Figure 112.1 Pathology associated with collie eye anomaly (CEA) including scleral ectasia, choroidal hypoplasia, abnormal vasculature, and posterior segment coloboma.

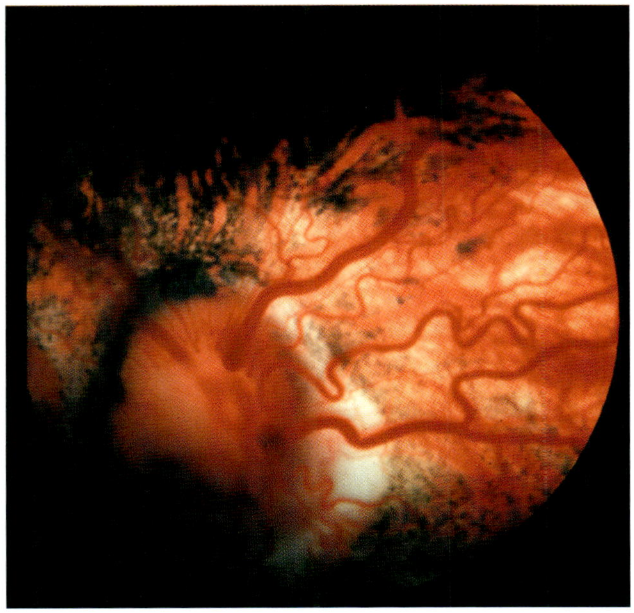

Figure 112.2 Pathology associated with collie eye anomaly (CEA) including scleral ectasia, choroidal hypoplasia, abnormal vasculature, and posterior segment coloboma.

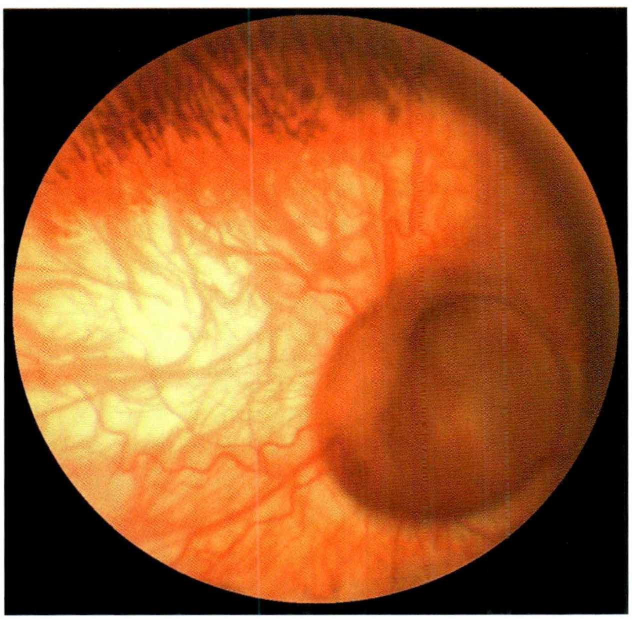

Figure 112.3 Pathology associated with collie eye anomaly (CEA) including scleral ectasia, choroidal hypoplasia, abnormal vasculature, and posterior segment coloboma.

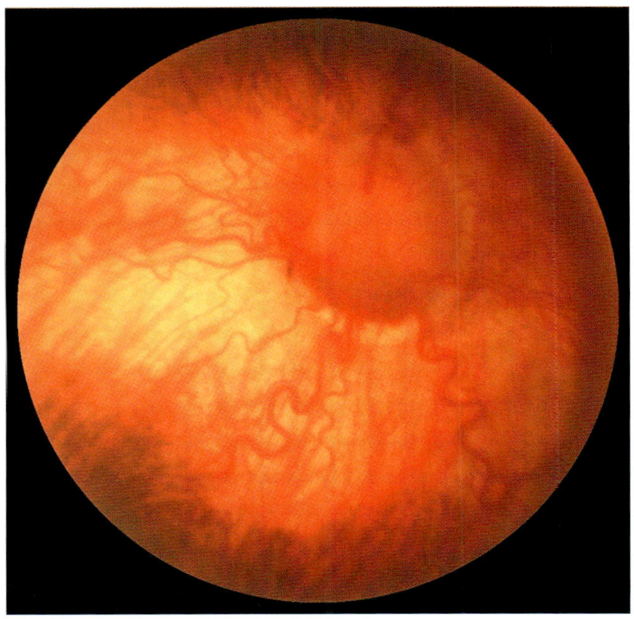

Figure 112.4 Pathology associated with collie eye anomaly (CEA) including scleral ectasia, choroidal hypoplasia, abnormal vasculature, and posterior segment coloboma.

CHAPTER 113
THE RETINAL ATROPHIES (RAs)

PRESENTATION

The retinal atrophies (RAs) represent a group of inherited (bilateral) retinal diseases, which result in photoreceptor dysfunction and death, leading to visual impairment and ultimately blindness. Various forms have been described as affecting a large (and increasing) number of dog breeds as well as some cat breeds. The classification of the RAs is complex; however, they may be simplified into early- and late-onset progressive retinal atrophy (PRA), congenital stationary night blindness (CSNB), cone degeneration ("day blindness"), and the feline RAs.

The early-onset (dysplastic) canine RAs include the following:

- Rod-cone dysplasia (RCD), notably affecting the Irish Setter, Miniature Schnauzer, Norwegian Elkhound, Dachshund, Cardigan Welsh Corgi, and Collies
- X-Linked PRA (XLPRA), notably affecting the Samoyed and Siberian Husky
- Early retinal degeneration (ERD), notably affecting the Norwegian Elkhound.

The late-onset (degenerative) canine RAs include the following:

- Progressive rod-cone degeneration (PRCD), notably affecting the Labrador Retriever, Chesapeake Bay Retriever, Nova Scotia Duck-Tolling Retriever, American Cocker Spaniel, American Eskimo, Australian Cattle Dog, Chinese Crested, Miniature Poodle, Toy Poodle, Akita, and Finnish Lapphund
- Dominant PRA, notably affecting the Old English and Bull Mastiff
- Retinal pigment epithelial dystrophy (RPED), notably affecting the Labrador Retriever, Golden Retriever, Chesapeake Bay Retriever and Collie breeds

These diseases typically manifest initially as relative mydriasis as well as loss of night-vision (nyctalopia). The onset of symptoms is variable, however, may be noticed in the early onset RAs between 6 weeks and 6 months of age (typically progressing to blindness by 1–5 years of age) and in the late onset RAs between 3 and 5 years of age (typically progressing to complete blindness by 6–8 years of age). Congenital stationary night blindness (CSNB), represents a condition in which affected dogs are congenitally night blind and may additionally develop decreased day vision over the course of several years. The Briard is notably reported as affected by this condition. Cone degeneration (also described as day blindness or hemeralopia), represents a condition in which affected dogs demonstrate early-onset and rapidly progressive loss of cone function so that visual function is lost under daylight conditions. The Alaskan Malamute and German Shorthaired Pointer are notably affected. The feline RAs are less well described; however, they largely follow the same natural course with early disease present by 1–2 years of age and advanced disease present by 3–6 years of age. Cat breeds known to be affected by various forms of retinal atrophy include the Abyssinian, Somali, Bengal, and Persian.

DIAGNOSIS AND TREATMENT

The diagnosis of the RAs may be made on the basis of multiple criteria, including clinical findings, funduscopic visualization (varying degrees of tapetal hyperreflectivity, vascular attenuation, and ONH degeneration), and/or ERG testing. Genetic testing is also available for multiple-breed-related RAs (www.optigen.com). Accurate gene-based testing facilitates breeding programs designed to help reduce the incidence of disease within a breed. Many patients will develop secondary cataracts over time. The administration of antioxidant-containing products has been advocated in an effort to slow the progression of disease; however, will not prevent blindness.

SELECTED REFERENCES

Clements PJ, Sargan DR, Gould DJ, Petersen-Jones SM. Recent advances in understanding the spectrum of canine generalised progressive retinal atrophy. *J Small Anim Pract* 1996;**37**(4):155–162. Review.

Downs LM, Hitti R, Pregnolato S, Mellersh CS. Genetic screening for PRA-associated mutations in multiple dog breeds shows that PRA is heterogeneous within and between breeds. *Vet Ophthalmol* 2014;**17**(2):126–130. DOI: 10.1111/vop.12122. Epub 2013 Nov 21.

Narfström K. Hereditary and congenital ocular disease in the cat. *J Feline Med Surg* 1999;**1**(3):135–141.

Petersen-Jones S. Advances in the molecular understanding of canine retinal diseases. *J Small Anim Pract* 2005;**46**(8):371–380.

Clinical Atlas of Canine and Feline Ophthalmic Disease, First Edition. Douglas Esson.

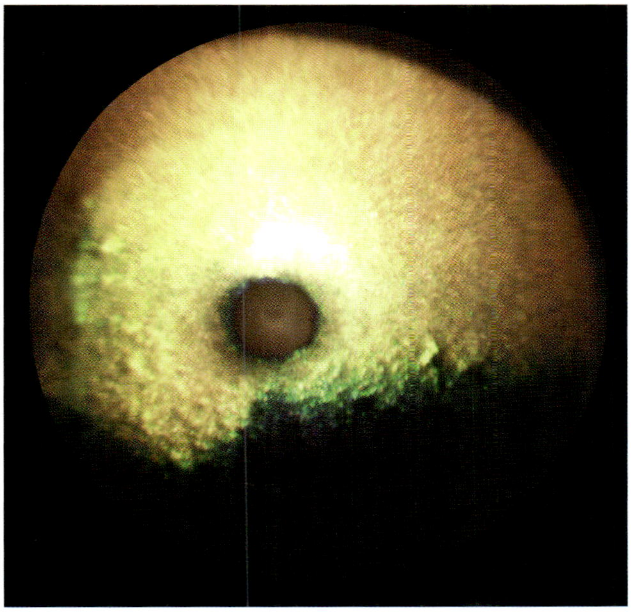

Figure 113.1 Funduscopic findings associated with retinal atrophy (RA), including tapetal hyperreflectivity and marked vascular attenuation.

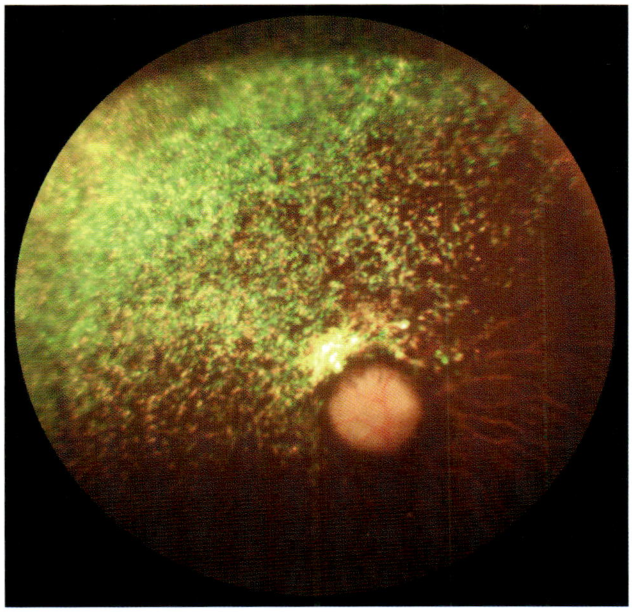

Figure 113.2 Funduscopic findings associated with retinal atrophy (RA), including tapetal hyperreflectivity and marked vascular attenuation.

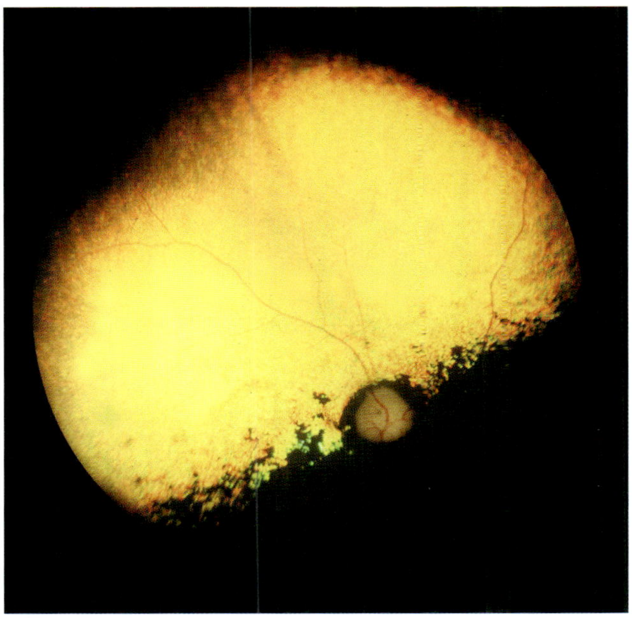

Figure 113.3 Funduscopic findings associated with retinal atrophy (RA), including tapetal hyperreflectivity and marked vascular attenuation.

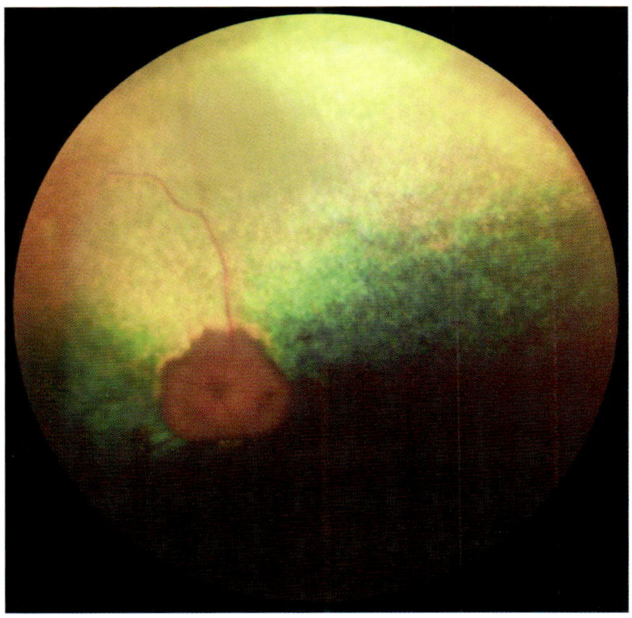

Figure 113.4 Funduscopic findings associated with retinal atrophy (RA), including tapetal hyperreflectivity and marked vascular attenuation.

CHAPTER 114
VITREAL DEGENERATION/HERNIATION

PRESENTATION

The vitreous body consists of a transparent hydrogel, which contains collagen and hyaluronic acid and occupies approximately 75% of the volume of the eye. The vitreous body supports both the lens and the neuroretina. Inherited factors as well as age-related degeneration may lead to pathological changes including vitreal syneresis, asteroid hyalosis (calcium/phospholipid bodies), cyst formation, hemorrhage, retinal tears, lenticular instability, vitreal herniation into the anterior chamber, and/or glaucoma. Clinically, degenerate vitreous may be noted to be herniating through the pupil into the anterior chamber, frequently containing fine melanin-rich granules and/or cells (notably in the Italian Greyhound, Boston Terrier, and Jack Russell Terrier) and/or to contain multiple, fine, gravity-dependent crystalline hyaloid bodies—sometimes referred to as synchysis scintillans (notably in the Shih Tzu, Miniature Poodle, and Bichon Frisé).

DIAGNOSIS AND TREATMENT

The diagnosis of vitreal degeneration is made on the basis of clinical findings, supported if necessary by B-mode ultrasonography. Treatment may or may not be indicated depending on the severity of changes present and where indicated may comprise topical (steroidal or nonsteroidal) anti-inflammatory therapy, the use of a miotic agent to stabilize subluxated lenses, the removal of luxated lens(es), retinopexy/retinal reattachment, and/or surgical vitrectomy.

Potential Drug-Side-Effects

Potential adverse effects associated with the use of topical corticosteroids include impaired wound healing and corneal degeneration.

SELECTED REFERENCES

Labruyère JJ, Hartley C, Rogers K, Wetherill G, McConnell JF, Dennis R. Ultrasonographic evaluation of vitreous degeneration in normal dogs. *Vet Radiol Ultrasound* 2008;**49**(2):165–171.

Papaioannou NG, Dubielzig RR. Histopathological and immunohistochemical features of vitreoretinopathy in Shih Tzu dogs. *J Comp Pathol* 2013;**148**(2–3):230–235. DOI: 10.1016/j.jcpa.2012.05.014. Epub 2012 Jul 20.

van der Woerdt A, Wilkie DA, Myer CW. Ultrasonographic abnormalities in the eyes of dogs with cataracts: 147 cases (1986–1992). *J Am Vet Med Assoc* 1993;**203**(6):838–841.

Wang M, Kador PF, Wyman M. Structure of asteroid bodies in the vitreous of galactose-fed dogs. *Mol Vis* 2006;**12**:283–289.

Clinical Atlas of Canine and Feline Ophthalmic Disease, First Edition. Douglas Esson.

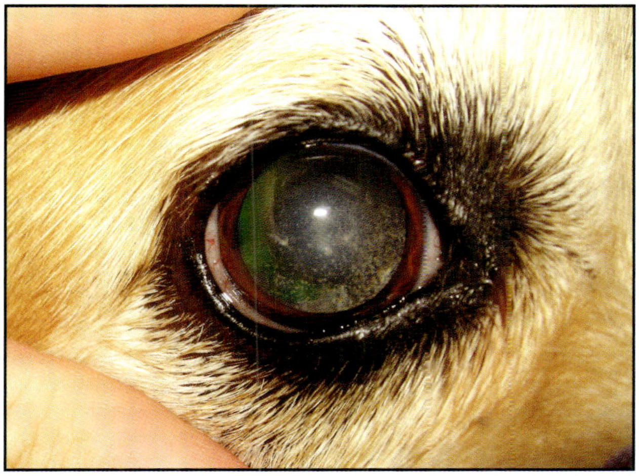

Figure 114.1 Vitreal degeneration. Asteroid hyalosis is notable.

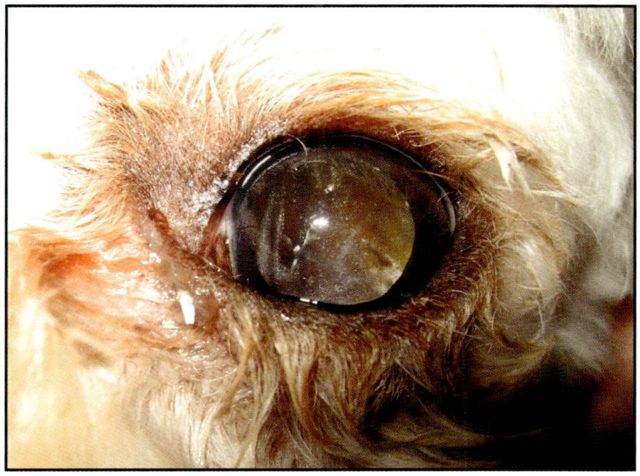

Figure 114.2 Vitreal degeneration. Asteroid hyalosis is notable.

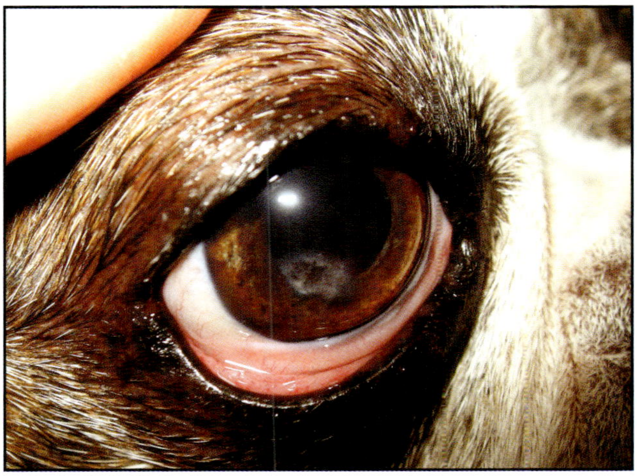

Figure 114.3 Vitreal degeneration. Herniated vitreous is visible in the anterior chamber.

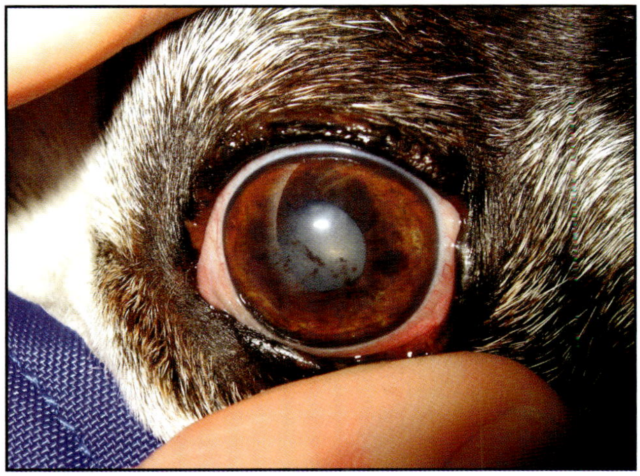

Figure 114.4 Vitreal degeneration. Herniated vitreous is visible in the anterior chamber.

CHAPTER 115
RETINAL TOXICITY

PRESENTATION

Sensitive neuroretinal tissues may be damaged by exposure to potentially harmful pharmacologic agents, frequently enrofloxacin in cats and ivermectin in dogs. Toxicity associated with enrofloxacin (and potentially other fluoroquinolones) in cats may result in varying degrees of visual impairment/blindness. This response appears to be idiosyncratic; however, it is more commonly encountered in association with significant overdose and/or rapid intravenous administration. Current recommendations are a maximum of 5 mg/kg Q 24 h. Funduscopic appearance is initially unremarkable; however, visible tapetal hyperreflectivity, vascular attenuation, and ONH degeneration ensue within days to weeks following exposure. Toxicity associated with ivermectin (and potentially other avermectins) may result in varying degrees of visual impairment/blindness as well as neurological defects, altered mentation, and/or thermal dysregulation. This response may be more commonly encountered in association with significant overdose (notably following the inadvertent ingestion of equine anthelminthic products) and/or long-term exposure (notably in association with the management of chronic dermal parasitic infestation). Collie breeds including the Australian Shepherd and Shetland Sheepdog are potentially more susceptible to ivermectin toxicity because of a hereditary defect associated with the MDR1 gene, which regulates molecular transport at the level of the blood–brain barrier. Doses as low as 100 μg/kg may be associated with toxicosis in predisposed breeds. Funduscopically, affected dogs may display varying combinations of papilledema and/or irregular to vermiform retinal edema.

DIAGNOSIS AND TREATMENT

The diagnosis of retinal toxicity is made on the basis of clinical findings and history. Electroretinography (ERG) may be used to evaluate photoreceptor function, and levels of specific agents (such as ivermectin) may be assessed by laboratory assay. Treatment comprises drug withdrawal and supportive care. Changes associated with enrofloxacin toxicity are generally irreversible. Those associated with ivermectin toxicity are frequently reversible.

SELECTED REFERENCES

Epstein SE, Hollingsworth SR. Ivermectin-induced blindness treated with intravenous lipid therapy in a dog. *J Vet Emerg Crit Care (San Antonio)* 2013;**23**(1):58–62. DOI: 10.1111/vec.12016. Epub 2013 Jan 14.

Gelatt KN, van der Woerdt A, Ketring KL, Andrew SE, Brooks DE, Biros DJ, Denis HM, Cutler TJ. Enrofloxacin-associated retinal degeneration in cats. *Vet Ophthalmol* 2001;**4**(2):99–106.

Kenny PJ, Vernau KM, Puschner B, Maggs DJ. Retinopathy associated with ivermectin toxicosis in two dogs. *J Am Vet Med Assoc* 2008;**233**(2):279–284. DOI: 10.2460/javma.233.2.279.

Wiebe V, Hamilton P. Fluoroquinolone-induced retinal degeneration in cats. *J Am Vet Med Assoc* 2002;**221**(11):1568–1571.

Clinical Atlas of Canine and Feline Ophthalmic Disease, First Edition. Douglas Esson.

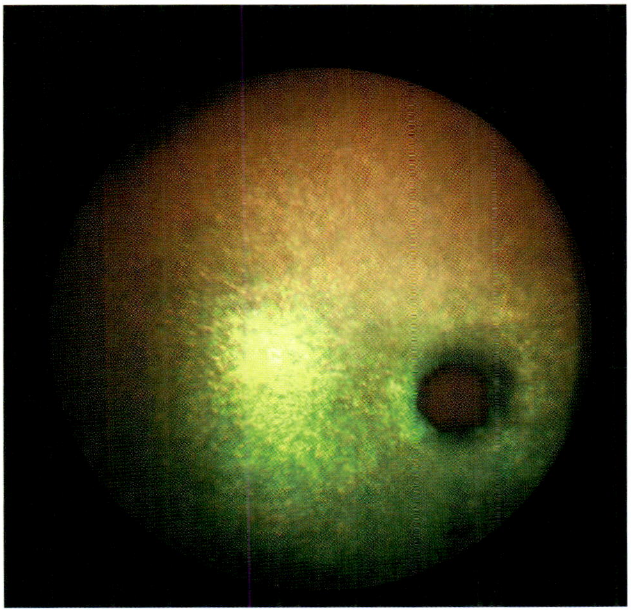

Figure 115.1 Funduscopic changes as a result of enrofloxacin toxicity. Changes include tapetal hyperreflectivity and vascular attenuation.

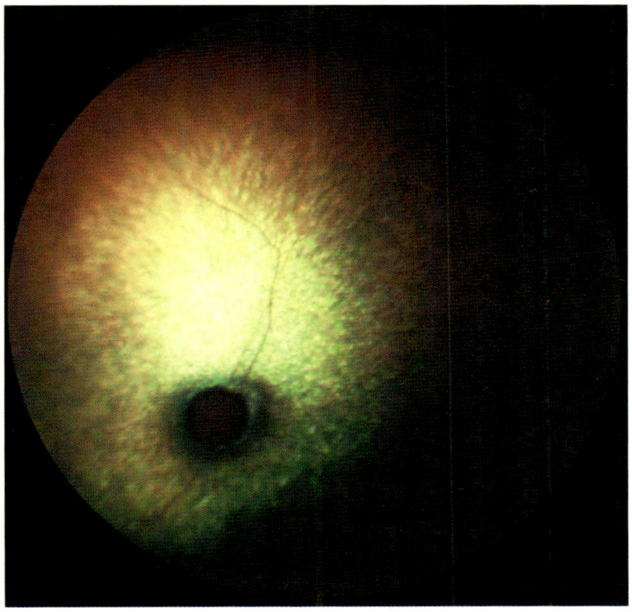

Figure 115.2 Funduscopic changes as a result of enrofloxacin toxicity. Changes include tapetal hyperreflectivity and vascular attenuation.

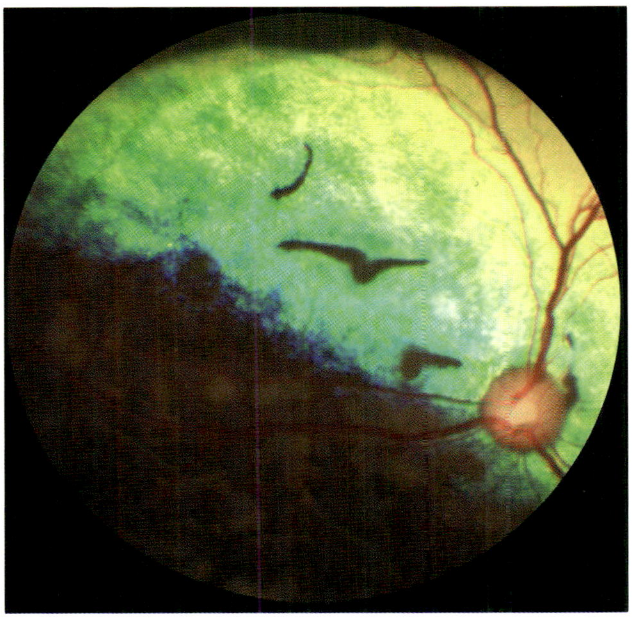

Figure 115.3 Funduscopic changes as a result of ivermectin toxicity. Changes include irregular linear to vermiform areas of retinal edema

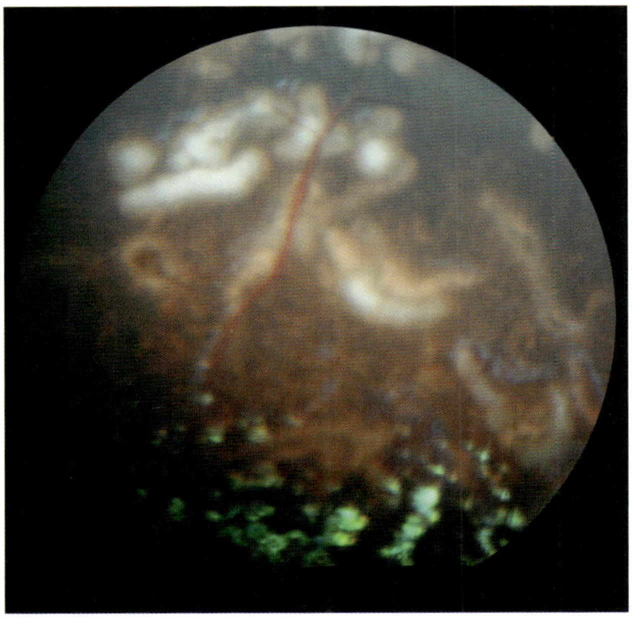

Figure 115.4 Funduscopic changes as a result of ivermectin toxicity. Changes include irregular linear to vermiform areas of retinal edema.

CHAPTER 116
SARDs/IMR

PRESENTATION

Sudden acquired retinal degeneration syndrome/immune-mediated retinitis (SARDs/IMR) describes a spectrum of disease resulting in acute-onset blindness, which is generally irreversible. The mechanism of photoreceptor death in SARDs/IMR appears to be immune (antibody)-mediated. Symptoms generally develop over the course of several days, with affected patients presenting with severe visual disturbance and disorientation. Clinically, although signs of functional vision are typically absent, sluggish and incomplete pupillary light reflexes (PLRs) are frequently elicited in the early stages of the disease. Ophthalmic examination (including funduscopic assessment) is otherwise initially unremarkable (although signs of generalized neuroretinal degeneration including tapetal hyperreflectivity and vascular attenuation become evident in the ensuing months). Affected animals are commonly middle-aged, female, small-breed dogs, which may additionally be overweight and/or exhibit symptoms of polyuria/polydipsia/polyphagia. Associations have been made with paraneoplastic syndromes, hyperadrenocorticism, and/or sex hormone imbalances. Commonly affected breeds include the Dachshund and Miniature Schnauzer.

DIAGNOSIS AND TREATMENT

The diagnosis of SARDs/IMR is made on the basis of presentation and clinical findings, supported by electroretinography (ERG), which additionally rules out central causes of blindness (see Central Blindness). Routine complete blood count (CBC)/chemistry analysis may indicate the presence of a stress leukogram and/or elevated levels of cholesterol and/or alkaline phosphatase. Attempted treatment of fully extinguished photoreceptor function is fruitless. In rare cases of peracute IMR (associated with a degree of residual visual and/or electroretinographic function), experimental treatment using immunomodulating therapy comprising systemic doxycycline, corticosteroids, and/or immunoglobulin therapy has been described.

Potential Drug-Side-Effects

Potential adverse effects associated with doxycycline, include gastrointestinal (GI) distress, photosensitivity, and hepatic damage. Potential adverse effects associated with the use of systemic cortiocosteroids include polyphagia, polydipsia, polyuria, hair coat changes, weight gain, pancreatitis, enteritis, muscular damage, hepatic impairment, and diabetes. Potential side effects associated with the use of immunoglobulins include severe anaphylaxis and/or death.

SELECTED REFERENCES

Grozdanic SD, Harper MM, Kecova H. Antibody-mediated retinopathies in canine patients: mechanism, diagnosis, and treatment modalities. *Vet Clin North Am Small Anim Pract* 2008;**38**(2):361–387, vii. DOI: 10.1016/j.cvsm.2007.12.003.

Keller RL, Kania SA, Hendrix DV, Ward DA, Abrams K. Evaluation of canine serum for the presence of antiretinal autoantibodies in sudden acquired retinal degeneration syndrome. *Vet Ophthalmol* 2006;**9**(3):195–200.

Miller PE, Galbreath EJ, Kehren JC, Steinberg H, Dubielzig RR. Photoreceptor cell death by apoptosis in dogs with sudden acquired retinal degeneration syndrome. *Am J Vet Res* 1998;**59**(2):149–152.

Montgomery KW, van der Woerdt A, Cottrill NB. Acute blindness in dogs: sudden acquired retinal degeneration syndrome versus neurological disease (140 cases, 2000–2006). *Vet Ophthalmol* 2008;**11**(5):314–320. DOI: 10.1111/j.1463-5224.2008.00652.x.

Stuckey JA, Pearce JW, Giuliano EA, Cohn LA, Bentley E, Rankin AJ, Gilmour MA, Lim CC, Allbaugh RA, Moore CP, Madsen RW. Long-term outcome of sudden acquired retinal degeneration syndrome in dogs. *J Am Vet Med Assoc* 2013;**243**(10):1425–1431. DOI: 10.2460/javma.243.10.1426.

Clinical Atlas of Canine and Feline Ophthalmic Disease, First Edition. Douglas Esson.

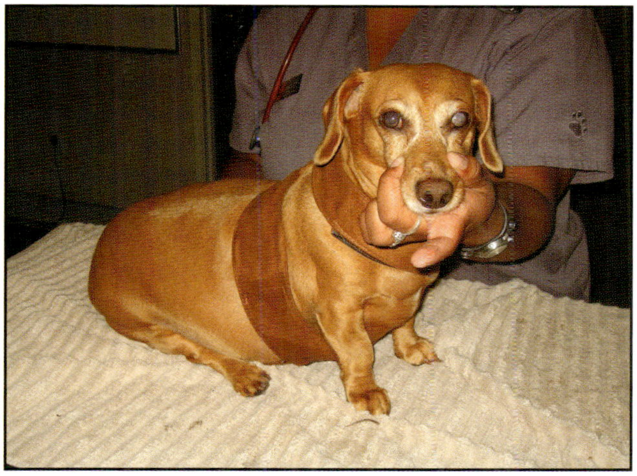

Figure 116.1 Clinical presentation associated with SARDs/IMR, comprising acute-onset dilated, poorly responsive pupils, and functional blindness in the absence of other significant ocular abnormalities.

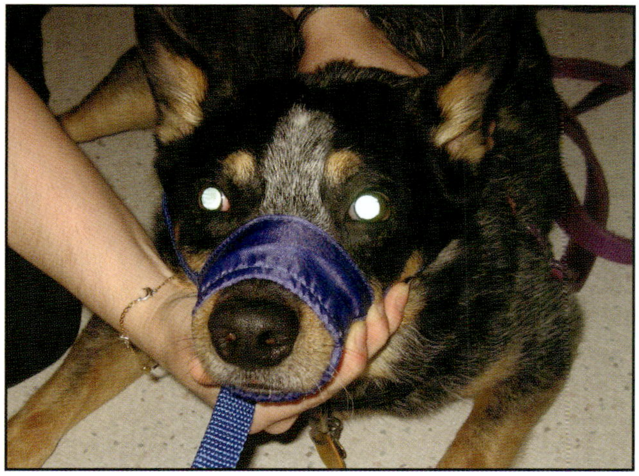

Figure 116.2 Clinical presentation associated with SARDs/IMR, comprising acute-onset dilated, poorly responsive pupils, and functional blindness in the absence of other significant ocular abnormalities.

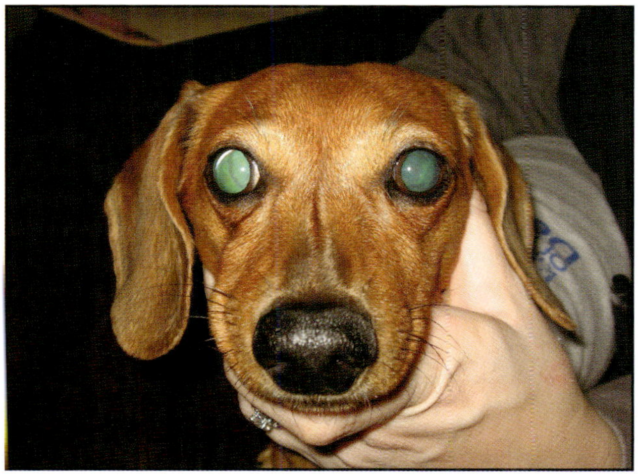

Figure 116.3 Clinical presentation associated with SARDs/IMR, comprising acute-onset dilated, poorly responsive pupils, and functional blindness in the absence of other significant ocular abnormalities.

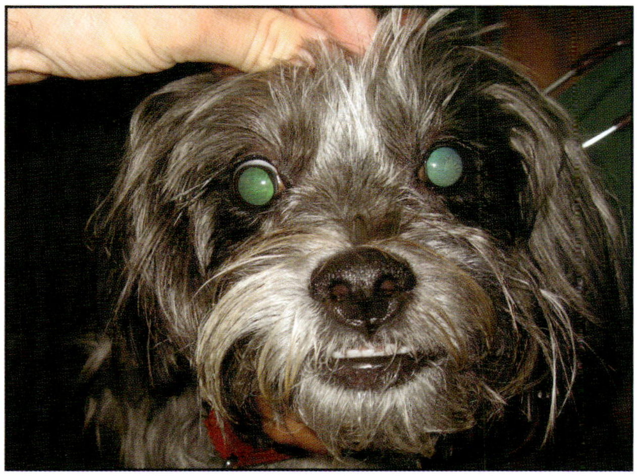

Figure 116.4 Clinical presentation associated with SARDs/IMR, comprising acute-onset dilated, poorly responsive pupils, and functional blindness in the absence of other significant ocular abnormalities.

CHAPTER 117
HYPERTENSIVE RETINOPATHY

PRESENTATION

Systemic hypertension may be primary in etiology or may occur secondary to underlying systemic disease (including renal or cardiovascular dysfunction), endocrinopathy (including hyperthyroidism, hyperadrenocorticism, diabetes mellitus), or neoplasia (including lymphoma, multiple myeloma and pheochromocytoma). Nonhypertensive, hemorrhagic retinopathy may also be associated with inflammatory, infectious, and/or neoplastic disease. Ocular changes are often the presenting symptom of systemic hypertension. Blood–ocular barrier breakdown results in variable combinations of subretinal fluid leakage, (pre, intra- or sub)retinal hemorrhage and/or detachment, hyphema, visual deficits/blindness and/or secondary glaucoma. Neurological symptoms may additionally be present. Ocular symptoms are usually bilateral; however, they are not necessarily symmetrical. Values indicative of hypertension are variable; however, systolic pressures above 160 mm Hg in cats and 140 mm Hg in dogs generally justify therapy, particularly when associated with clinical symptoms.

DIAGNOSIS AND TREATMENT

The diagnosis of hypertensive retinopathy is made based on clinical findings as well as ancillary testing, notably blood-pressure measurement. Treatment comprises addressing underlying disease where present. Blood pressure may be directly regulated, typically using amlodipine, and/or an angiotensin-converting enzyme (ACE) inhibitor where indicated, with close, regular monitoring of blood pressure being advised. Retinal hemorrhage will typically resolve, and retinal detachment may spontaneously reattach (notably in cats), depending on the chronicity and severity of the preexisting detachment. Surgical reattachment may also be considered in select cases, once underlying pathology has been addressed.

Potential Drug-Side-Effects

Adverse effects potentially associated with the use of amlodipine include lethargy. Adverse effects potentially associated with the use of ACE inhibitors include lethargy, gastrointestinal (GI) distress, and renal dysfunction.

SELECTED REFERENCES

Jepson RE. Feline systemic hypertension: classification and pathogenesis. *J Feline Med Surg* 2011;**13**(1):25–34. DOI: 10.1016/j.jfms.2010.11.007. Review.

Leblanc NL, Stepien RL, Bentley E. Ocular lesions associated with systemic hypertension in dogs: 65 cases (2005–2007). *J Am Vet Med Assoc* 2011;**238**(7):915–921.

Stepien RL. Feline systemic hypertension: diagnosis and management. *J Feline Med Surg* 2011;**13**(1):35–43. DOI: 10.1016/j.jfms.2010.11.008. Review.

Clinical Atlas of Canine and Feline Ophthalmic Disease, First Edition. Douglas Esson.

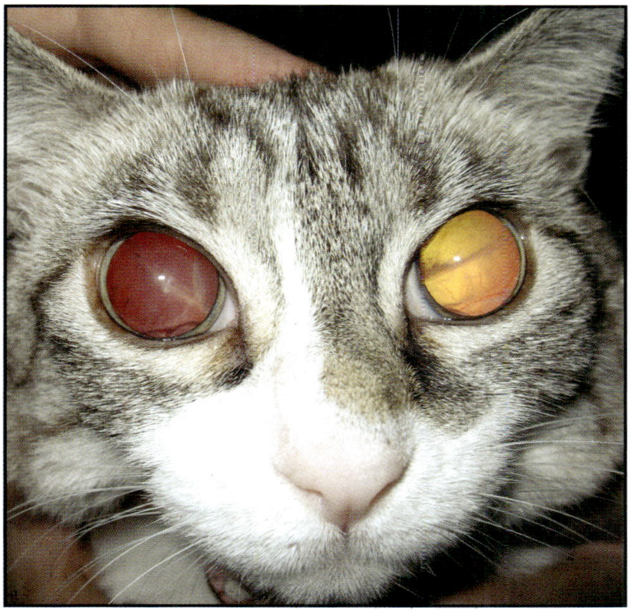

Figure 117.1 Typical clinical presentation associated with feline hypertensive retinopathy.

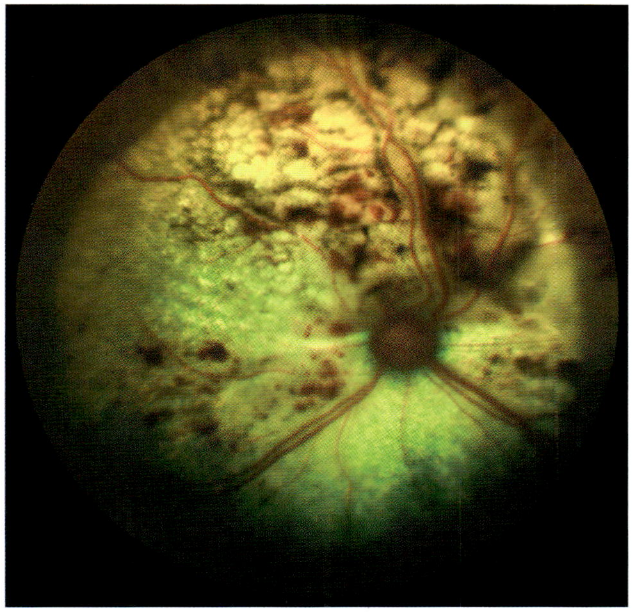

Figure 117.2 Funduscopic findings associated with feline hypertensive retinopathy. Retinal hemorrhages are notable.

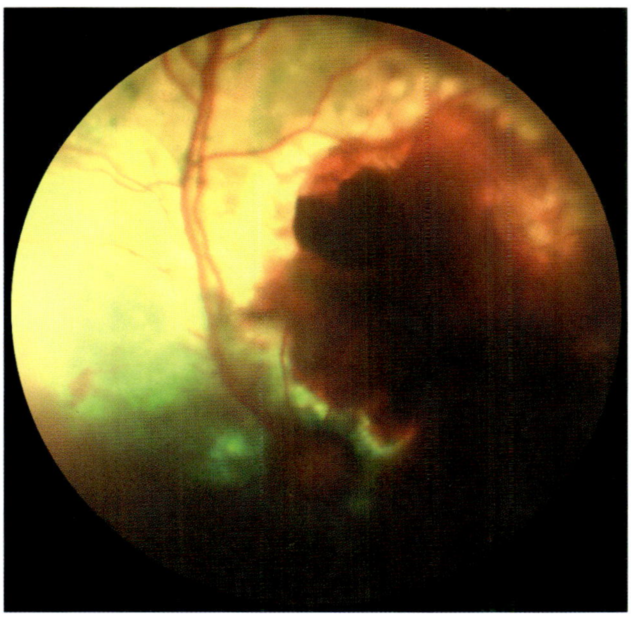

Figure 117.3 Funduscopic findings associated with feline hypertensive retinopathy. Vitreoretinal hemorrhage is notable.

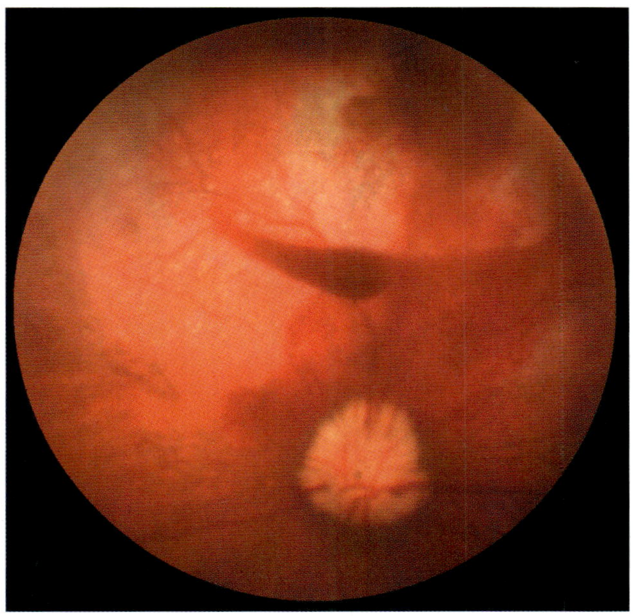

Figure 117.4 Funduscopic findings associated with canine hypertensive retinopathy. Vitreoretinal hemorrhage is notable.

CHAPTER 118
FELINE CHORIORETINITIS

PRESENTATION

The uveal tract is composed of the anterior (iris and ciliary body) and posterior (choroid) tissues. These tissues contain components of the "blood–ocular barrier," which prevents the passage of significant amounts of protein into the aqueous humor. The term uveitis describes inflammation of any of these tissues and is typically associated with variable breakdown of the blood–ocular barrier. The spectrum of clinical symptoms potentially associated with feline chorioretinitis (posterior uveitis) may include a variable degree of anterior uveitis (see also Feline Anterior Uveitis) vitritis, chorioretinal inflammation (marked by edema, exudation, hemorrhage, and/or retinal detachment), visual impairment, and/or blindness. Initially, intraocular pressures are typically decreased in patients affected by uveitis; however, secondary glaucoma may occur as a later complication. One or both eyes may be affected. Bilateral uveitis should prompt concern for the presence of systemic disease.

DIAGNOSIS AND TREATMENT

The diagnosis of chorioretinitis is made on the basis of clinical findings. Potential etiologies include trauma, systemic disease, exposure to infectious organisms, the presence of (local or systemic) neoplasia, and/or hereditary factors. Infectious etiologies which may be associated with the development of chorioretinitis in cats include viral (notably FeLV, FIV, FIP, FHV), protozoal (notably *Toxoplasma gondii*), bacterial (notably *Bartonealla* spp in cats), and fungal (notably *cryptococcus*, *coccidioides*, *aspergillus*, *blastomyces*, and *histoplasma*) organisms. Frustratingly, however, the precise etiology of uveitis remains unclear in a significant number of cases. In addition, clinical uveitis may be recurrent and or chronic in its behavior. Treatment encompasses addressing underlying systemic, infectious, or neoplastic disease. In addition, topical and/or systemic anti-inflammatory therapy (nonsteroidal or steroidal) is typically warranted. Long-term treatment may be indicated in order to minimize the risk of secondary glaucoma. Clindamycin generally represents a suitable empirical/initial antimicrobial choice.

Potential Drug-Side-Effects

Potential side effects associated with the use of clindamycin include gastrointestinal (GI) distress.

SELECTED REFERENCES

Colitz CM. Feline uveitis: diagnosis and treatment. *Clin Tech Small Anim Pract* 2005;**20**(2):117–120.

van der Woerdt A. Management of intraocular inflammatory disease. *Clin Tech Small Anim Pract* 2001;**16**(1):58–61.

Townsend WM. Canine and feline uveitis. *Vet Clin North Am Small Anim Pract* 2008;**38**(2):323–346, vii. DOI: 10.1016/j.cvsm.2007.12.004.

Clinical Atlas of Canine and Feline Ophthalmic Disease, First Edition. Douglas Esson.

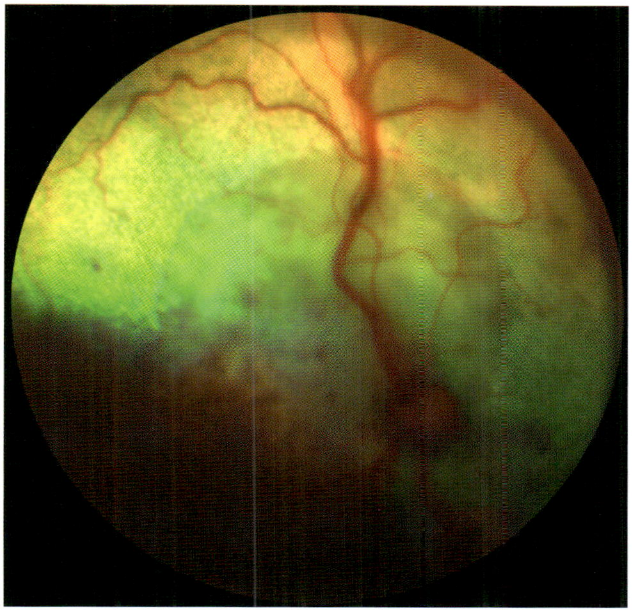

Figure 118.1 Funduscopic changes in association with active feline chorioretinitis due to *toxoplasmosis*.

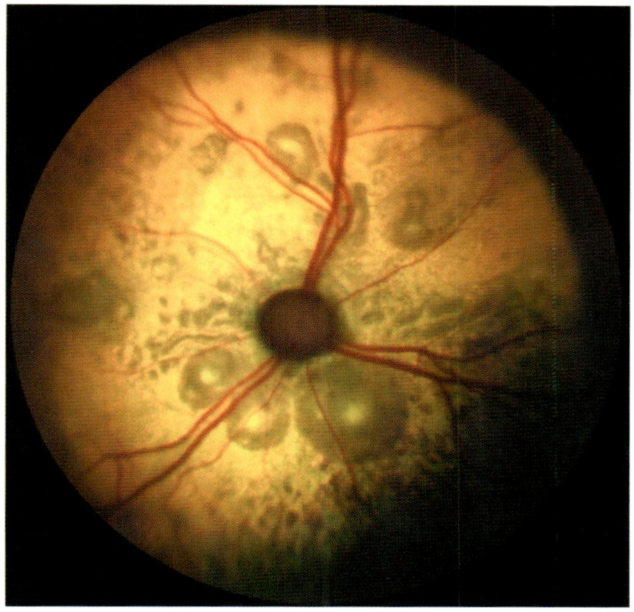

Figure 118.2 Funduscopic changes in association with active feline chorioretinitis due to *cryptococcosis*.

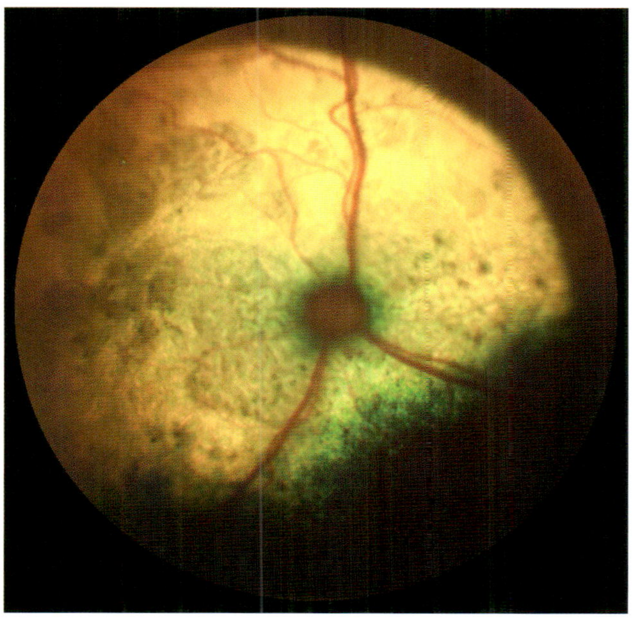

Figure 118.3 Funduscopic changes in association with active feline chorioretinitis due to *FeLV*.

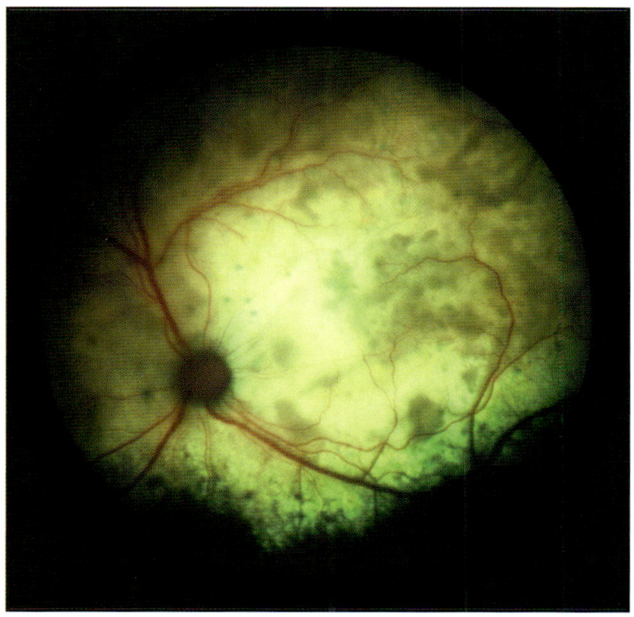

Figure 118.4 Funduscopic changes in association with active feline chorioretinitis due to *bartonellosis*.

CHAPTER 119
CANINE CHORIORETINITIS

PRESENTATION

The uveal tract is composed of the anterior (iris and ciliary body) and posterior (choroid) tissues. These tissues contain components of the "blood–ocular barrier," which prevents the passage of significant amounts of protein into the aqueous humor. The term uveitis describes inflammation of any of these tissues and is typically associated with variable breakdown of the blood–ocular barrier. The spectrum of clinical symptoms potentially associated with canine chorioretinitis (posterior uveitis) may include a variable degree of anterior uveitis (see also Canine Anterior Uveitis) vitritis, chorioretinal inflammation (marked by edema, exudation, hemorrhage, and/or retinal detachment), visual impairment, and/or blindness. Initially, intraocular pressures are typically decreased in patients affected by uveitis; however, secondary glaucoma may occur as a complication. One or both eyes may be affected. Bilateral uveitis should prompt concern for the presence of systemic disease.

DIAGNOSIS AND TREATMENT

The diagnosis of chorioretinitis is made on the basis of clinical findings. Potential etiologies include trauma, systemic disease, exposure to infectious organisms, the presence of (local or systemic) neoplasia and/or hereditary factors. Infectious etiologies that may be associated with the development of chorioretinitis in dogs include viral (notably canine adenovirus-1 and canine parvovirus), protozoal (notably Toxoplasma gondii), bacterial (notably *Ehrlichia* canis, Rickettsia *rickettsia*, Leptospira spp and *Borrelia* spp) and fungal (notably *coccidioides*, aspergillus, blastomyces and histoplasma) organisms. Frustratingly, however, the precise etiology of uveitis remains idiopathic in a significant number of cases. In addition, clinical uveitis may be recurrent and or chronic in its behavior. Treatment encompasses addressing underlying systemic, infectious, or neoplastic disease. In addition, topical and/or systemic anti-inflammatory therapy (non-steroidal or steroidal) is typically warranted. Long-term treatment may be indicated in order to minimize the risk of secondary glaucoma. Mydriatic agents (atropine/tropicamide) should be used with caution where indicated. Doxycycline generally represents a suitable empirical/initial antimicrobial choice.

Potential Drug-Side-Effects

Potential side effects associated with the use of doxycycline, include gastrointestinal (GI) distress.

SELECTED REFERENCES

Peiffer RL, Cook CS, Möller I. Therapeutic strategies involving antimicrobial treatment of ophthalmic disease in small animals. *J Am Vet Med Assoc* 1984;**185**(10):1172–1175.

Massa KL, Gilger BC, Miller TL, Davidson MG. Causes of uveitis in dogs: 102 cases (1989–2000). *Vet Ophthalmol* 2002;**5**(2):93–98.

Townsend WM. Canine and feline uveitis. *Vet Clin North Am Small Anim Pract* 2008;**38**(2):323–346, vii. DOI: 10.1016/j.cvsm.2007.12.004.

Clinical Atlas of Canine and Feline Ophthalmic Disease, First Edition. Douglas Esson.

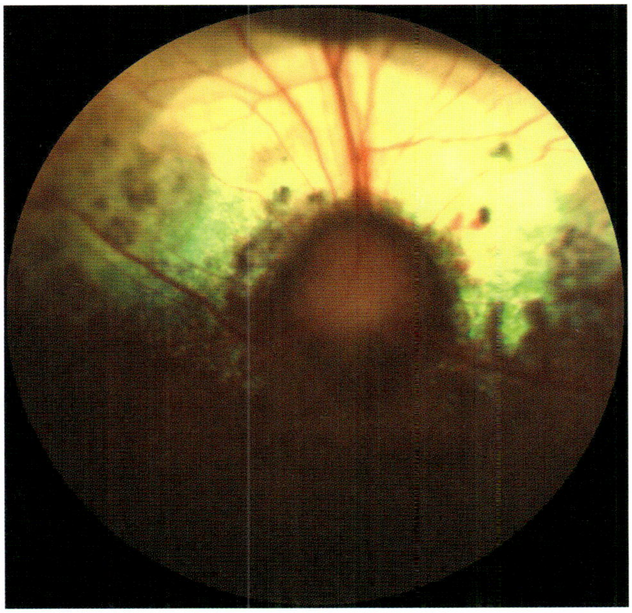

Figure 119.1 Funduscopic changes in association with active canine chorioretinitis due to *toxoplasmosis*.

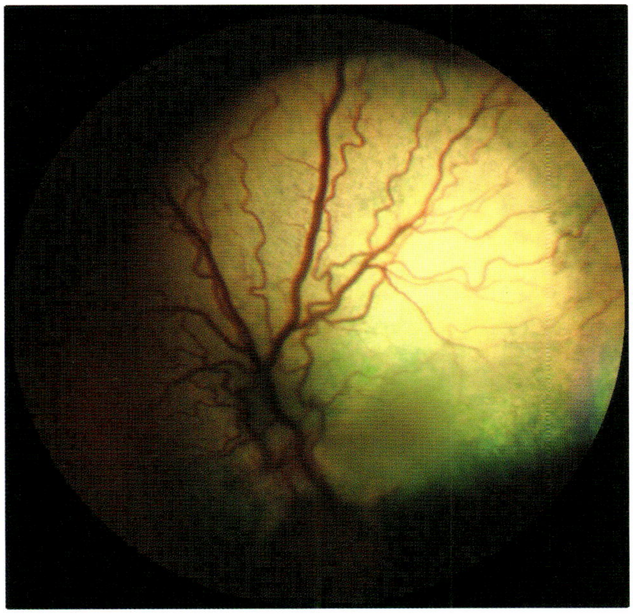

Figure 119.2 Funduscopic changes in association with active canine chorioretinitis due to *coccidioidomycosis*.

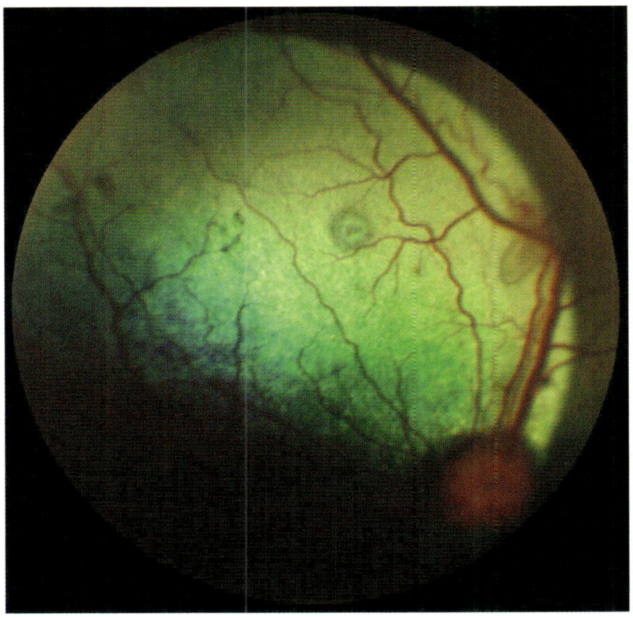

Figure 119.3 Funduscopic changes in association with active canine chorioretinitis due to *blastomycosis*.

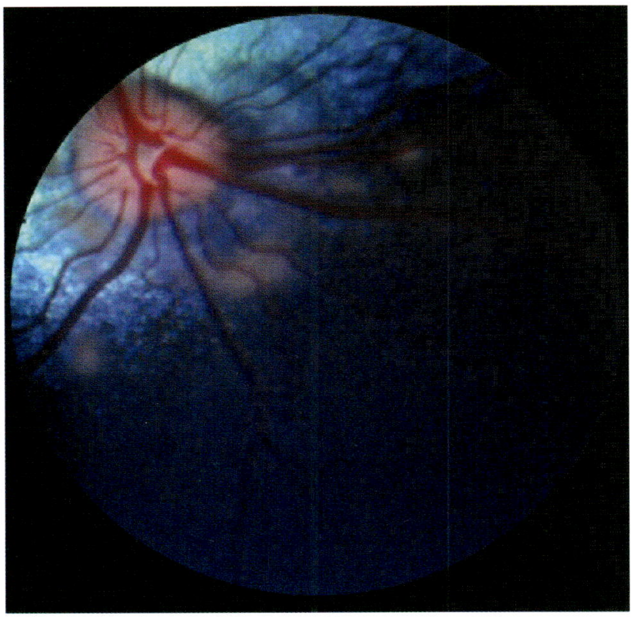

Figure 119.4 Funduscopic changes in association with active canine chorioretinitis due to *ehrlichiosis*.

CHAPTER 120
RETINAL PIGMENT EPITHELIAL DYSTROPHY (RPED)

PRESENTATION

Retinal pigment epithelial dystrophy (RPED) describes a disease of the retinal pigment epithelium, marked by the pathological accumulation of lipofuscin and may be associated with more widespread secondary retinal degeneration. This condition has also been referred to as central progressive retinal atrophy (CPRA). Clinically, this disease manifests as decreased visual function (which may progress to outright blindness), subtle neurological defects (notably proprioceptive deficits), and/or secondary cataract formation. Funduscopically, disease presentation is characterized by the (bilateral) presence of scattered tan to brown foci, which may coalesce with time. More generalized secondary retinal degeneration typically ensues. Similarities between this disease and deficiencies in the availability and absorption/metabolism of vitamin E have also been noted. Commonly affected breeds include the Labrador Retriever, Golden Retriever, Cocker Spaniel, Briard, and the Collie breeds, notably in European populations.

DIAGNOSIS AND TREATMENT

The diagnosis of retinal pigment epithelial dystrophy is made based on clinical and funduscopic findings. The supplementation of large doses of oral vitamin E (600–900 iu bid) has been advocated and may help limit disease progression.

SELECTED REFERENCES

Lightfoot RM, Cabral L, Gooch L, Bedford PG, Boulton ME. Retinal pigment epithelial dystrophy in Briard dogs. *Res Vet Sci* 1996;**60**(1):17–23.

McLellan GJ, Bedford PG. Oral vitamin E absorption in English Cocker Spaniels with familial vitamin E deficiency and retinal pigment epithelial dystrophy. *Vet Ophthalmol* 2012;**15**(Suppl 2):48–56. DOI: 10.1111/j.1463-5224.2012.01049.x. Epub 2012 Jul 25.

McLellan GJ, Cappello R, Mayhew IG, Elks R, Lybaert P, Watté C, Bedford PG. Clinical and pathological observations in English cocker spaniels with primary metabolic vitamin E deficiency and retinal pigment epithelial dystrophy. *Vet Rec* 2003;**153**(10):287–292.

Clinical Atlas of Canine and Feline Ophthalmic Disease, First Edition. Douglas Esson.

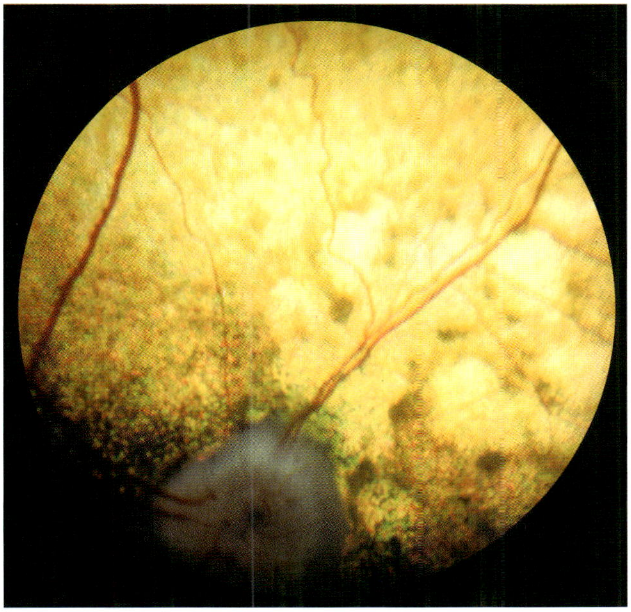

Figure 120.1 Funduscopic changes associated with retinal pigment epithelial dystrophy (RPED). Multiple discrete areas representing lipofuscin accumulation are visible.

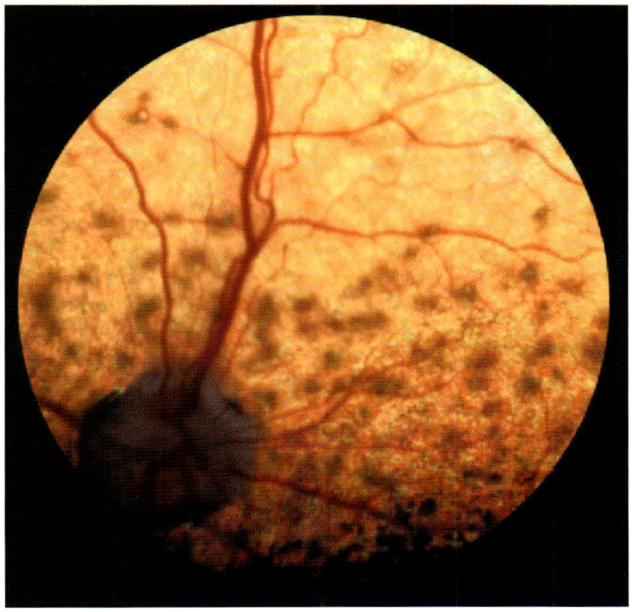

Figure 120.2 Funduscopic changes associated with retinal pigment epithelial dystrophy (RPED). Multiple discrete areas representing lipofuscin accumulation are visible.

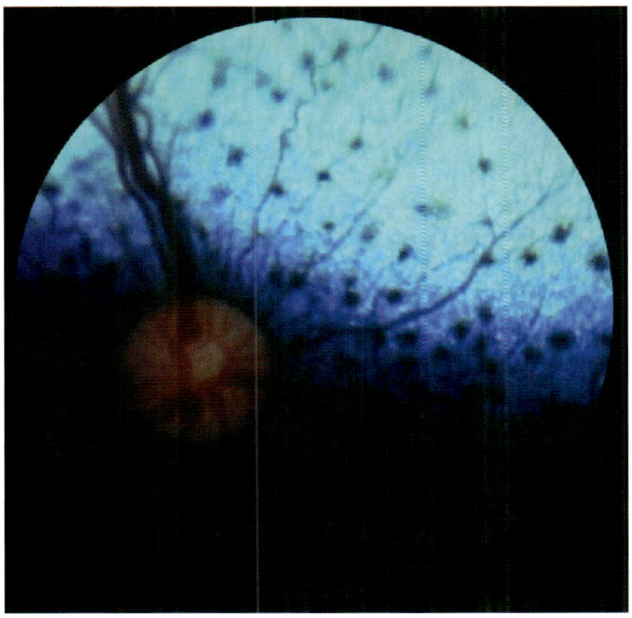

Figure 120.3 Funduscopic changes associated with retinal pigment epithelial dystrophy (RPED). Multiple discrete areas representing lipofuscin accumulation are visible.

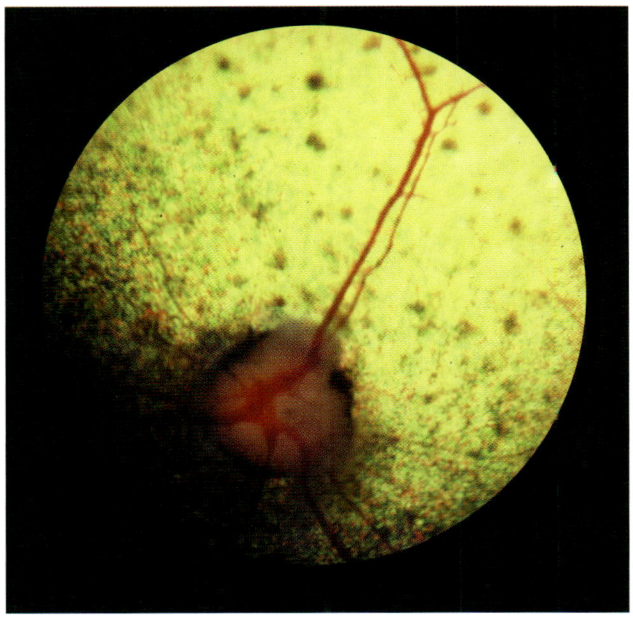

Figure 120.4 Funduscopic changes associated with retinal pigment epithelial dystrophy (RPED). Multiple discrete areas representing lipofuscin accumulation are visible.

CHAPTER 121
UVEODERMATOLOGIC SYNDROME (UDS)-ASSOCIATED CHORIORETINITIS

PRESENTATION

Canine uveodermatologic syndrome (UDS) represents an immune-mediated disease, predominantly affecting melanocytic tissues, likely hereditary in etiology and exhibiting many similarities to Vogt-Koyanagi-Harada (VKH) disease in humans. This condition has consequently also been referred to as *VKH-like disease*. Ocular symptoms associated with UDS may include any combination of anterior uveitis, chorioretinitis, or panuveitis, frequently marked by pigment loss. Secondary changes may include any combination of cataract formation, retinal detachment, hyphema, and/or glaucoma. Typically, both eyes are affected to a variable degree. Additional symptoms may include any combination of periocular, mucocutaneous, oral and/or nasal vitiligo (loss of pigment), poliosis (whitening of hair), and/or ulcerative dermatitis. Typically, these symptoms are relatively bilaterally symmetrical in appearance (see also Autoimmune Blepharitis and Uveodermatologic Syndrome (UDS)-Associated Uveitis). Commonly affected breeds include the Akita, Siberian Husky, Samoyed, Chow Chow, German Shepherd, and Shetland Sheepdog.

DIAGNOSIS AND TREATMENT

The diagnosis of UDS is made on the basis of a combination of signalment and clinical findings. Where representative adnexal or dermal changes are present, the harvesting of a small incisional skin biopsy for histopathological interpretation may support the diagnosis. Treatment usually comprises aggressive, long-term anti-inflammatory and/or immune-modulating therapy. Typically, this involves the topical and systemic administration of corticosteroids with or without the adjunctive use of additional agents including cyclosporine and/or azathioprine.

Potential Drug-Side-Effects

Potential adverse effects associated with the use of topical corticosteroids include impaired wound healing and corneal degeneration. Potential adverse effects associated with the use of systemic corticosteroids include polyphagia, polydipsia, polyuria, hair coat changes, weight gain, pancreatitis, enteritis, muscular damage, hepatic impairment, and diabetes. Potential adverse effects associated with the use of azathioprine include gastrointestinal (GI) distress, pancreatitis, hepatotoxicity, and myelosuppression. Potential adverse affects associated with the use of cyclosporine include hypersensitivity and GI distress.

SELECTED REFERENCES

Angles JM, Famula TR, Pedersen NC. Uveodermatologic (VKH-like) syndrome in American Akita dogs is associated with an increased frequency of DQA1*00201. *Tissue Antigens* 2005;**66**(6):656–665.

Carter WJ, Crispin SM, Gould DJ, Day MJ. An immunohistochemical study of uveodermatologic syndrome in two Japanese Akita dogs. *Vet Ophthalmol* 2005;**8**(1):17–24.

Horikawa T, Vaughan RK, Sargent SJ, Toops EE, Locke EP. Pathology in practice. Uveodermatologic syndrome. *J Am Vet Med Assoc* 2013;**242**(6):759–761. DOI: 10.2460/javma.242.6.759.

Clinical Atlas of Canine and Feline Ophthalmic Disease, First Edition. Douglas Esson.

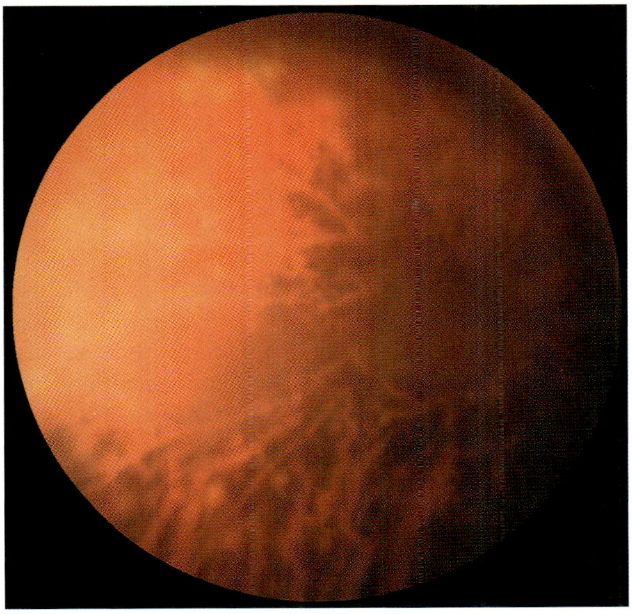

Figure 121.1 Funduscopic changes due to canine uveodermatologic syndrome (UDS). Notable are focal to coalescing areas displaying loss of choriodal pigment.

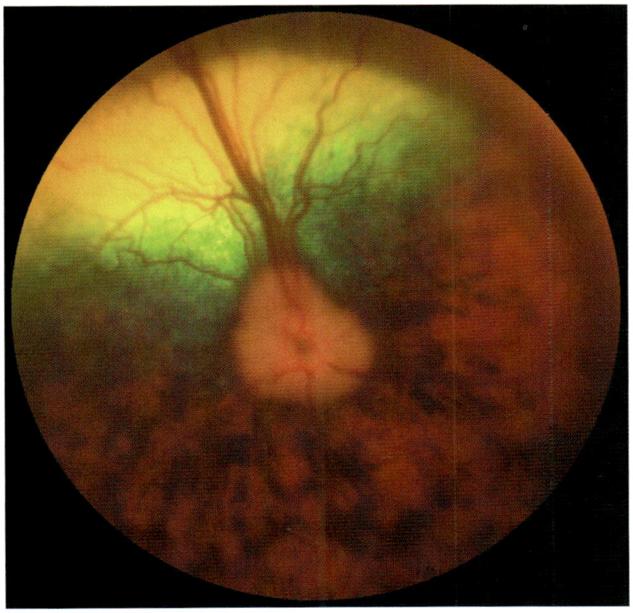

Figure 121.2 Funduscopic changes due to canine uveodermatologic syndrome (UDS). Notable are focal to coalescing areas displaying loss of choriodal pigment.

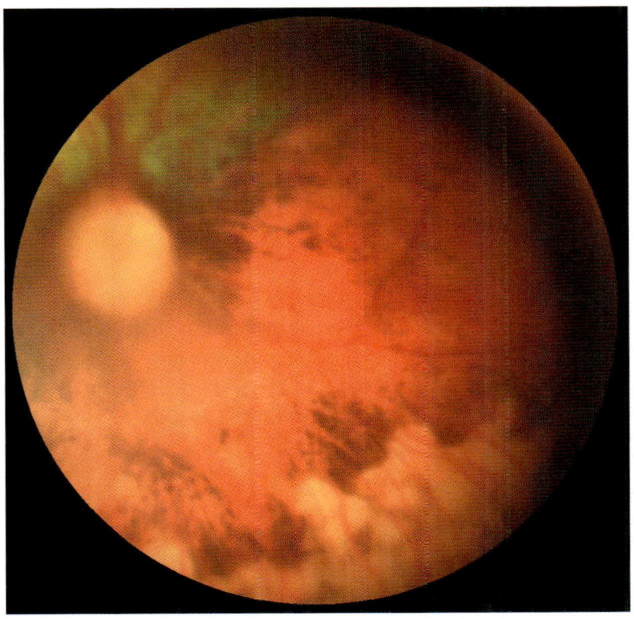

Figure 121.3 Funduscopic changes due to canine uveodermatologic syndrome (UDS). Notable are focal to coalescing areas displaying loss of choriodal pigment.

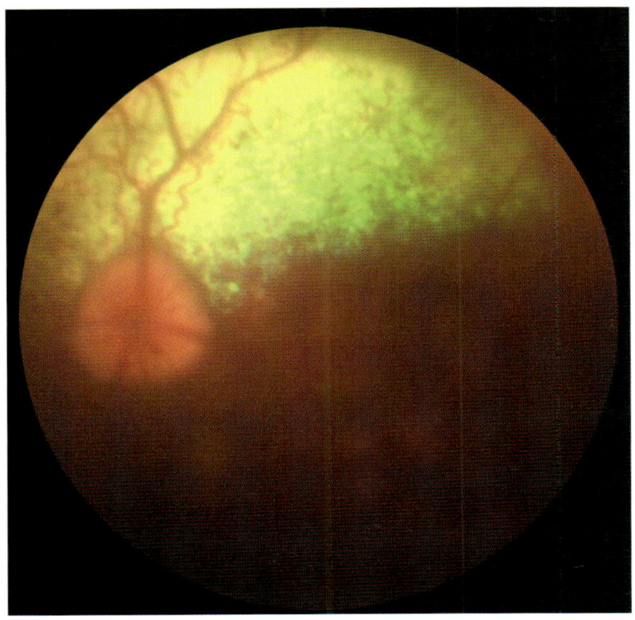

Figure 121.4 Funduscopic changes due to canine uveodermatologic syndrome (UDS). Notable are focal to coalescing areas displaying loss of choriodal pigment.

CHAPTER 122
PRIMARY (BULLOUS) RETINAL DETACHMENT

PRESENTATION

Primary, bullous retinal detachment represents a separation of the neurosensory retina from the underlying retinal pigment epithelium (RPE) due to subretinal fluid accumulation. This process is suspected to be immune-mediated in etiology. Clinical symptoms typically comprise bilaterally dilated poorly, or nonresponsive pupils in association with acute-onset blindness. Retinal tissue may be noted to be "billowing" forward posterior to the level of the pupils. Funduscopically, complete or multiple areas of (non-hemorrhagic) bullous detachment are noted. Commonly affected breeds include the German Shepherd, Australian Shepherd, and Labrador Retriever.

DIAGNOSIS AND TREATMENT

The diagnosis of bullous retinal detachment is made on the basis of clinical findings (including funduscopy), supported if necessary by B-mode ultrasonography. Bullous detachments are typically responsive to medical therapy comprising anti-inflammatory to immunosuppressive doses of systemic corticosteroids. The term steroid-responsive retinal detachment has also been used to describe this condition. Underlying systemic pathology should be ruled out through routine complete blood count (CBC)/chemistry and infectious titer testing, imaging, and the measurement of systemic blood pressure. Where a positive response to therapy is achieved, the withdrawal of corticosteroids should be pursued cautiously, with some patients requiring long-term treatment.

Potential Drug-Side-Effects

Potential adverse effects associated with the use of systemic corticosteroids include polyphagia, polydipsia, polyuria, hair coat changes, weight gain, pancreatitis, gastrointestinal (GI) distress, muscle damage, hepatic impairment, and diabetes.

SELECTED REFERENCES

Andrew SE, Abrams KL, Brooks DE, Kublis PS. Clinical features of steroid responsive retinal detachments in twenty-two dogs. *Vet Comp Ophthalmol* 1997;7:82–87.

Grahn BH, Wolfer J. Diagnostic ophthalmology. Bilateral multifocal serous retinal detachments. *Can Vet J* 1997;**38**(4):250–251.

Wolfer J, Grahn B, Arrington K. Diagnostic ophthalmology. Bilateral, bullous retinal detachment. *Can Vet J* 1998;**39**(1):57–58.

Clinical Atlas of Canine and Feline Ophthalmic Disease, First Edition. Douglas Esson.

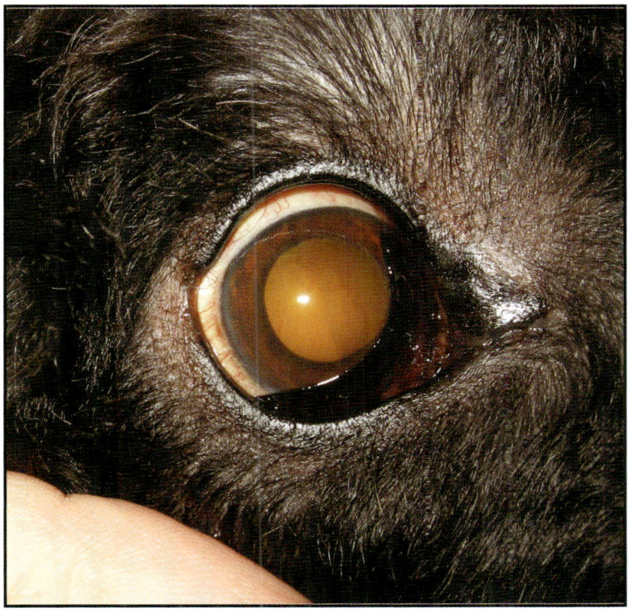

Figure 122.1 Ocular findings associated with primary (bullous) retinal detachment. Bullous retinal detachment can frequently be diagnosed by simple external examination, as shown in this figure.

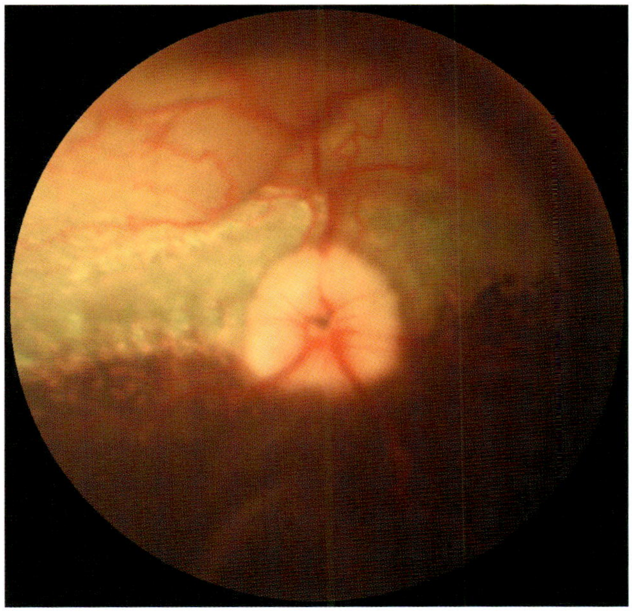

Figure 122.2 Funduscopic findings associated with primary (bullous) retinal detachment.

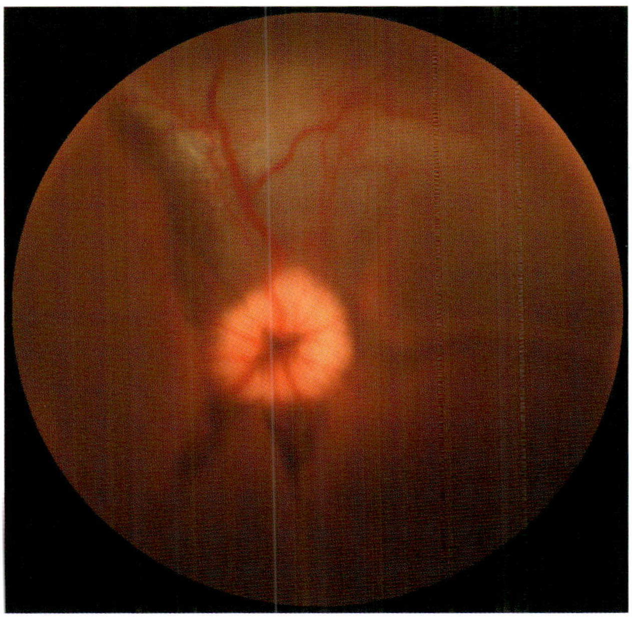

Figure 122.3 Funduscopic findings associated with primary (bullous) retinal detachment.

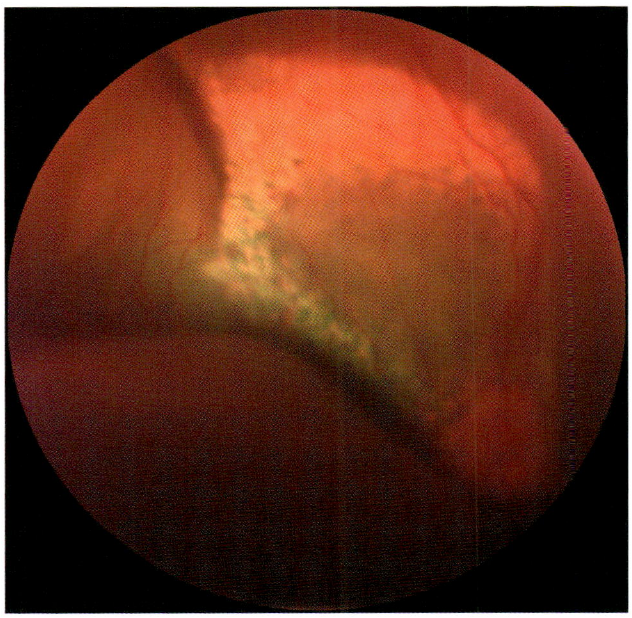

Figure 122.4 Funduscopic findings associated with primary (bullous) retinal detachment.

CHAPTER 123
RHEGMATOGENOUS RETINAL DETACHMENT (RRD)

PRESENTATION

Rhegmatogenous retinal detachment represents a separation of the neurosensory retina from the underlying retinal pigment epithelium (RPE) stemming from a break in the retinal tissue. Rhegmatogenous detachments may be

- primary (spontaneous)—particularly around the ora ciliaris retinae and frequently in association with vitreoretinal degeneration
- secondary—arising as a result of inflammation and/or trauma.

Clinical symptoms may include dilated, poorly responsive pupil(s), vitreous degeneration, herniation, and/or hemorrhage visual deficits and/or blindness. Funduscopically retinal tears and/or folds may be visualized; however, accurate visualization is frequently challenging. Symptoms may be unilateral or bilateral. Frequently affected breeds include the Shih Tzu, Bichon Frisé, Italian Greyhound, Yorkshire Terrier, Jack Russell Terrier, and Labrador Retriever.

DIAGNOSIS AND TREATMENT

The diagnosis of rhegmatogenous retinal detachment is made on the basis of clinical findings (including funduscopy), supported if necessary by B-mode ultrasonography. Medical therapy is unlikely to result in resolution of rhegmatogenous retinal detachment. Where pathology is relatively recent (1–3 weeks) and significant secondary complications have not developed, surgical options include the following:

- Transpupillary laser "barrier" retinopexy—most suitable for cases involving limited pathology such as small tears or holes or lesions associated with geographic retinal dysplasia;
- Complete retinal reattachment, typically encompassing endoscopic retinopexy, vitrectomy, and silicone oil exchange.

SELECTED REFERENCES

Grahn BH, Barnes LD, Breaux CB, Sandmeyer LS. Chronic retinal detachment and giant retinal tears in 34 dogs: outcome comparison of no treatment, topical medical therapy, and retinal reattachment after vitrectomy. *Can Vet J* 2007;**48**(10):1031–1039.

Papaioannou NG, Dubielzig RR. Histopathological and immunohistochemical features of vitreoretinopathy in Shih Tzu dogs. *J Comp Pathol* 2013;**148**(2–3):230–235. DOI: 10.1016/j.jcpa.2012.05.014. Epub 2012 Jul 20.

Steele KA, Sisler S, Gerding PA. Outcome of retinal reattachment surgery in dogs: a retrospective study of 145 cases. *Vet Ophthalmol* 2012;**15**(Suppl 2):35–40. DOI: 10.1111/j.1463-5224.2012.01009.x. Epub 2012 Mar 29.

Vainisi SJ, Wolfer JC. Canine retinal surgery. *Vet Ophthalmol* 2004;**7**(5):291–306.

Clinical Atlas of Canine and Feline Ophthalmic Disease, First Edition. Douglas Esson.

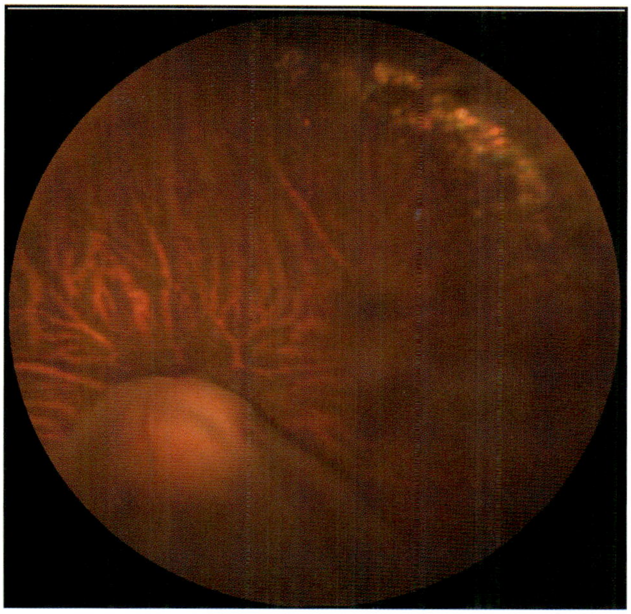

Figure 123.1 Complete peripheral rhegmatogenous detachment such that the neuroretina remains anchored around the optic nerve head (sometimes described as a *hanging veil* detachment).

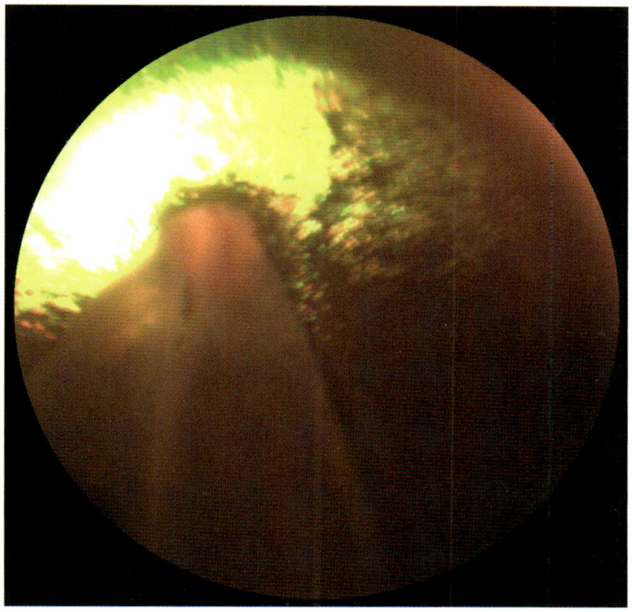

Figure 123.2 Complete peripheral rhegmatogenous detachment such that the neuroretina remains anchored around the optic nerve head (sometimes described as a *hanging veil* detachment).

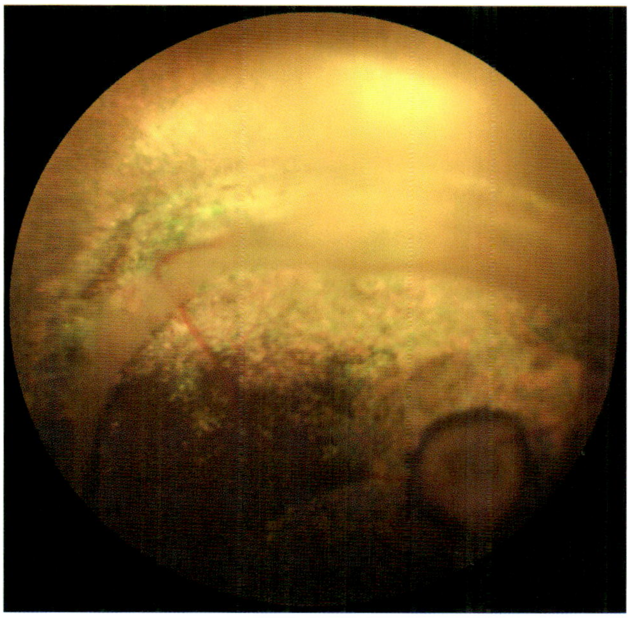

Figure 123.3 Retinal detachment in association with a giant retinal tear.

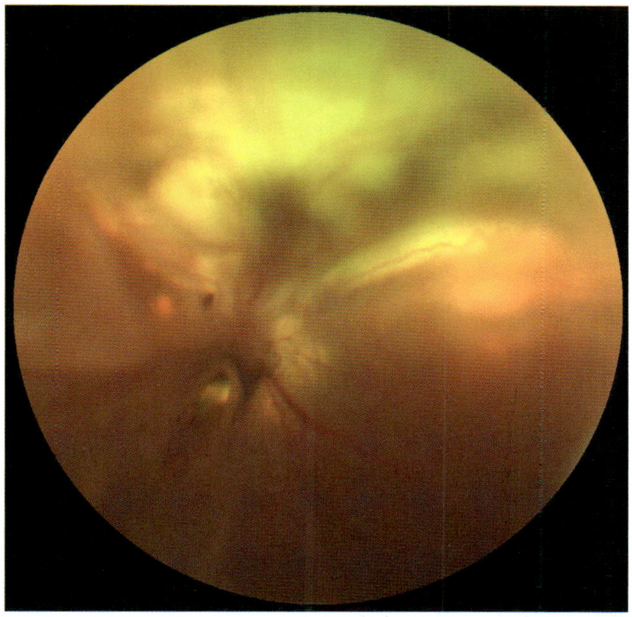

Figure 123.4 Retinal detachment in association with a small retinal tear.

CHAPTER 124
CHORIORETINAL LYMPHOMA

PRESENTATION

Lymphoma affecting the posterior segment occurs with the highest frequency in combination with systemic neoplasia, although, in some cases, ocular changes may precede systemic symptoms. One, or more commonly both, eye(s) may be affected and associated ocular findings may include any combination of visual deficits, anterior or panuveitis, retinal hemorrhage and/or detachment, and/or glaucoma (see also Feline Chorioretinitis, Canine Chorioretinitis, and Uveal Lymphoma). Systemic symptoms may include any combination of weight loss, lethargy, inappetence, gastrointestinal (GI) distress, pyrexia, lymphadenopathy, organomegaly, hypercalcemia, and/or anemia. Both canine and feline species of any breed or crossed breed may be affected.

DIAGNOSIS AND TREATMENT

The diagnosis of lymphoma may be made on the basis of clinical findings, ancillary imaging, cytological/histological interpretation, polymerase chain reaction (PCR) analysis of samples obtained by aqueocentesis as well as lymph node and/or affected organ aspiration/biopsy. Treatment comprises topical anti-inflammatory therapy (typically utilizing a corticosteroid) as well as systemic chemotherapy. Associated ophthalmic changes such as elevated intraocular pressure should be addressed as appropriate. Staging via local lymph node (and/or organ/bone marrow) aspiration, three-view radiography, and complete blood count (CBC)/chemistry analysis is recommended before initiation of systemic chemotherapy. Diagnostic testing for infectious viruses including FeLV, FIV, and FIP is additionally recommended in feline patients. Individual chemotherapeutic protocols are most ideally designed by a veterinary oncologist; however, they typically include a variable combination of prednisone, vincristine, cyclophosphamide, and/or doxyrubicin.

Potential Drug-Side-Effects

Potential adverse effects associated with the use of systemic cortiocosteroids include polyphagia, polydipsia, polyuria, hair coat changes, weight gain, pancreatitis, gastrointestinal (GI) distress, muscle damage, hepatic impairment, and diabetes. Potential adverse effects associated with the use of vincristine include stomatitis, GI distress, neuropathy, hepatopathy, and myelosuppression. Potential adverse effects associated with the use of cyclophospamide include GI distress, pancreatitis, hepatotoxicity, and myelosuppression. Potential adverse affects associated with the use of doxyrubicin include hypersensitivity, GI distress, cardiac dysfunction, and myelosuppression.

The prognosis varies depending on the extent of disease present before initiating therapy.

SELECTED REFERENCES

Massa KL, Gilger BC, Miller TL, Davidson MG. Causes of uveitis in dogs: 102 cases (1989–2000). *Vet Ophthalmol* 2002;**5**(2):93–98.

Nerschbach V, Eule JC, Eberle N, Höinghaus R, Betz D. Ocular manifestation of lymphoma in newly diagnosed cats. *Vet Comp Oncol* 2013. DOI: 10.1111/vco.12061.

Ota-Kuroki J, Ragsdale JM, Bawa B, Wakamatsu N, Kuroki K. Intraocular and periocular lymphoma in dogs and cats: a retrospective review of 21 cases (2001–2012). *Vet Ophthalmol* 2013. DOI: 10.1111/vop.12106.

Rutley M, MacDonald V. Managing the canine lymphosarcoma patient in general practice. *Can Vet J* 2007;**48**(9):977–979.

Clinical Atlas of Canine and Feline Ophthalmic Disease, First Edition. Douglas Esson.

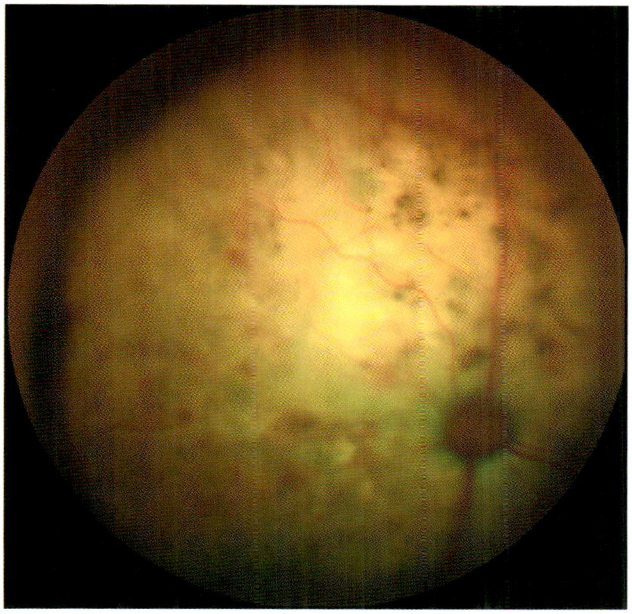

Figure 124.1 Funduscopic findings associated with chorioretinal lymphoma, including chorioretinitis, exudation, sub-retinal infiltration and hemorrhage.

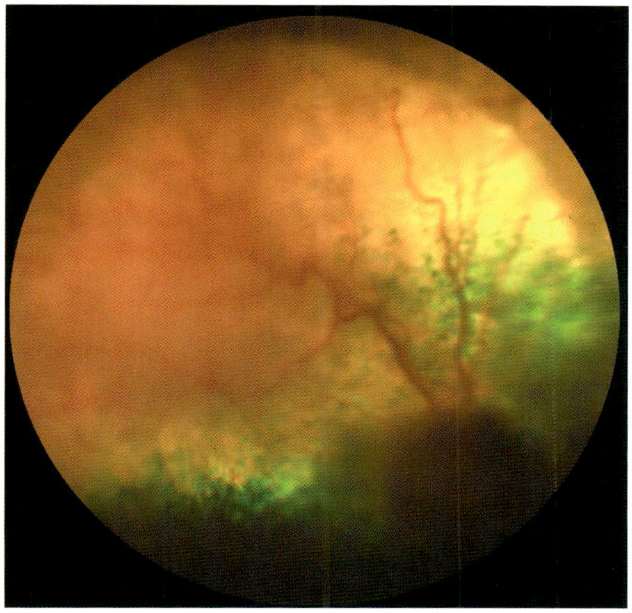

Figure 124.2 Funduscopic findings associated with chorioretinal lymphoma, including chorioretinitis, exudation, sub-retinal infiltration and hemorrhage.

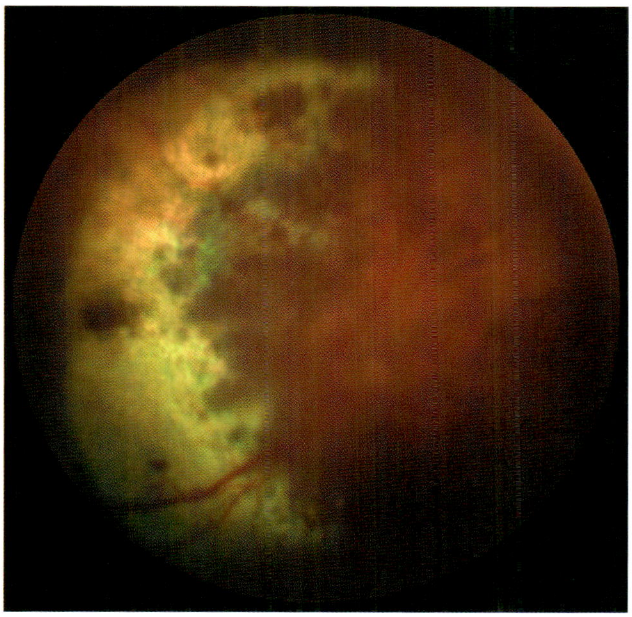

Figure 124.3 Funduscopic findings associated with chorioretinal lymphoma, including chorioretinitis, exudation, sub-retinal infiltration and hemorrhage.

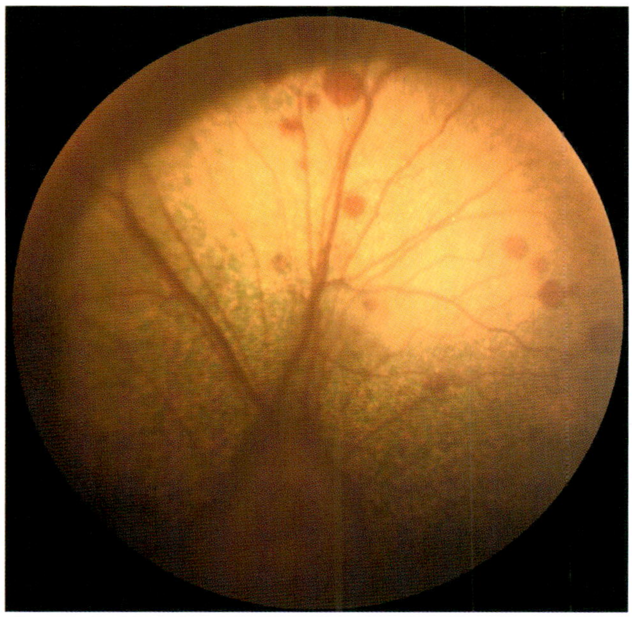

Figure 124.4 Funduscopic findings associated with chorioretinal lymphoma, including chorioretinitis, exudation, sub-retinal infiltration and hemorrhage.

CHAPTER 125
MYELOMA

PRESENTATION

The neoplastic proliferation of plasma cells may result in solitary or multiple plasmacytomas (typically affecting osseous and/or soft tissue), as well as multiple myeloma (typically associated with bone marrow as well as generalized symptoms that may include any combination of lethargy, discomfort, osteolysis, pathologic fractures, and/or renal dysfunction). Ophthalmic findings may include any combination of visual deficits, anterior uveitis, chorioretinitis, retinal hemorrhage, retinal detachment, and/or secondary glaucoma. Ancillary laboratory findings may include hyperglobulinemia, anemia, thrombocytopenia, neutropenia, and/or hypercalcemia. Commonly affected breeds include the Cocker Spaniel, the German Shepherd, and the Boxer.

DIAGNOSIS AND TREATMENT

The diagnosis of myeloma is made on the basis of clinical findings as well as serum electrophoresis and/or bone marrow evaluation. Treatment comprises surgical excision where possible as well as case-specific chemotherapy and/or radiation therapy. Commonly employed chemotherapeutic agents include prednisone, melphalan, and cyclophosphamide.

Potential Drug-Side-Effects

Potential adverse effects associated with the use of systemic corticosteroids include polyphagia, polydipsia, polyuria, hair coat changes, weight gain, pancreatitis, enteritis, muscular damage, hepatic impairment, and diabetes. Potential adverse effects associated with the use of melphalan include gastrointestinal (GI) distress and myelosuppression. Potential adverse effects associated with the use of cyclophosphamide include GI distress, myelosuppression, and hemorrhagic cystitis.

SELECTED REFERENCES

Breuer W, Colbatzky F, Platz S, Hermanns W. Immunoglobulin-producing tumours in dogs and cats. *J Comp Pathol* 1993;**109**(3):203–216.

Hendrix DV, Gelatt KN, Smith PJ, Brooks DE, Whittaker CJ, Chmielewski NT. Ophthalmic disease as the presenting complaint in five dogs with multiple myeloma. *J Am Anim Hosp Assoc* 1998;**34**(2):121–128.

Patel RT, Caceres A, French AF, McManus PM. Multiple myeloma in 16 cats: a retrospective study. *Vet Clin Pathol* 2005;**34**(4):341–352.

Clinical Atlas of Canine and Feline Ophthalmic Disease, First Edition. Douglas Esson.

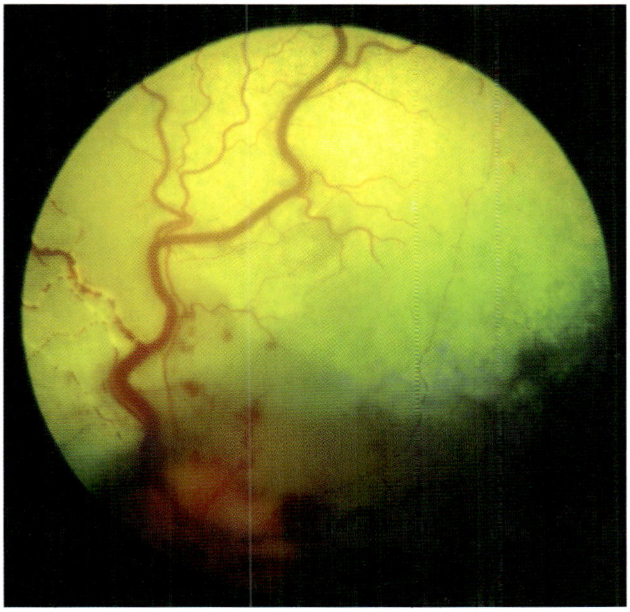

Figure 125.1 Funduscopic changes associated with multiple myeloma including chorioretinitis, exudation, hemorrhage and papillitis. Vascular congestion marked by "box-carring" is notable.

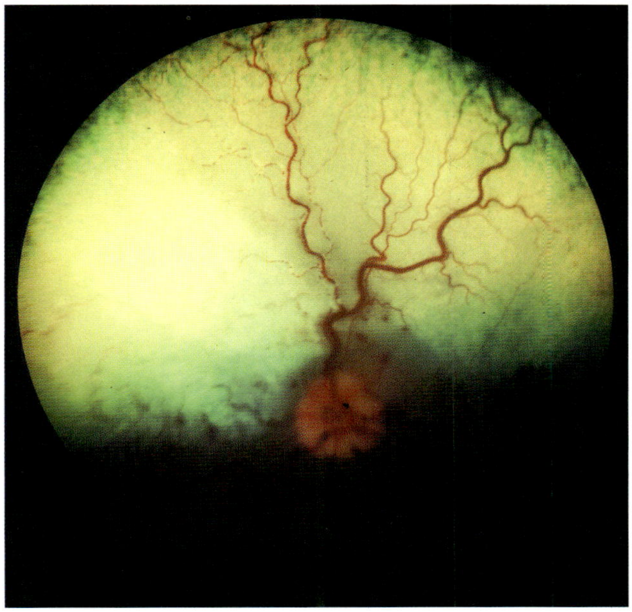

Figure 125.2 Funduscopic changes associated with multiple myeloma including chorioretinitis, exudation, hemorrhage and papillitis. Vascular congestion marked by "box-carring" is notable.

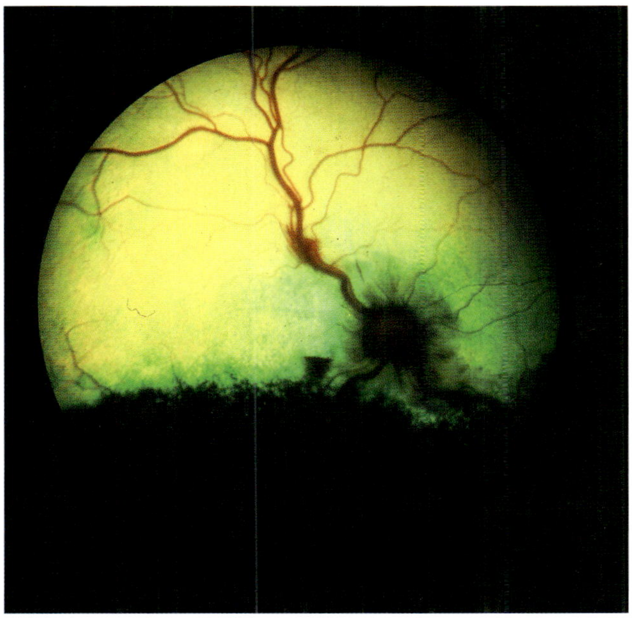

Figure 125.3 Funduscopic changes associated with multiple myeloma including chorioretinitis, exudation, hemorrhage and papillitis.

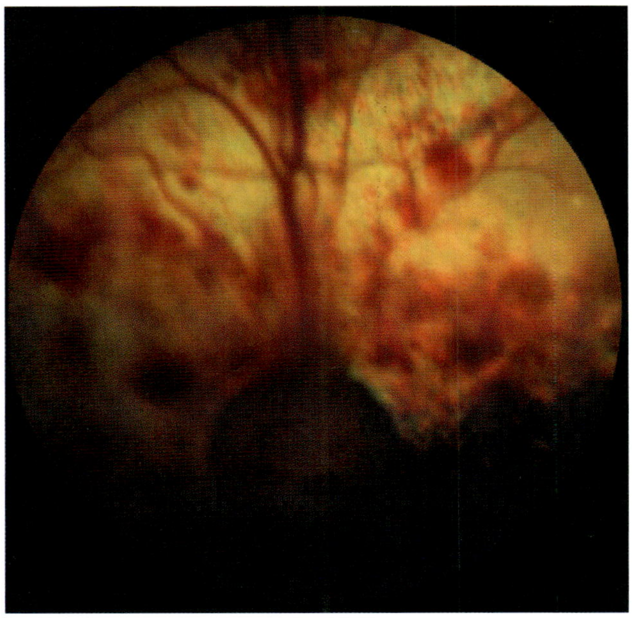

Figure 125.4 Funduscopic changes associated with multiple myeloma including chorioretinitis, exudation, extensive hemorrhage and papillitis.

Section 8

Diseases of the Globe and Orbit

CHAPTER 126
MICROPHTHALMIA

PRESENTATION

Congenital microphthalmia describes an abnormally small globe, generally noted in combination with a smaller palpebral fissure and orbit. The degree of microphthalmia varies considerably, extending from only a mild decrease in size of a functional globe to rare cases of anophthalmos, in which there is a complete absence of ocular tissue. Changes are generally bilateral. Commonly affected breeds include the Collie breeds, notably the Rough Collie.

DIAGNOSIS AND TREATMENT

The diagnosis of microphthalmia is made on the basis of clinical findings, supported if necessary by B-mode ultrasonography. The major differential is phthisis bulbus (see also Phthisis Bulbus), which, unlike congenital microphthalmia, is the result of prior ocular inflammation. There is no treatment for microphthalmia; however, associated cataracts, if present, may be surgically addressed where indicated. In severe cases, secondary conjunctivitis may require either medical management using a topical anti-inflammatory agent or surgical management via the enucleation of residual ocular tissues.

SELECTED REFERENCES

Dell M. Severe bilateral microphthalmos in a Pomeranian pup. *Can Vet J* 2010;**51**(12):1405–1407.

Gelatt KN, Samuelson DA, Barrie KP, Das ND, Wolf ED, Bauer JE, Andresen TL. Biometry and clinical characteristics of congenital cataracts and microphthalmia in the Miniature Schnauzer. *J Am Vet Med Assoc* 1983;**183**(1):99–102.

Kern TJ. Persistent hyperplastic primary vitreous and microphthalmia in a dog. *J Am Vet Med Assoc* 1981;**178**(11):1169–1171. No abstract available.

Priester WA. Congenital ocular defects in cattle, horses, cats, and dogs. *J Am Vet Med Assoc* 1972;**160**(11):1504–1511. No abstract available.

Clinical Atlas of Canine and Feline Ophthalmic Disease, First Edition. Douglas Esson.

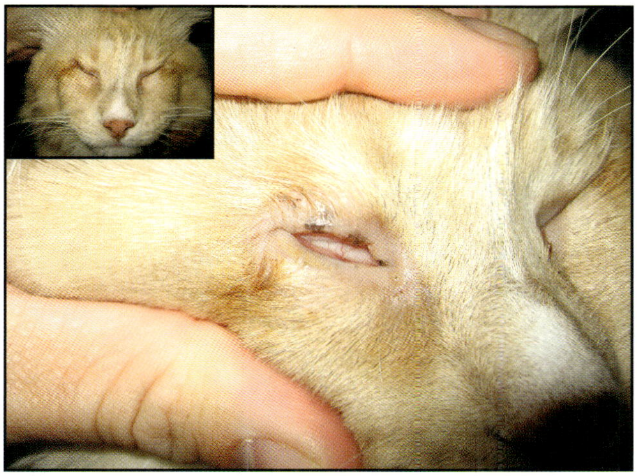

Figure 126.1 Clinical findings associated with congenital microphthalmos. Inset demonstrates bilateral changes.

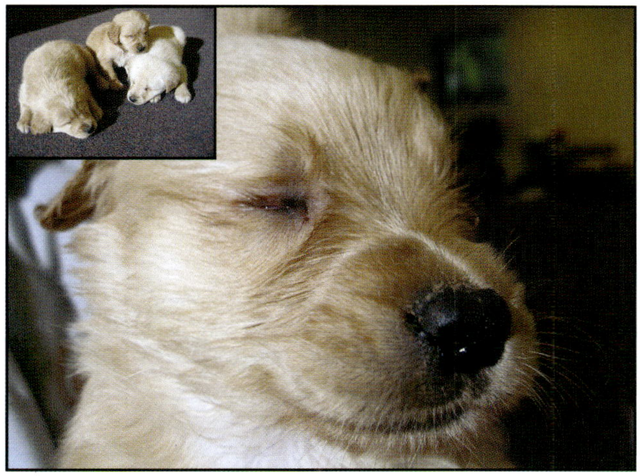

Figure 126.2 Clinical findings associated with congenital microphthalmos. Inset demonstrates multiple affected littermates.

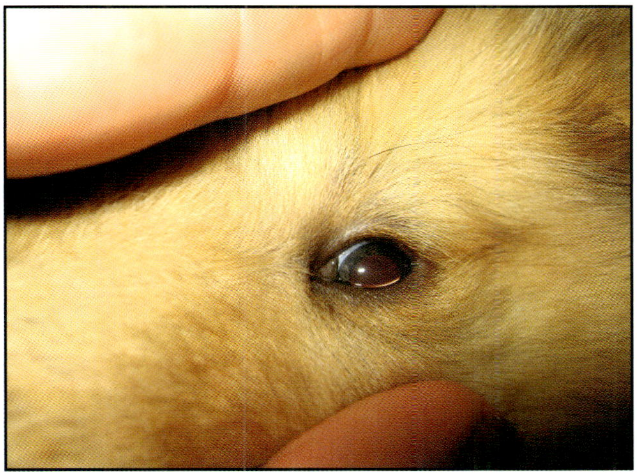

Figure 126.3 Clinical findings associated with congenital microphthalmos.

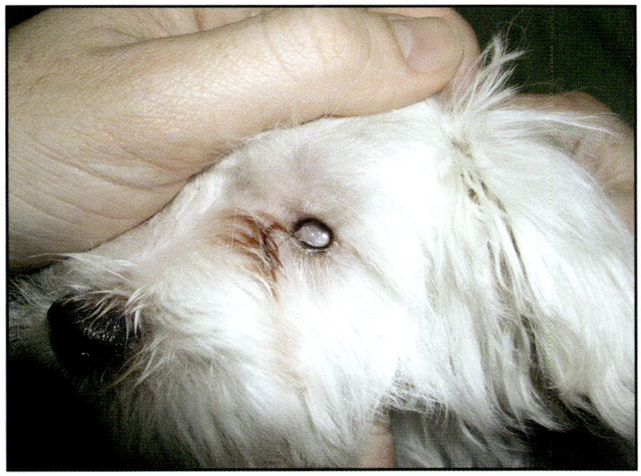

Figure 126.4 Clinical findings associated with congenital microphthalmos.

CHAPTER 127
PHTHISIS BULBUS

PRESENTATION

Phthisis bulbus describes a "shrunken" eye, typically as a result of severe and/or chronic intraocular inflammation, infection, aqueous humor leakage, and/or trauma. Clinically, affected globes are blind and may display reduced size, corneal fibrosis, uveal adhesions, cataracts, and/or retinal detachment. Both canine and feline species of any breed or crossed breed may be affected.

DIAGNOSIS AND TREATMENT

The diagnosis of phthisis bulbus is made on the basis of clinical findings, supported if necessary by B-mode ultrasonography. The major differential is congenital microphthalmia (see also Microphthalmia). Treatment of this condition may comprise benign neglect in comfortable patients, the medical management of secondary conjunctivitis, if present, or enucleation if severe secondary inflammation, infection, and/or discomfort ensue.

SELECTED REFERENCES

Busse C, Hartley C, Kafarnik C, Pivetta M. Ocular alkaline injury in four dogs—presentation, treatment, and follow-up—a case series. *Vet Ophthalmol* 2014. DOI: 10.1111/vop.12171.

Duke FD, Strong TD, Bentley E, Dubielzig RR. Canine ocular tumors following ciliary body ablation with intravitreal gentamicin. *Vet Ophthalmol* 2013;**16**(2):159–162. DOI: 10.1111/j.1463-5224.2012.01050.x. Epub 2012 Jul 19.

van der Woerdt A, Nasisse MP, Davidson MG. Lens-induced uveitis in dogs: 151 cases (1985–1990). *J Am Vet Med Assoc* 1992;**201**(6):921–926.

Clinical Atlas of Canine and Feline Ophthalmic Disease, First Edition. Douglas Esson.

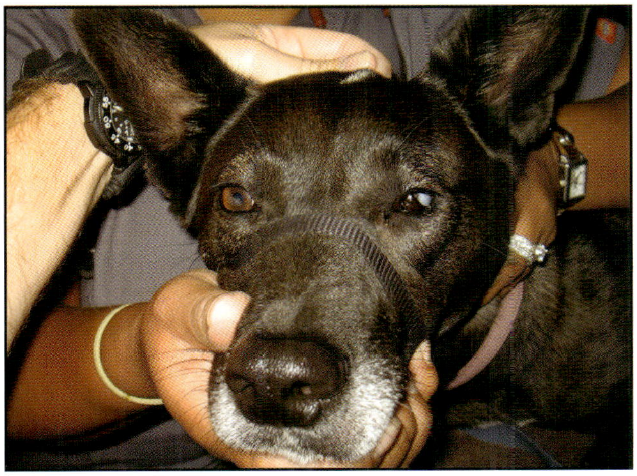

Figure 127.1 Clinical findings associated with phthisis bulbus as a result of previous intraocular inflammation.

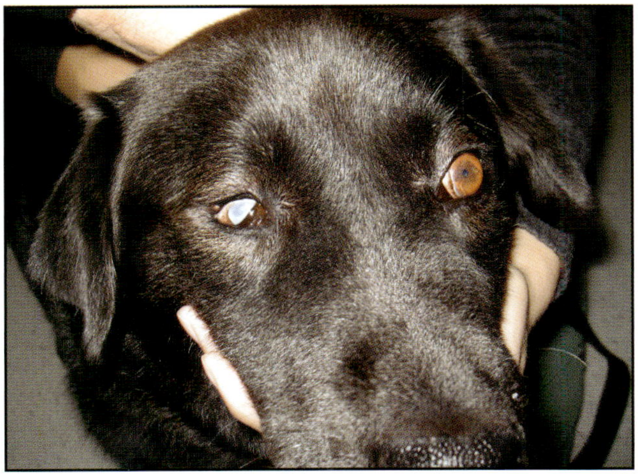

Figure 127.2 Clinical findings associated with phthisis bulbus as a result of previous intraocular inflammation.

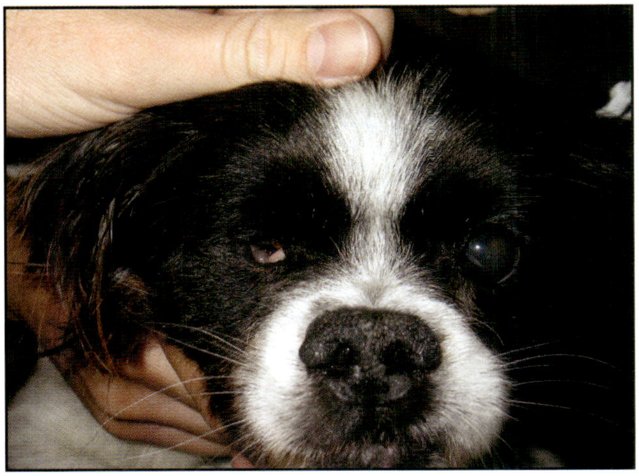

Figure 127.3 Clinical findings associated with phthisis bulbus as a result of previous intraocular inflammation.

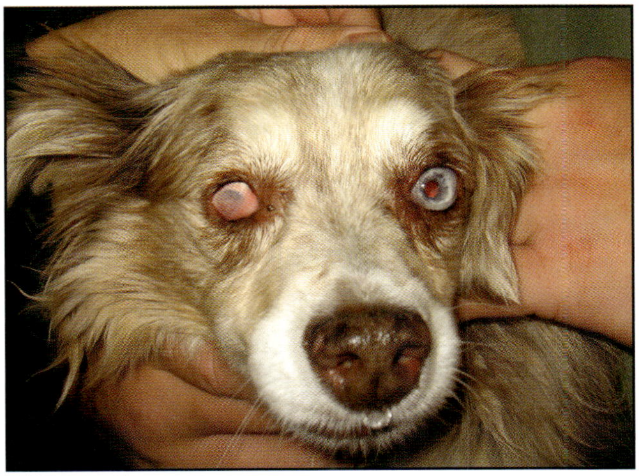

Figure 127.4 Clinical findings associated with phthisis bulbus as a result of previous intraocular inflammation.

CHAPTER 128
ORBITAL CELLULITIS

PRESENTATION

Orbital cellulitis (and/or abscessation) describes inflammation of any of the periocular tissues. Findings may include blepharospasm, conjunctivitis, chemosis, third eyelid elevation, ocular discharge, deviation of the globe from its normal position, secondary exposure keratitis, periocular swelling/fluctuance, and/or difficulty opening the mouth as a result of pressure placed on inflamed retrobulbar soft tissues by the ramus of the mandible. Symptoms typically develop relatively rapidly (over the course of several days). This process may result from trauma, penetrating wounds, extension of inflammation/infection from adjacent tissues (such as dental disease), the presence of foreign material and/or neoplasia (see also Orbital Foreign Bodies and Retrobulbar Neoplasia). Canine and feline species of any breed or crossed breed may be affected.

DIAGNOSIS AND TREATMENT

Evaluating patients affected by orbital cellulitis can be challenging as result of patient discomfort and sedation or anesthesia is frequently required in order to fully assess affected structures. The diagnosis is made on the basis of clinical findings in conjunction (where indicated) with adjunctive diagnostics including complete blood count (CBC)/chemistry analysis, ultrasonography, radiography, and/or magnetic resonance imaging. Diagnostic samples may support initial clinical finings, including culture and sensitivity testing where the presence of infectious organisms is suspected as well as cytology (fine-needle aspiration (FNA)) and/or histopathology (biopsy) where appropriate. Therapy comprises the institution of drainage where abscessation has developed as well as the institution of systemic (broad-spectrum) antimicrobial and anti-inflammatory therapy. Anti-inflammatory therapy typically comprises the use of corticosteroids where not contraindicated.

Potential Drug-Side-Effects

Potential adverse effects associated with the use of systemic corticosteroid include polyphagia, polydipsia, polyuria, hair coat changes, weight gain, pancreatitis, gastrointestinal (GI) distress, muscle damage, hepatic impairment, and diabetes.

Corneal protection in order to avoid exposure keratitis should be considered through the use of topical lubricating agents and/or (where indicated) the placement of temporary tarsorrhaphy sutures. The use of a protective Elizabethan collar will prevent self-trauma until healing is complete.

SELECTED REFERENCES

Armour MD, Broome M, Dell'Anna G, Blades NJ, Esson DW. A review of orbital and intracranial magnetic resonance imaging in 79 canine and 13 feline patients (2004–2010). *Vet Ophthalmol* 2011;**14**(4):215–226. DOI: 10.1111/j.1463-5224.2010.00865.x. Epub 2011 Apr 18.

Dennis R. Use of magnetic resonance imaging for the investigation of orbital disease in small animals. *J Small Anim Pract* 2000;**41**(4):145–155.

Tovar MC, Huguet E, Gomezi MA. Orbital cellulitis and intraocular abscess caused by migrating grass in a cat. *Vet Ophthalmol* 2005;**8**(5):353–356.

Wang AL, Ledbetter EC, Kern TJ. Orbital abscess bacterial isolates and in vitro antimicrobial susceptibility patterns in dogs and cats. *Vet Ophthalmol* 2009;**12**(2):91–96. DOI: 10.1111/j.1463-5224.2008.00687.x.

Clinical Atlas of Canine and Feline Ophthalmic Disease, First Edition. Douglas Esson.

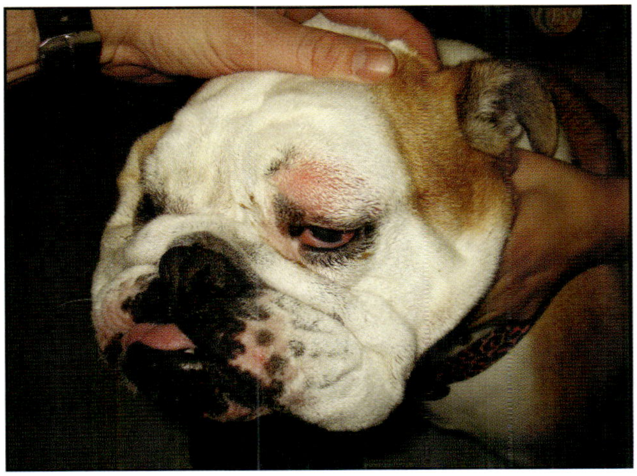

Figure 128.1 Clinical findings associated with orbital cellulitis.

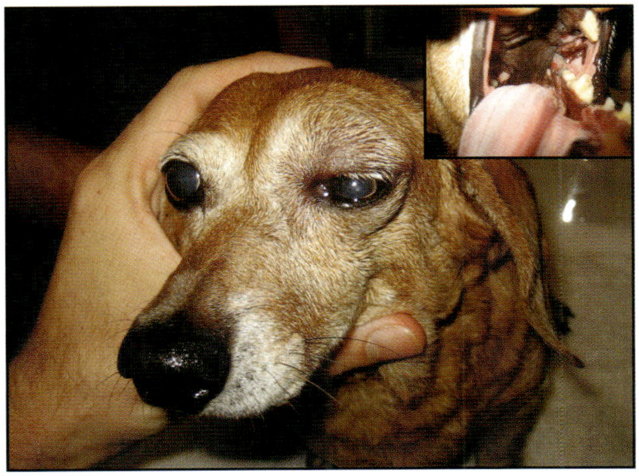

Figure 128.2 Clinical findings associated with orbital cellulitis. Inset demonstrates changes in the adjacent oral cavity.

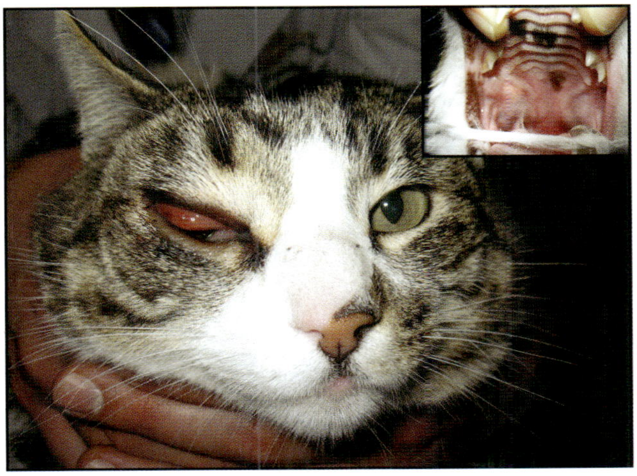

Figure 128.3 Clinical findings associated with orbital cellulitis. Inset demonstrates changes in the adjacent oral cavity.

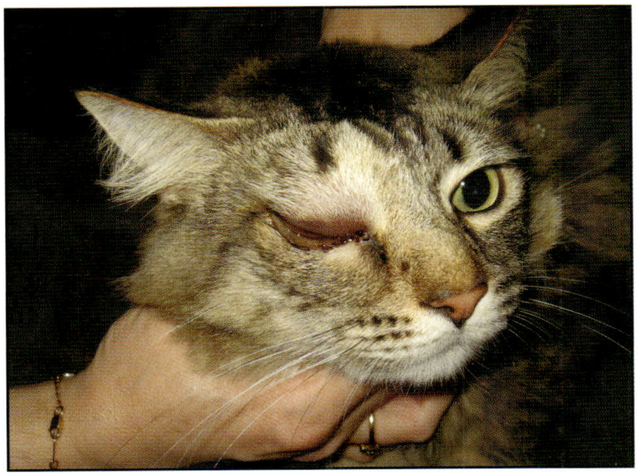

Figure 128.4 Clinical findings associated with orbital cellulitis.

CHAPTER 129
EXTRAOCULAR MYOSITIS (EOM)

PRESENTATION

Extraocular myositis (EOM) describes a primary (lymphocyte-mediated) inflammatory process affecting the extra ocular muscles in dogs. Clinical symptoms comprise acute-onset, bilateral, symmetrical exophthalmos. Despite their startling appearance, patients are typically visual, normotensive, and relatively comfortable. Young, large-breed dogs are commonly affected, notably the Golden Retriever.

DIAGNOSIS AND TREATMENT

The diagnosis is made on the basis of clinical findings, notably exophthalmos secondary to swelling of the extraocular muscles. Biopsy of affected muscles is only rarely indicated because of the significant risk of serious iatrogenic trauma and subsequent fibrosis. In contrast to orbital myositis, antibodies directed against type 2M fibers are not typically detected. Chronic or untreated cases may develop secondary fibrosis of the extraocular muscles, leading to significant strabismus. Treatment encompasses systemic immunosuppressive therapy, typically comprising corticosteroids, azathioprine, and/or cyclosporine. Therapy can frequently be tapered once symptoms are controlled; however, long-term treatment may be required.

Potential Drug-Side-Effects

Potential adverse effects associated with the use of systemic corticosteroids include polyphagia, polydipsia, polyuria, hair coat changes, weight gain, pancreatitis, enteritis, muscular damage, hepatic impairment, and diabetes. Potential adverse effects associated with the use of azathioprine include gastrointestinal (GI) distress, pancreatitis, hepatotoxicity, and myelosuppression. Potential adverse affects associated with the use of cyclosporine include hypersensitivity and GI distress.

SELECTED REFERENCES

Allgoewer I, Blair M, Basher T, Davidson M, Hamilton H, Jandeck C, Ward D, Wolfer J, Shelton GD. Extraocular muscle myositis and restrictive strabismus in 10 dogs. *Vet Ophthalmol* 2000;**3**(1):21–26.

Carpenter JL, Schmidt GM, Moore FM, Albert DM, Abrams KL, Elner VM. Canine bilateral extraocular polymyositis. *Vet Pathol* 1989;**26**(6):510–512.

Williams DL (2008) Extraocular myositis in the dog. *Vet Clin North Am Small Anim Pract* **38**(2):347–359, vii. doi: 10.1016/j.cvsm.2007.11.010. Review.

Clinical Atlas of Canine and Feline Ophthalmic Disease, First Edition. Douglas Esson.

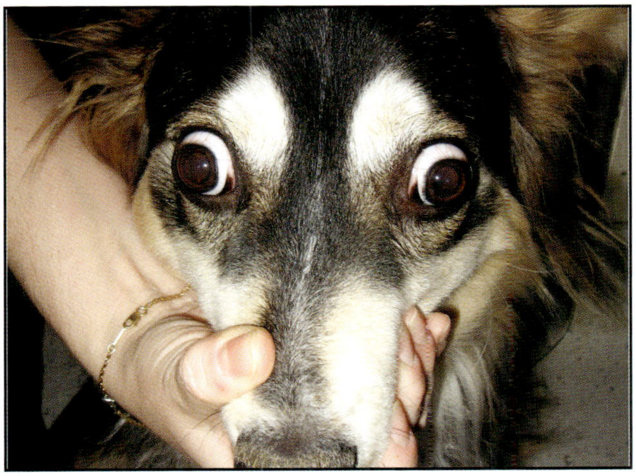

Figure 129.1 Clinical findings associated with extraocular myositis.

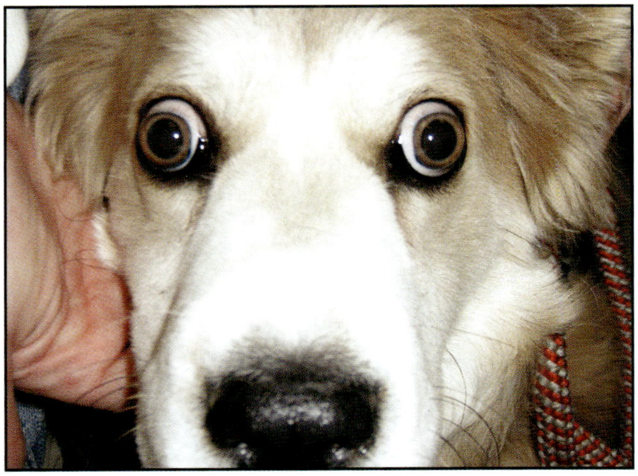

Figure 129.2 Clinical findings associated with extraocular myositis.

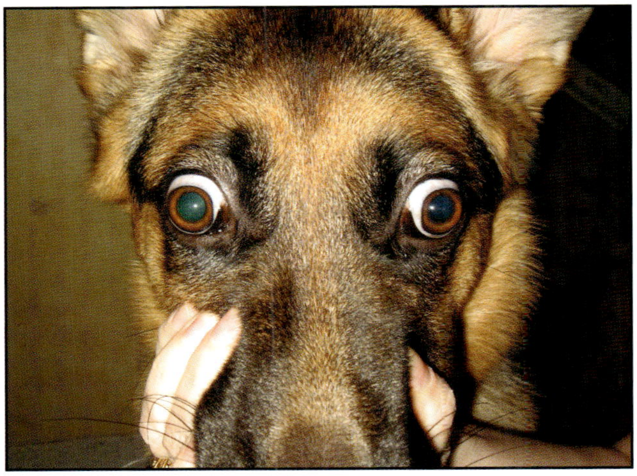

Figure 129.3 Clinical findings associated with extraocular myositis.

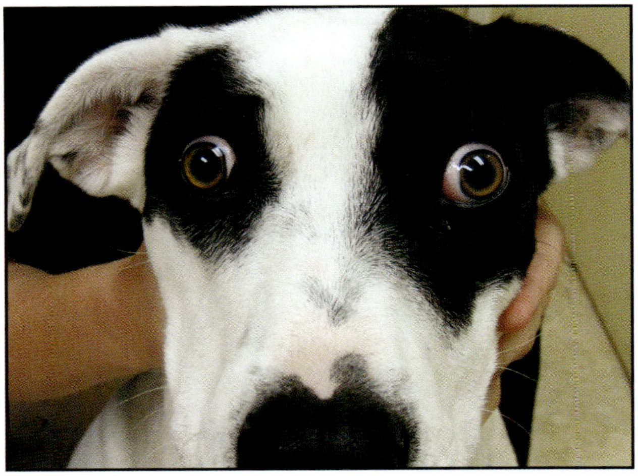

Figure 129.4 Clinical findings associated with extraocular myositis.

CHAPTER 130
ZYGOMATIC SIALOADENITIS

PRESENTATION

Zygomatic sialoadenitis (and/or associated zygomatic salivary mucocoele) describes an inflammatory process affecting the zygomatic salivary gland. Potential causes include bacterial infection, immune-mediated inflammation, and/or trauma. Clinically, affected patients may display any combination of conjunctivitis, ocular discharge, third eyelid elevation, exophthalmos, globe deviation, and/or difficulty opening the mouth. Commonly affected breeds include the Labrador Retriever and Golden Retriever.

DIAGNOSIS AND TREATMENT

The diagnosis of zygomatic sialoadenitis is made on the basis of clinical findings, orbital magnetic resonance imaging, and cytological or histological evaluation of fine-needle aspiration (FNA) or biopsy samples of affected tissue. Differentials for sialoadenitis represent orbital cellulitis and neoplasia (including neoplasia of the zygomatic salivary gland itself) and (see also Orbital Cellulitis and Retrobulbar Neoplasia). Treatment may comprise medical (systemic antimicrobial and anti-inflammatory therapy) and/or surgical resection of affected tissue.

SELECTED REFERENCES

Adams P, Halfacree ZJ, Lamb CR, Smith KC, Baines SJ. Zygomatic salivary mucocoele in a Lhasa apso following maxillary tooth extraction. *Vet Rec* 2011;**168**(17):458. DOI: 10.1136/vr.c6878. Epub 2011 Mar 17.

Bartoe JT, Brightman AH, Davidson HJ. Modified lateral orbitotomy for vision-sparing excision of a zygomatic mucocele in a dog. *Vet Ophthalmol* 2007;**10**(2):127–131.

Boland L, Gomes E, Payen G, Bouvy B, Poncet C. Salivary gland diseases in the dog: three cases diagnosed by MRI. *J Am Anim Hosp Assoc* 2013;**49**(5):333–337. DOI: 10.5326/JAAHA-MS-5882. Epub 2013 Jul 16.

McGill S, Lester N, McLachlan A, Mansfield C. Concurrent sialocoele and necrotising sialadenitis in a dog. *J Small Anim Pract* 2009;**50**(3):151–156. DOI: 10.1111/j.1748-5827.2009.00706.x.

Philp HS, Rhodes M, Parry A, Baines SJ (2012) Canine zygomatic salivary mucocoele following suspected oropharyngeal penetrating stick injury. *Vet Rec* **171**(16):402. doi: 10.1136/vr.100892. Epub 2012 Aug 18.

Clinical Atlas of Canine and Feline Ophthalmic Disease, First Edition. Douglas Esson.

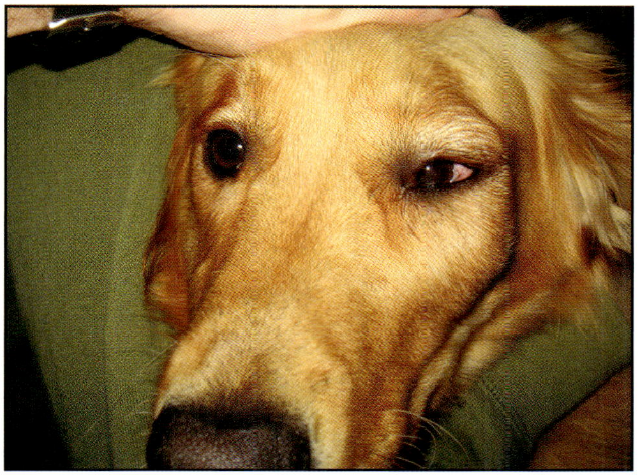

Figure 130.1 Typical clinical presentation associated with zygomatic sialoadenitis.

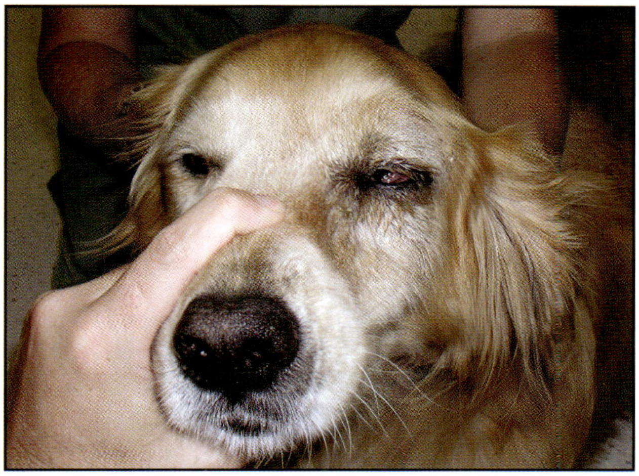

Figure 130.2 Typical clinical presentation associated with zygomatic sialoadenitis.

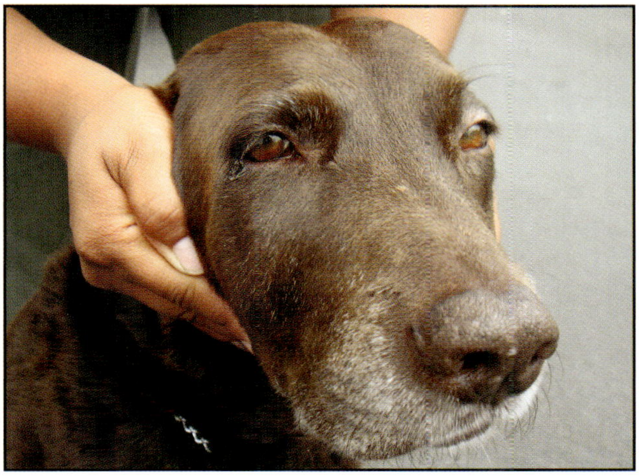

Figure 130.3 Typical clinical presentation associated with zygomatic sialoadenitis.

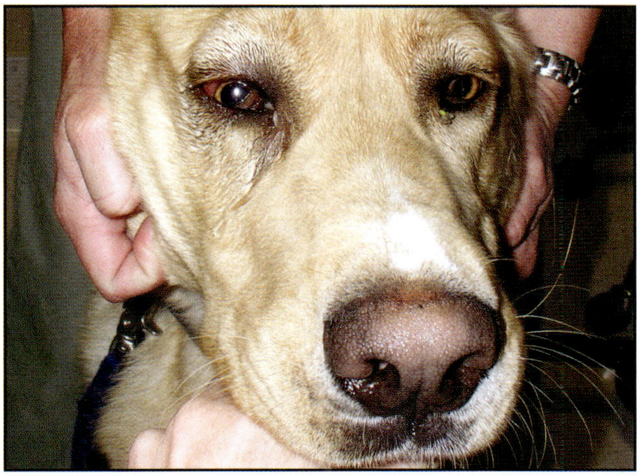

Figure 130.4 Typical clinical presentation associated with zygomatic sialoadenitis.

CHAPTER 131
ORBITAL FAT PAD PROLAPSE

PRESENTATION

Occasionally, a partial prolapse of the orbital fat pad may be noted in dogs, and less commonly in cats. Fat prolapse results from either congenital or traumatic weakness associated with orbital soft tissues. Clinically, a fat prolapse presents as a smooth, pink to cream-colored, fluctuant, nonpainful swelling adjacent to the globe. Manipulation of the globe may exacerbate symptoms. Symptoms are commonly unilateral. Canine and feline species of any breed or crossed breed may be affected.

DIAGNOSIS AND TREATMENT

A tentative diagnosis of orbital fat pad prolapse is made on the basis of clinical findings. The diagnosis may be confirmed by cytological or histological evaluation of representative fine-needle aspirate or biopsy samples respectively. The major differential for fat pad prolapse is represented by neoplastic tissue, notably benign hibernomas. If indicated, prolapsed tissue may be surgically excised and surrounding soft tissue imbricated. Postoperative care comprises routine systemic and/or topical antimicrobial and/or anti-inflammatory therapy as well as the use of a protective Elizabethan collar to prevent self-trauma.

SELECTED REFERENCES

Boydell P, Paterson S, Pike R. Orbital fat prolapse in the dog. *J Small Anim Pract* 1996;**37**(2):61–63.

Cho J. Surgery of the globe and orbit. *Top Companion Anim Med* 2008;**23**(1):23–37. DOI: 10.1053/j.ctsap.2007.12.004.

McNab AA. Subconjunctival fat prolapse. *Aust N Z J Ophthalmol* 1999;**27**(1):33–36.

Ravi M, Schobert CS, Kiupel M, Dubielzig RR. Clinical, morphologic, and immunohistochemical features of canine orbital hibernomas. *Vet Pathol* 2014;**51**(3):563–568. DOI: 10.1177/0300985813493913. Epub 2013 Jun 21.

Clinical Atlas of Canine and Feline Ophthalmic Disease, First Edition. Douglas Esson.

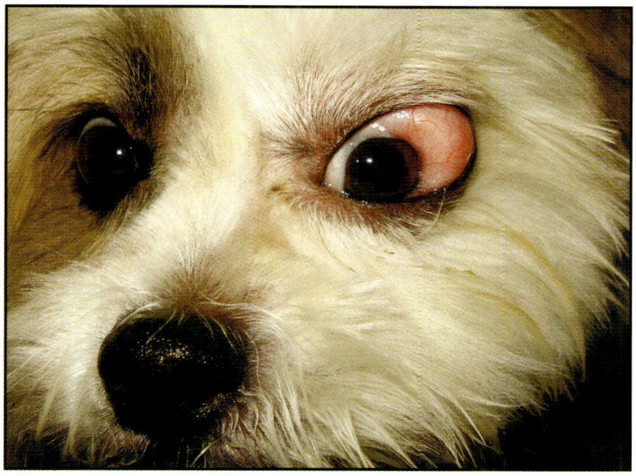

Figure 131.1 Clinical presentation associated with prolapsed orbital fat.

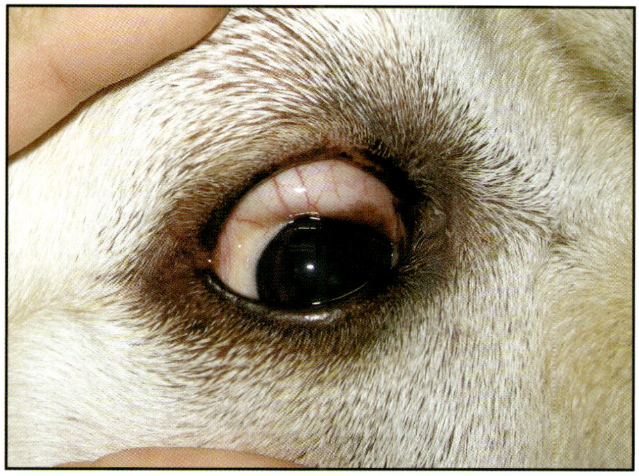

Figure 131.2 Clinical presentation associated with prolapsed orbital fat.

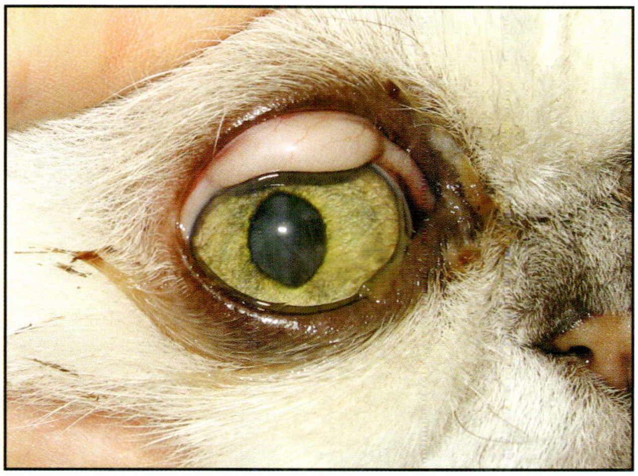

Figure 131.3 Clinical presentation associated with prolapsed orbital fat.

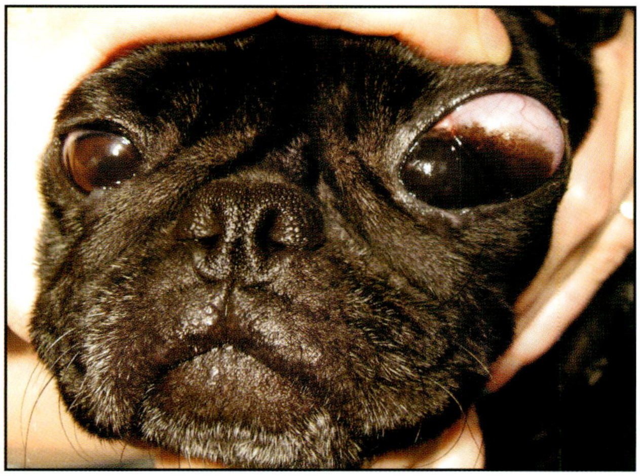

Figure 131.4 Clinical presentation associated with prolapsed orbital fat.

CHAPTER 132
ORBITAL FOREIGN BODIES

PRESENTATION

The orbit comprises the bones of the skull adjacent to the globe, temporal, masseter and pterygoid muscles, and the periorbital fascia. Foreign material may enter the orbit, including plant-based material (notably retrobulbar "stick injuries," which gain entry to the orbit via the oral cavity and "foxtails" which gain entry to the orbit via the fornix), and metallic objects (notably air gun pellets). Clinical symptoms may include any combination of blepharospasm, conjunctivitis, chemosis, third eyelid elevation, ocular discharge, deviation of the globe from its normal position, secondary exposure keratitis, and/or periocular swelling. Symptoms typically develop relatively rapidly (over the course of hours to days) and are typically unilateral.

DIAGNOSIS AND TREATMENT

Evaluating patients affected by orbital inflammation and/or the presence of foreign material can be challenging as a result of patient discomfort and sedation or anesthesia is frequently required in order to fully assess affected structures. The diagnosis is made on the basis of clinical findings in conjunction (where indicated) with adjunctive diagnostics including ultrasonography, radiography, and/or magnetic resonance imaging of affected tissues. Plant-based foreign bodies can be challenging to identify, MRI being most useful in this regard and surgical exploration sometimes being required. Metallic foreign bodies are easily identified using conventional radiography. Differentials include orbital cellulitis and retrobulbar neoplasia (see also Orbital Cellulitis and Retrobulbar Neoplasia) Therapy comprises the removal of reactive or organic foreign material (as well as the institution of drainage where abscessation has developed) and the institution of systemic (broad-spectrum) antimicrobial and anti-inflammatory therapy. Anti-inflammatory therapy typically comprises the use of corticosteroids where possible. Corneoscleral repair and/or lens extraction may be indicated depending on the extent of injury. Severely traumatized globes or those displaying endophthalmitis (see also Endophthalmitis/Panophthalmitis), may require enucleation.

Potential Drug-Side-Effects

Potential adverse effects associated with the use of systemic prednisone include polyphagia, polydipsia, polyuria, hair coat changes, weight gain, pancreatitis, gastrointestinal (GI) distress, muscle damage, hepatic impairment, and diabetes.

Corneal protection in order to avoid exposure keratitis should be considered through the use of topical lubricating agents and/or (where indicated) the placement of temporary tarsorrhaphy sutures.

SELECTED REFERENCES

Håkansson NW, Håkansson BW. Transfrontal orbitotomy in the dog: an adaptable three-step approach to the orbit. *Vet Ophthalmol* 2010;**13**(6):377–383. DOI: 10.1111/j.1463-5224.2010.00830.x.

Welihozkiy A, Pirie CG, Pizzirani S. Scleral and suprachoroidal foreign body in a dog—a case report. *Vet Ophthalmol* 2011;**14**(5):345–351. DOI: 10.1111/j.1463-5224.2011.00922.x. Epub 2011 Jul 12.

Woolfson JM, Wesley RE. Magnetic resonance imaging and computed tomographic scanning of fresh (green) wood foreign bodies in dog orbits. *Ophthal Plast Reconstr Surg* 1990;**6**(4):237–240.

Clinical Atlas of Canine and Feline Ophthalmic Disease, First Edition. Douglas Esson.

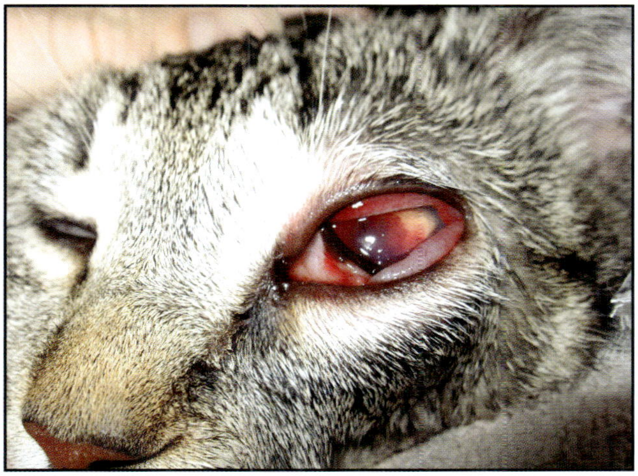

Figure 132.1 Clinical presentation associated with penetrating orbital and ocular trauma as a result of a metallic air gun pellet.

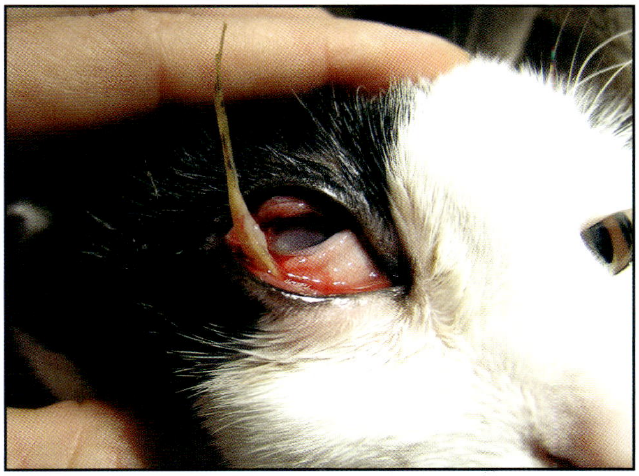

Figure 132.2 Clinical presentation associated with the presence of a grass awn, embedded in the orbital tissues.

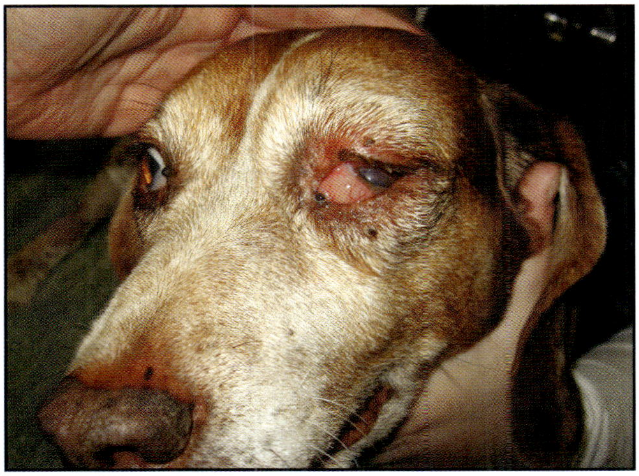

Figure 132.3 Clinical presentation associated with an oral (plant based) penetrating injury.

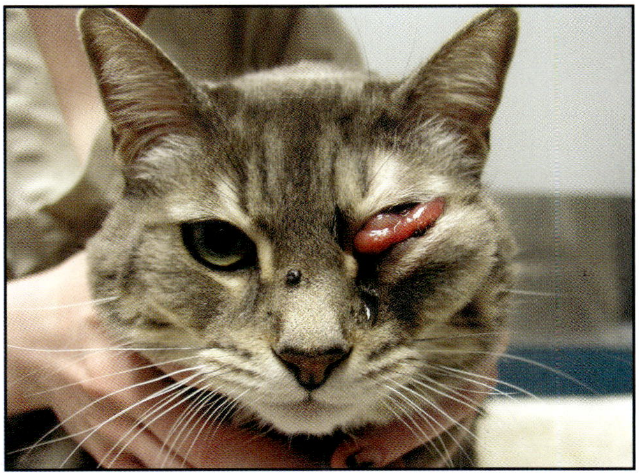

Figure 132.4 Clinical presentation associated with the presence of a cat claw embedded in scleral and orbital tissues.

CHAPTER 133
ENDOPHTHALMITIS/PANOPHTHALMITIS

PRESENTATION

The term endophthalmitis describes inflammation of the internal tissues of the eye. The term panophthalmitis describes inflammation of the internal tissues as well as external layers of the eye. Panophthalmitis is frequently associated with inflammation of adjacent orbital tissues. Both conditions may result from trauma, infection (external or internal), penetrating wounds, foreign material, postsurgical complication, the extension of neoplasia, or the extension of uncontrolled inflammation from other parts of the eye such as the lens or uvea. Affected patients may display any combination of blepharospasm, conjunctivitis, chemosis, periocular swelling, third eyelid elevation, ocular discharge, keratitis and/or clinically apparent uveitis/chorioretinitis

DIAGNOSIS AND TREATMENT

Evaluating patients affected by endophthalmitis/panophthalmitis can be challenging as result of patient discomfort and sedation or anesthesia may be required in order to fully assess affected structures. The diagnosis is made on the basis of clinical findings in conjunction (where indicated) with complete blood count (CBC)/chemistry analysis, ultrasonography, radiography, and/or magnetic resonance imaging of affected tissues. Diagnostic samples may support diagnostic findings, including culture and sensitivity testing where the presence of infectious organisms is suspected as well as cytology (fine-needle aspiration (FNA)) and/or histopathology (biopsy) where appropriate. Therapy comprises the institution of drainage where abscessation has developed, as well as the institution of aggressive topical, subconjunctival, intraocular, and/or systemic (broad spectrum) antimicrobial therapy. Systemic anti-inflammatory therapy typically comprises the use of corticosteroids where possible. Severely and/or chronically inflamed globes frequently require enucleation.

Potential Drug-Side-Effects

Potential adverse effects associated with the use of systemic prednisone include polyphagia, polydipsia, polyuria, hair coat changes, weight gain, pancreatitis, gastrointestinal (GI) distress, muscle damage, hepatic impairment, and diabetes.

The use of a protective Elizabethan collar will prevent self-trauma until healing is complete.

SELECTED REFERENCES

Bell CM, Pot SA, Dubielzig RR. Septic implantation syndrome in dogs and cats: a distinct pattern of endophthalmitis with lenticular abscess. *Vet Ophthalmol* 2013;**16**(3):180–185. DOI: 10.1111/j.1463-5224.2012.01046.x. Epub 2012 Jul 19.

Hendrix DV, Rohrbach BW, Bochsler PN, English RV. Comparison of histologic lesions of endophthalmitis induced by Blastomyces dermatitidis in untreated and treated dogs: 36 cases (1986–2001). *J Am Vet Med Assoc* 2004;**224**(8):1317–1322.

Ledbetter EC, Landry MP, Stokol T, Kern TJ, Messick JB. Brucella canis endophthalmitis in 3 dogs: clinical features, diagnosis, and treatment. *Vet Ophthalmol* 2009;**12**(3):183–191. DOI: 10.1111/j.1463-5224.2009.00690.x.

Scott EM, Esson DW, Fritz KJ, Dubielzig RR. Major breed distribution of canine patients enucleated or eviscerated due to glaucoma following routine cataract surgery as well as common histopathologic findings within enucleated globes. *Vet Ophthalmol* 2013;**16**(Suppl 1):64–72. DOI: 10.1111/vop.12034. Epub 2013 Feb 13.

Clinical Atlas of Canine and Feline Ophthalmic Disease, First Edition. Douglas Esson.

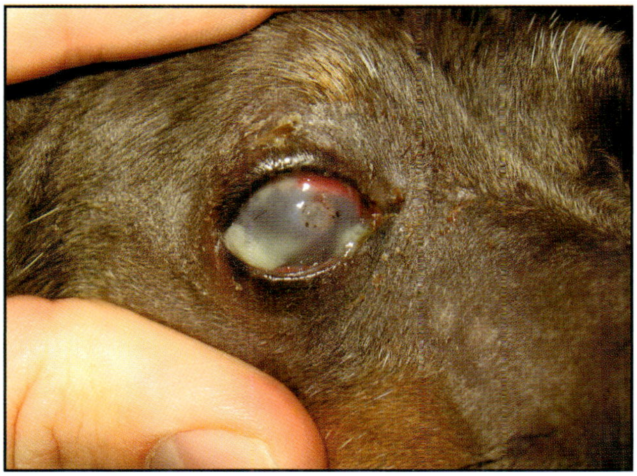

Figure 133.1 Clinical presentation associated with endophthalmitis.

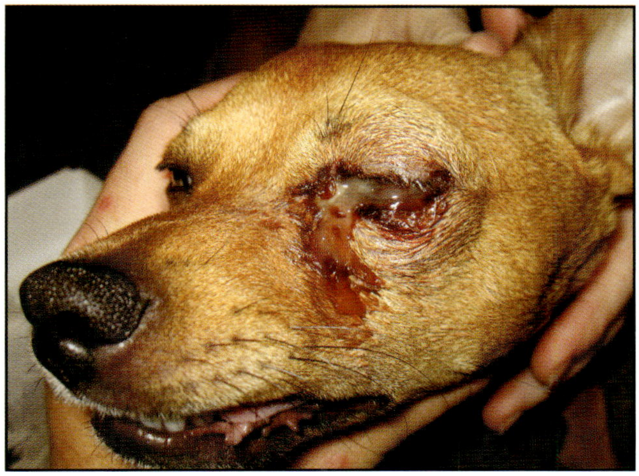

Figure 133.2 Clinical presentation associated with panophthalmitis.

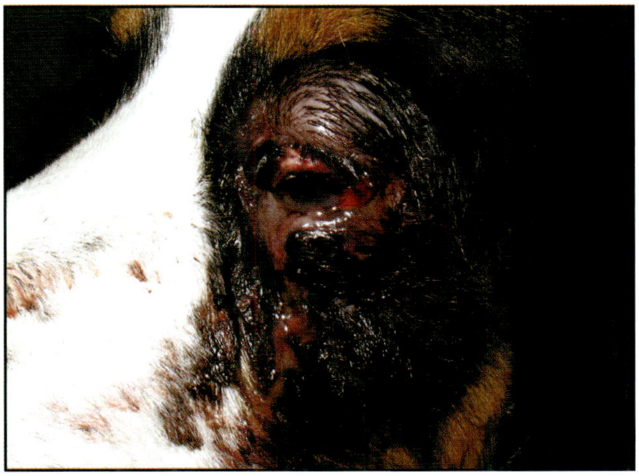

Figure 133.3 Clinical presentation associated with panophthalmitis.

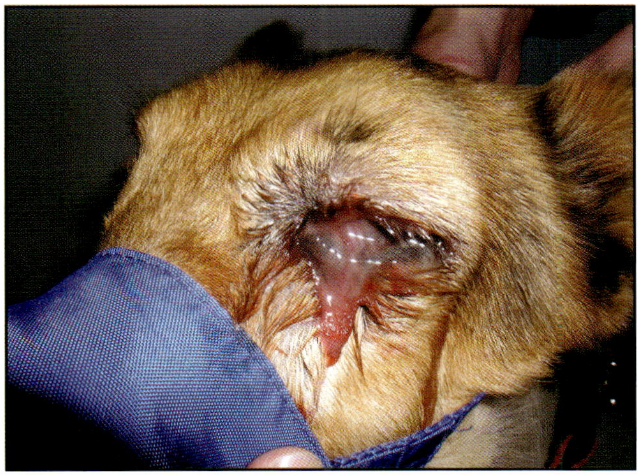

Figure 133.4 Clinical presentation associated with panophthalmitis.

CHAPTER 134
PROPTOSIS OF THE GLOBE

PRESENTATION

Proptosis describes partial or complete anterior dislocation of the globe from its normal position within the orbit, typically as a result of trauma. Secondary entrapment by severely swollen periorbital tissue is common. Other associated symptoms may include subconjunctival hemorrhage, episcleral hemorrhage, hyphema, and/or exposure keratopathy. Negative prognostic indicators include the following:

- Multiple extraocular muscular avulsions
- Corneoscleral rupture
- Hyphema

Positive prognostic indicators include the following:

- Significantly brachycephalic conformation
- Minimal globe displacement
- Miotic pupil and/or the presence of a pupillary light reflex (PLR)

Proptosis occurs most commonly in brachycephalic breeds, notably the Shih Tzu, Pug, and Lhasa Apso.

DIAGNOSIS AND TREATMENT

Initial treatment of ocular proptosis encompasses addressing potentially life-threatening injuries and stabilizing the patient. Consideration should be given to enucleating severely traumatized globes, which are unlikely to be salvageable. The ocular surface should be moistened with physiologic fluids, before globe replacement under general anesthesia. Severe eyelid swelling may necessitate canthotomy in order to facilitate globe replacement. Temporary tarsorrhaphy sutures are typically placed following proptosis reduction and left in place for 10–14 days. Care should be taken to avoid corneal abrasion and to allow for the resolution of eyelid swelling, which will occur in the days following repair. Postoperative care comprises routine (systemic) antimicrobial, anti-inflammatory, and analgesic therapy. The use of a protective Elizabethan collar will prevent self-trauma. Where possible, the goal of proptosis reduction is both vision and globe salvage; however, in some cases it may be possible to salvage the globe but not vision. Potential complications following proptosis include permanent strabismus (commonly as a result of medial rectus muscle avulsion), ulcerative keratitis, keratoconjunctivitis sicca (KCS), neuroretinal degeneration, and/or phthisis bulbus (see also Phthisis Bulbus).

SELECTED REFERENCES

Cho J. Surgery of the globe and orbit. *Top Companion Anim Med* 2008;**23**(1):23–37. DOI: 10.1053/j.ctsap.2007.12.004.

Gilger BC, Hamilton HL, Wilkie DA, van der Woerdt A, McLaughlin SA, Whitley RD. Traumatic ocular proptoses in dogs and cats: 84 cases (1980–1993). *J Am Vet Med Assoc* 1995;**206**(8):1186–1190.

Mandell DC, Holt E. Ophthalmic emergencies. *Vet Clin North Am Small Anim Pract* 2005;**35**(2):455–80, vii–viii.

Clinical Atlas of Canine and Feline Ophthalmic Disease, First Edition. Douglas Esson.

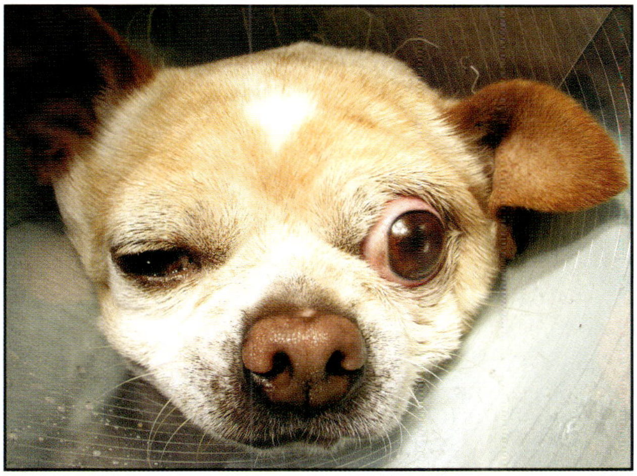

Figure 134.1 Clinical presentation associated with mild to moderate proptosis of the globe.

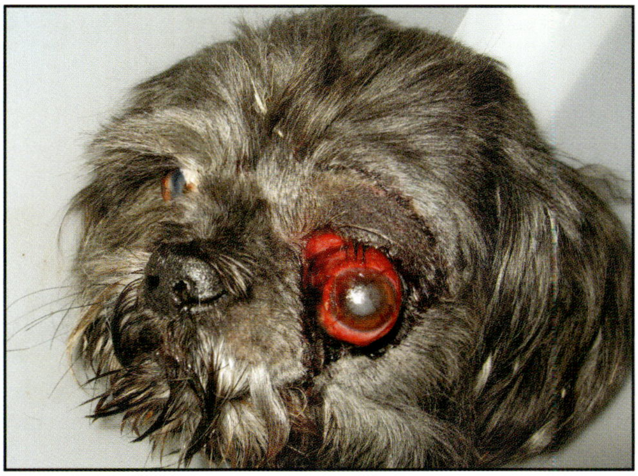

Figure 134.2 Clinical presentation associated with severe proptosis of the globe.

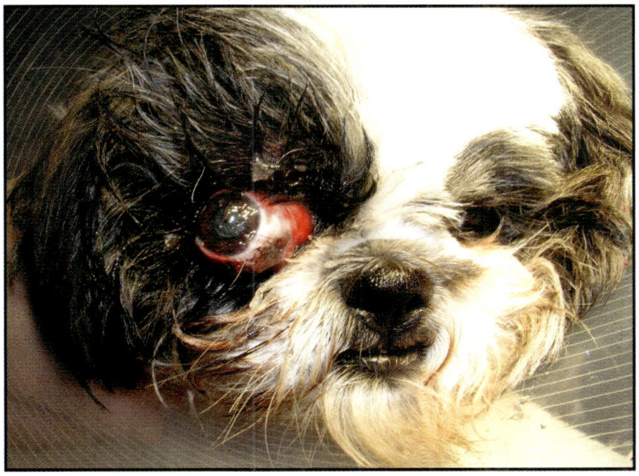

Figure 134.3 Clinical presentation associated with severe proptosis of the globe.

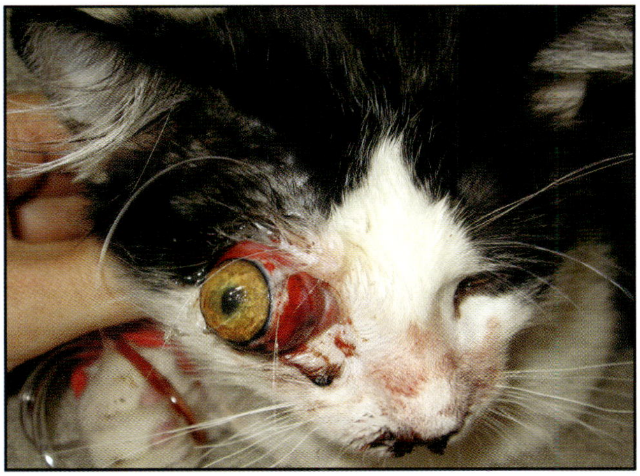

Figure 134.4 Clinical presentation associated with catastrophic proptosis of the globe.

CHAPTER 135
PERIPHERAL NERVE SHEATH TUMOR (PNST)

PRESENTATION

Peripheral nerve sheath tumors (PNSTs) represent a spindyloid neoplastic proliferation of the perineural connective tissues. These tumors include schwannomas, neurogenic sarcomas, neurofibromas, and neurofibrosarcomas and may affect a wide range of soft tissues including the orbital, adnexal, and ocular structures. Clinically, lesions appear as slowly progressive, firm, nonpainful swellings of the orbit, fornix, or eyelids. Secondary conjunctivitis and/or deviation of the globe may be associated with their development. Canine and feline species of any breed or crossed breed may be affected.

DIAGNOSIS AND TREATMENT

The diagnosis of PNST is made on the basis of clinical findings in conjunction with histopathological interpretation of biopsy samples. The extent of the lesion and involvement of local tissues may be further assessed by imaging in the form of magnetic resonance imaging (MRI) or computed tomography (CT). Pretreatment staging via thoracic radiography and regional lymph node aspiration is recommended. Treatment comprises wide surgical resection where possible, followed by radiation therapy, chemotherapy, and/or metronomic therapy (the combination of a nonsteroidal anti-inflammatory drug (NSAID) and alkylating agent to inhibit vascular growth) where indicated. Individual chemotherapeutic protocols are most ideally designed by a veterinary oncologist; however, they typically include a variable combination of prednisone, vincristine, cyclophosphamide, and/or doxorubicin.

Potential Drug-Side-Effects

Potential adverse effects associated with the use of systemic prednisone include polyphagia, polydipsia, polyuria, hair coat changes, weight gain, pancreatitis, gastrointestinal (GI) distress, muscle damage, hepatic impairment, and diabetes. Potential adverse effects associated with the use of vincristine include stomatitis, GI distress, neuropathy, hepatopathy, and myelosuppression. Potential adverse effects associated with the use of cyclophosphamide include GI distress, pancreatitis, hepatotoxicity, and myelosuppression. Potential adverse affects associated with the use of doxorubicin include hypersensitivity, GI distress, cardiac dysfunction, and myelosuppression.

SELECTED REFERENCES

Evans PM, Lynch GL, Dubielzig RR. Anterior uveal spindle cell tumor in a cat. *Vet Ophthalmol* 2010;**13**(6):387–390. DOI: 10.1111/j.1463-5224.2010.00837.x.

Hoffman A, Blocker T, Dubielzig R, Ehrhart EJ. Feline periocular peripheral nerve sheath tumor: a case series. *Vet Ophthalmol* 2005;**8**(3):153–158.

Newkirk KM, Rohrbach BW. A retrospective study of eyelid tumors from 43 cats. *Vet Pathol* 2009;**46**(5):916–927. DOI: 10.1354/vp.08-VP-0205-N-FL. Epub 2009 May 9.

Clinical Atlas of Canine and Feline Ophthalmic Disease, First Edition. Douglas Esson.

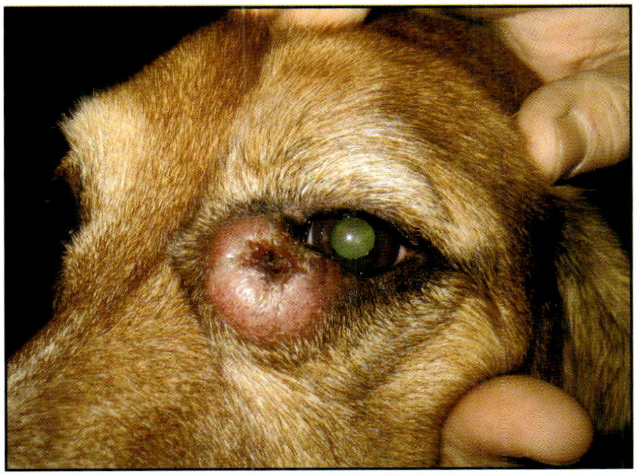

Figure 135.1 Clinical presentation associated with the presence of a peripheral nerve sheath tumor.

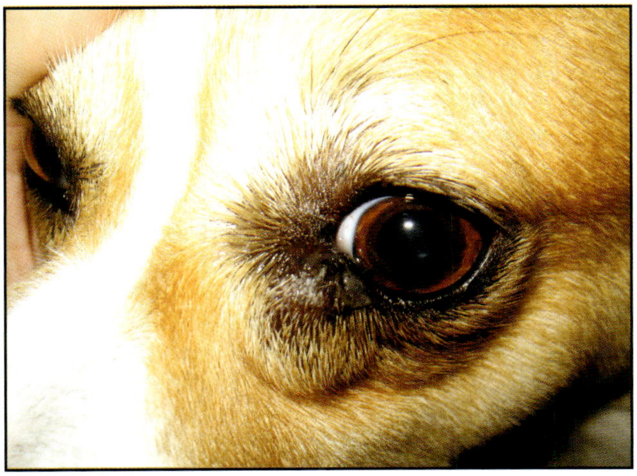

Figure 135.2 Clinical presentation associated with the presence of a peripheral nerve sheath tumor.

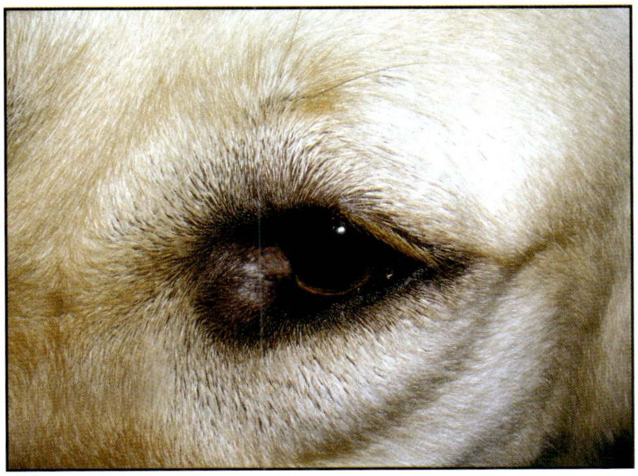

Figure 135.3 Clinical presentation associated with the presence of a peripheral nerve sheath tumor.

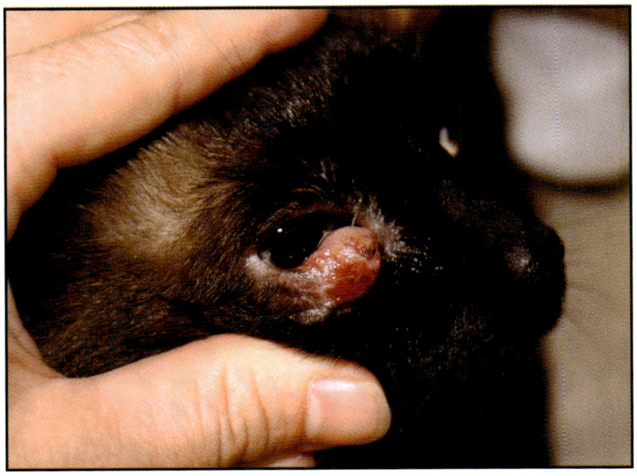

Figure 135.4 Clinical presentation associated with the presence of a peripheral nerve sheath tumor.

CHAPTER 136
RETROBULBAR NEOPLASIA

PRESENTATION

Retrobulbar neoplasia (with or without associated orbital inflammation) is not uncommon, with most orbital neoplasms being both primary and malignant. Prevalent tumor types include carcinoma (squamous cell carcinoma and adenocarcinoma), sarcoma (spindle cell sarcoma, fibrosarcoma, hemangiosarcoma, multilobular orbital sarcoma, osteosarcoma, and chondrosarcoma), meningioma, and lymphoma. Clinical findings may include blepharospasm, conjunctivitis, chemosis, third eyelid elevation, ocular discharge, deviation of the globe from its normal position, secondary exposure keratitis, periocular swelling/fluctuance, difficulty opening the mouth and visual and/or neurological defects. Symptoms typically develop relatively slowly (over the course of weeks to months), with most patients remaining comfortable until changes are significantly advanced. Affected patients are typically older. Canine and feline species of any breed or crossed breed may be affected.

DIAGNOSIS AND TREATMENT

Diagnostic modalities useful for the investigation of orbital disease include radiography, ultrasonography, computed tomography, and/or magnetic resonance imaging. The diagnosis is made on the basis of cytological or histopathological evaluation of samples harvested by fine-needle aspiration (FNA) or biopsy, typically post-imaging. The major differential represents orbital inflammatory disease (see also Orbital Cellulitis and Zygomatic Sialoadenitis). Treatment may include any combination of surgical resection where possible (potentially involving enucleation/exenteration), systemic chemotherapy and/or radiation therapy based on the tumor type present. Anti-inflammatory therapy typically comprises the use of corticosteroids where not contraindicated.

Potential Drug-Side-Effects

Potential adverse effects associated with the use of systemic corticosteroids include polyphagia, polydipsia, polyuria, hair coat changes, weight gain, pancreatitis, gastrointestinal (GI) distress, muscle damage, hepatic impairment, and diabetes.

Corneal protection in order to avoid exposure keratitis should be considered through the use of topical lubricating agents and/or (where indicated) the placement of temporary tarsorrhaphy sutures.

SELECTED REFERENCES

Armour MD, Broome M, Dell'Anna G, Blades NJ, Esson DW. A review of orbital and intracranial magnetic resonance imaging in 79 canine and 13 feline patients (2004–2010). *Vet Ophthalmol* 2011;**14**(4):215–226. DOI: 10.1111/j.1463-5224.2010.00865.xEpub 2011 Apr 18.

Attali-Soussay K, Jegou JP, Clerc B. Retrobulbar tumors in dogs and cats: 25 cases. *Vet Ophthalmol* 2001;**4**(1):19–27.

Cho J. Surgery of the globe and orbit. *Top Companion Anim Med* 2008;**23**(1):23–37. DOI: 10.1053/j.ctsap.2007.12.004. Review.

Hendrix DV, Gelatt KN. Diagnosis, treatment and outcome of orbital neoplasia in dogs: a retrospective study of 44 cases. *J Small Anim Pract* 2000;**41**(3):105–108.

Mason DR, Lamb CR, McLellan GJ. Ultrasonographic findings in 50 dogs with retrobulbar disease. *J Am Anim Hosp Assoc* 2001; **37**(6):557–562.

Clinical Atlas of Canine and Feline Ophthalmic Disease, First Edition. Douglas Esson.

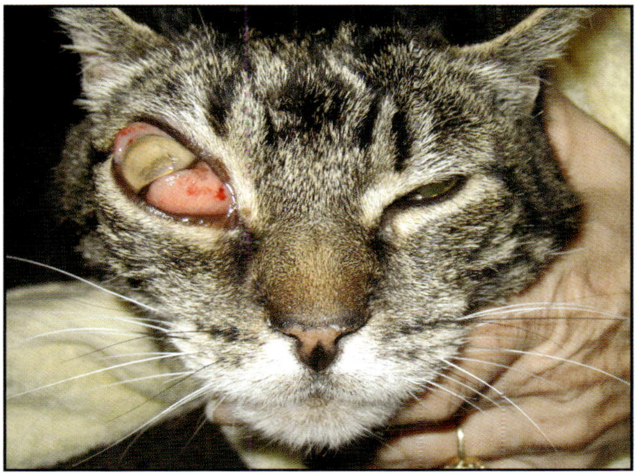

Figure 136.1 Clinical presentation associated with retrobulbar neoplasia (squamous cell carcinoma).

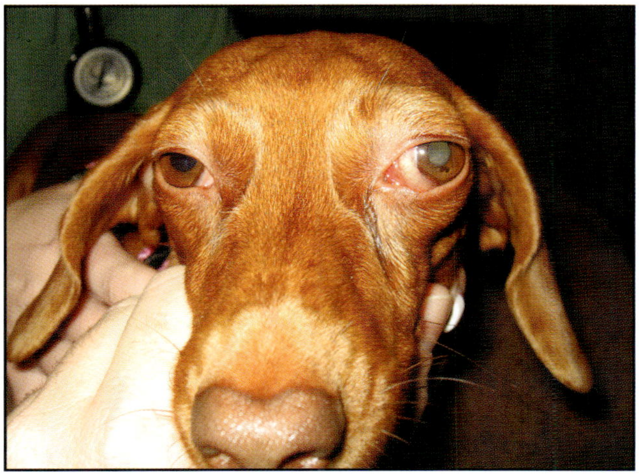

Figure 136.2 Clinical presentation associated with retrobulbar neoplasia (adenocarcinoma).

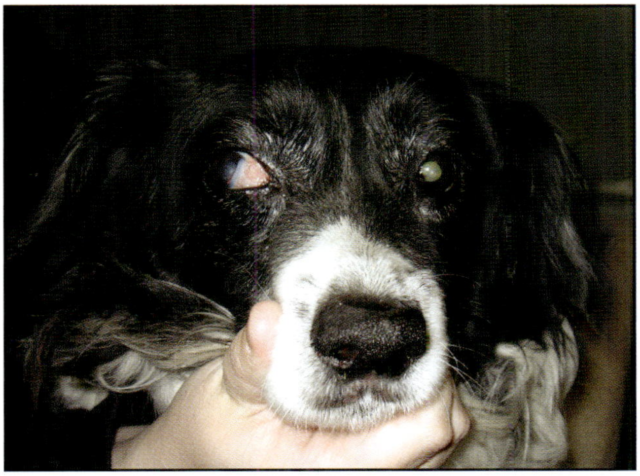

Figure 136.3 Clinical presentation associated with retrobulbar neoplasia (fibrosarcoma).

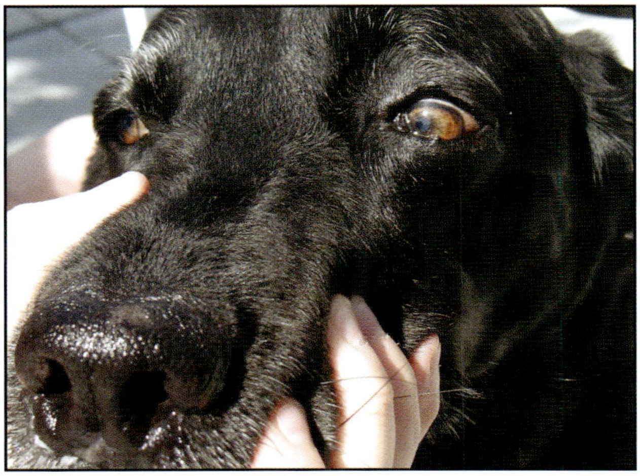

Figure 136.4 Clinical presentation associated with retrobulbar neoplasia (osteosarcoma).

Section 9

The Glaucomas

CHAPTER 137
CONGENITAL GLAUCOMA

PRESENTATION

Congenital glaucoma describes severe malformation of the aqueous drainage tracts, which are both hereditary and congenital (i.e., present at birth). As a result, affected animals display severe, bilateral, ocular pathology, very early in life (generally within weeks to months). Symptoms may include any combination of corneal edema, secondary ulcerative keratitis, episcleral injection, buphthalmos, optic nerve damage, and/or blindness. In some cases, additional ocular abnormalities may be present. Canine and feline species of any breed or crossed breed may be affected; however, this condition is uncommon.

DIAGNOSIS AND TREATMENT

Although treatment of affected animals may be attempted, vision salvage is generally not possible and typically, a (bilateral) surgical procedure of comfort is ultimately required (enucleation, cryoablation, intrascleral prosthesis, or chemical ciliary body ablation).

SELECTED REFERENCES

Glaze MB. Congenital and hereditary ocular abnormalities in cats. *Clin Tech Small Anim Pract* 2005;**20**(2):74–82.

Reinstein S, Rankin A, Allbaugh R. Canine glaucoma: pathophysiology and diagnosis. *Compend Contin Educ Vet* 2009;**31**(10):450–452; quiz 452–453.

Strom AR, Hässig M, Iburg TM, Spiess BM. Epidemiology of canine glaucoma presented to University of Zurich from 1995 to 2009. Part 1: Congenital and primary glaucoma (4 and 123 cases). *Vet Ophthalmol* 2011;**14**(2):121–126. DOI: 10.1111/j.1463-5224.2010.00855.x.

Clinical Atlas of Canine and Feline Ophthalmic Disease, First Edition. Douglas Esson.

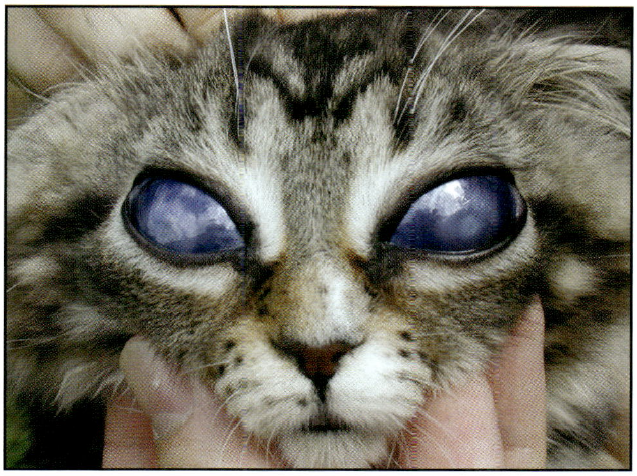

Figure 137.1 Clinical presentation associated with congenital glaucoma. Notable is the degree of buphthalmos present.

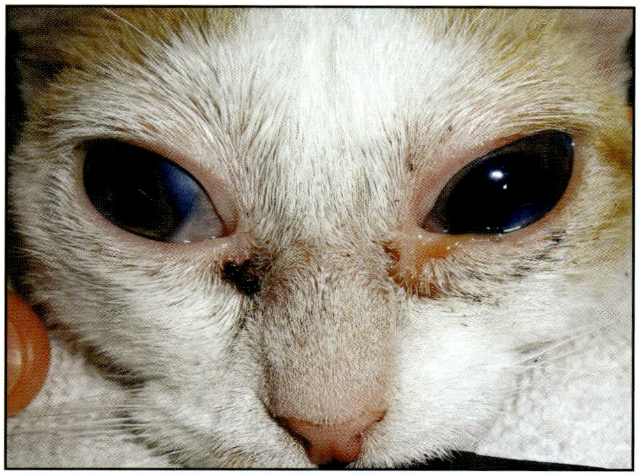

Figure 137.2 Clinical presentation associated with congenital glaucoma. Notable is the degree of buphthalmos present.

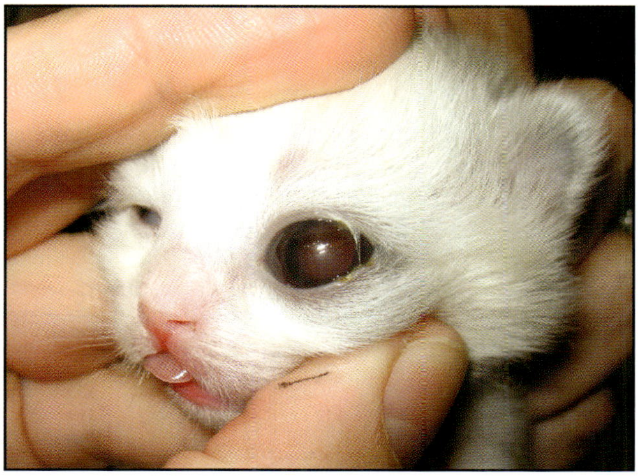

Figure 137.3 Clinical presentation associated with congenital glaucoma. Notable is the degree of buphthalmos present.

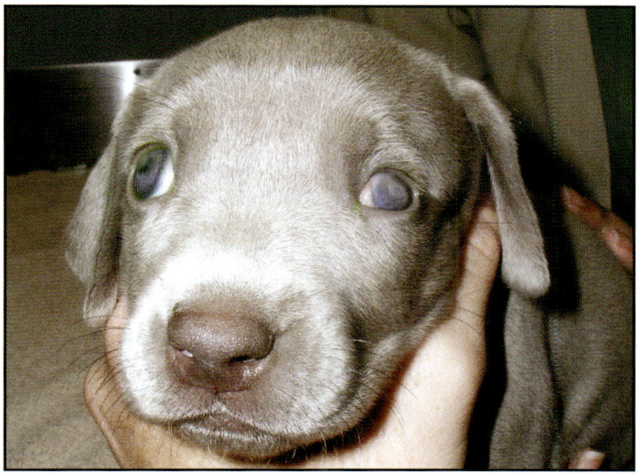

Figure 137.4 Clinical presentation associated with congenital glaucoma. Notable is the degree of buphthalmos present.

CHAPTER 138
PRIMARY GLAUCOMA

PRESENTATION

Primary glaucoma describes pathology associated with a hereditary predisposition for elevated intraocular pressure (IOP) and/or optic nerve (ON) degeneration. Although the underlying changes (comprising trabecular meshwork atrophy) generally develop over the course of many years, the presentation of primary glaucoma is typically peracute, frequently developing within just a few hours as a result of ciliary cleft collapse. Symptoms may include any combination of ocular discomfort, blepharospasm, corneal edema, episcleral injection, third eyelid elevation, miosis or mydriasis, visual deficits, and/or blindness. Chronically affected patients may display buphthalmos with time (see also Buphthalmos). Primary glaucoma has been described in association with numerous canine (as well as a limited number of feline) breeds, notably the Cocker Spaniel, Siberian Husky, Basset Hound, Boston Terrier, Bouvier des Flandres, Shiba Inu, Chow Chow, and Shar Pei.

DIAGNOSIS AND TREATMENT

The diagnosis of primary glaucoma is made on the basis of clinical findings as well as evaluation of IOP using a tonometer. Accurate "digital" tonometry is not possible. Adjunctive diagnostics include further evaluation of the external iridocorneal angle structures (via "gonioscopy") and/or the deeper trabecular meshwork and ciliary cleft (via high resolution ultrasonography). Effective treatment depends on prompt identification of symptoms and typically encompasses the rapid lowering of IOP using intravenous mannitol (with or without the administration of concurrent anti-inflammatory therapy in the form of a corticosteroid). Following the initial stabilization of IOP, more definitive control can be achieved by a combination of medical and/or surgical management using procedures to decrease aqueous production and/or maximize its outflow. Potentially beneficial agents when treating glaucoma include the prostaglandin analogues (such as latanoprost), the carbonic anhydrase-inhibitors (such as dorzolamide) and parasympathomimetic agents (such as demecarium bromide). Long-term adjunctive medical therapy is likely to be required in order to maintain control over IOP as well as to combat subsequent degeneration of ON tissue. Pharmacologic "neuroprotection" (using a variety of potentially beneficial anti-inflammatory, calcium channel blocking and/or receptor antagonist agents) in order to minimize ongoing ON damage in visual eyes is also indicated. Patients that develop primary glaucoma in one eye are at significant risk for the subsequent development of similar pathology in their contralateral eye. Irreversibly blind, painful, and/or buphthalmic eyes should be addressed through a procedure of comfort (enucleation, cryoablation, intrascleral prosthesis, or chemical ciliary body ablation).

Potential Drug-Side-Effects

Potential complications associated with the use of Mannitol include electrolyte imbalance, cardiopulmonary overload and gastrointestinal (GI) distress. Potential complications associated with the use of prostaglandin analogues include local irritation and discomfort secondary to profound miosis. Potential complications associated with the use of topical carbonic anhydrase-inhibitors include local irritation. Potential complications associated with the use of demecarium bromide include ocular discomfort and gastrointestinal (GI) distress.

SELECTED REFERENCES

Jacobi S, Dubielzig RR. Feline primary open angle glaucoma. *Vet Ophthalmol* 2008;**11**(3):162–165. DOI: 10.1111/j.1463-5224.2008.00614.x.

Reinstein S, Rankin A, Allbaugh R. Canine glaucoma: pathophysiology and diagnosis. *Compend Contin Educ Vet* 2009;**31**(10):450–452; quiz 452–453. Review.

Clinical Atlas of Canine and Feline Ophthalmic Disease, First Edition. Douglas Esson.

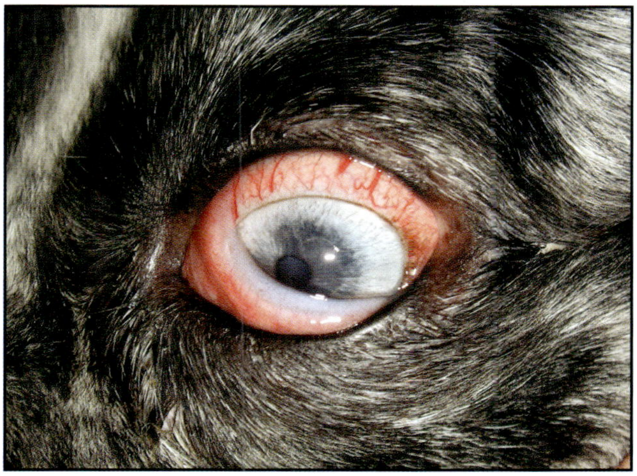

Figure 138.1 Clinical presentation associated with primary glaucoma. Episcleral injection is notable.

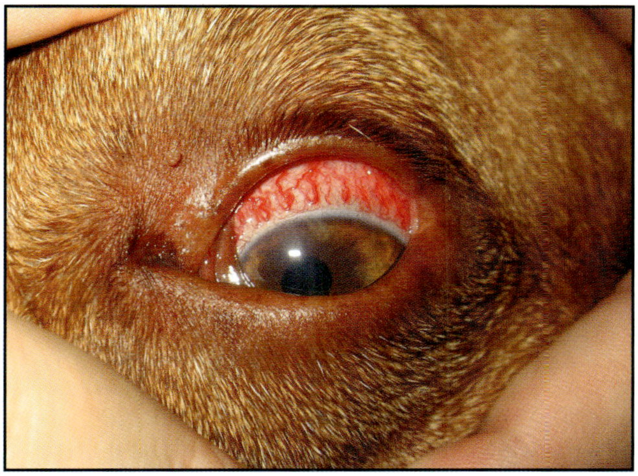

Figure 138.2 Clinical presentation associated with primary glaucoma. Episcleral injection is notable.

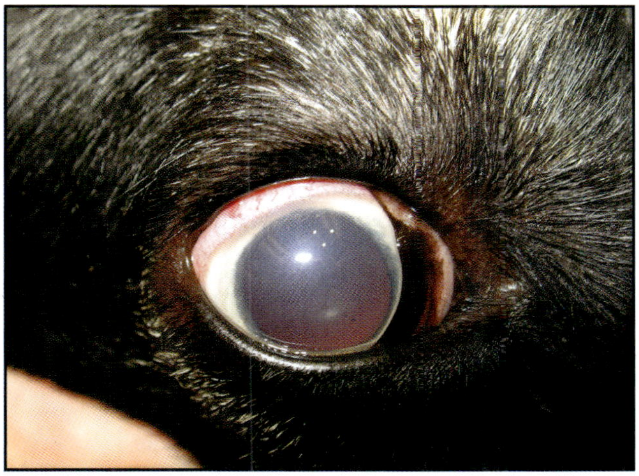

Figure 138.3 Clinical presentation associated with primary glaucoma. Corneal edema is notable.

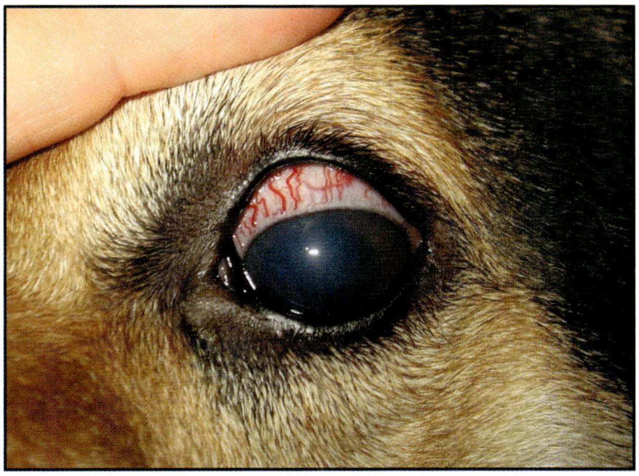

Figure 138.4 Clinical presentation associated with primary glaucoma. Episcleral injection and corneal edema are notable.

CHAPTER 139
SECONDARY (POSTINFLAMMATORY) GLAUCOMA

PRESENTATION

Secondary glaucoma describes elevated intraocular pressure associated with underlying ocular and/or systemic disease. Common causes of secondary glaucoma include lenticular (sub)luxation (anterior or posterior), ocular and/or systemic neoplasia, severe or chronic uveitis, retinal detachment, lens-induced uveitis, iris bombé, Golden Retriever-associated uveitis, uveodermatologic syndrome (see also Anterior Lens Luxation, Posterior Lens Luxation, Uveal Adenoma/Adenocarcinoma, Uveal Melanoma, Uveal Lymphoma, Feline Anterior Uveitis, Canine Anterior Uveitis, Phacolytic Uveitis, Phacoclastic Uveitis, Golden Retriever-Associated Uveitis and Glaucoma, and Uveodermatological Syndrome). Secondary glaucoma may develop acutely, subacutely, or chronically and may affect one or both eyes. Symptoms may include any combination of ocular discomfort, blepharospasm, corneal edema, episcleral injection, third eyelid elevation, miosis or mydriasis, uveitis, visual deficits, and/or blindness. Chronically affected may display buphthalmos with time (see also Buphthalmos).

DIAGNOSIS AND TREATMENT

The diagnosis of glaucoma is made on the basis of clinical findings as well as evaluation of intraocular pressure using a tonometer. Accurate "digital" tonometry is not possible. Adjunctive diagnostics may include further evaluation of the intraocular structures using B-mode ultrasonography. Effective treatment depends on prompt identification of symptoms and typically encompasses the rapid lowering of intraocular pressure (IOP) using intravenous mannitol (with or without the administration of concurrent anti-inflammatory therapy in the form of a corticosteroid). Underlying causes of secondary glaucoma including ocular/systemic inflammation, immune deviation, lenticular stability, and/or neoplasia should specifically be addressed if identified. The use of miotic agents should be avoided when anterior lenticular (sub)luxation is present or suspected as their use may exacerbate symptoms. Following the initial stabilization of IOP, more definitive control can be achieved by a combination of medical and/or surgical management using procedures to decrease aqueous production and/or maximize its outflow. Potentially beneficial agents when treating glaucoma include the prostaglandin analogues (such as latanoprost), the carbonic anhydrase-inhibitors (such as dorzolamide) and parasympathomimetic agents (such as demecarium bromide). Pharmacologic "neuroprotection" (using a variety of potentially beneficial anti-inflammatory, calcium channel blocking, and/or receptor antagonist agents) in order to minimize ongoing optic nerve damage in visual eyes is also indicated. Irreversibly blind, painful, and/or buphthalmic eyes should be addressed through a procedure of comfort (enucleation, cryoablation, intrascleral prosthesis, or chemical ciliary body ablation).

Potential Drug-Side-Effects

Potential complications associated with the use of Mannitol include electrolyte imbalance, cardiopulmonary overload and gastrointestinal (GI) distress. Potential complications associated with the use of prostaglandin analogues include local irritation and discomfort secondary to profound miosis. Potential complications associated with the use of topical carbonic anhydrase-inhibitors include local irritation. Potential complications associated with the use of demecarium bromide include ocular discomfort and gastrointestinal (GI) distress.

SELECTED REFERENCES

Gelatt KN, MacKay EO. Secondary glaucomas in the dog in North America. *Vet Ophthalmol* 2004;7(4):245–259.

Clinical Atlas of Canine and Feline Ophthalmic Disease, First Edition. Douglas Esson.

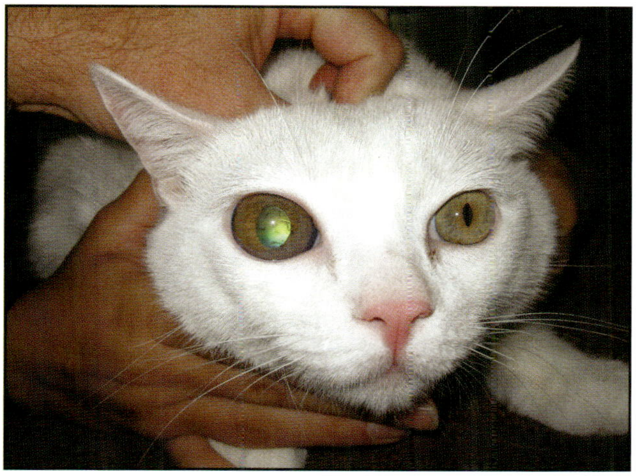

Figure 139.1 Clinical presentation associated with secondary glaucoma as a result of chronic lymphoplasmacytic uveitis.

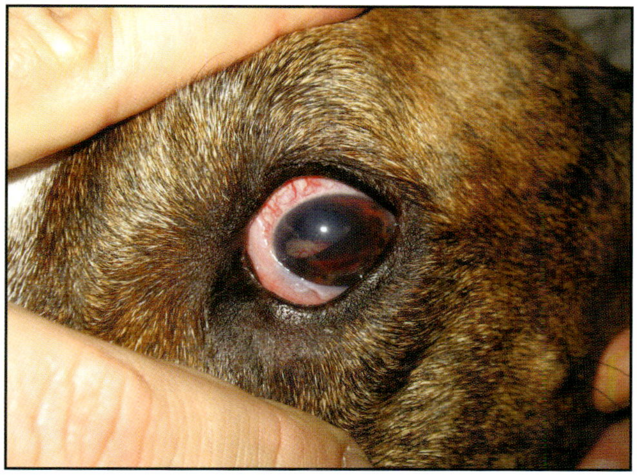

Figure 139.2 Clinical presentation associated with secondary glaucoma as a result of intraocular neoplasia.

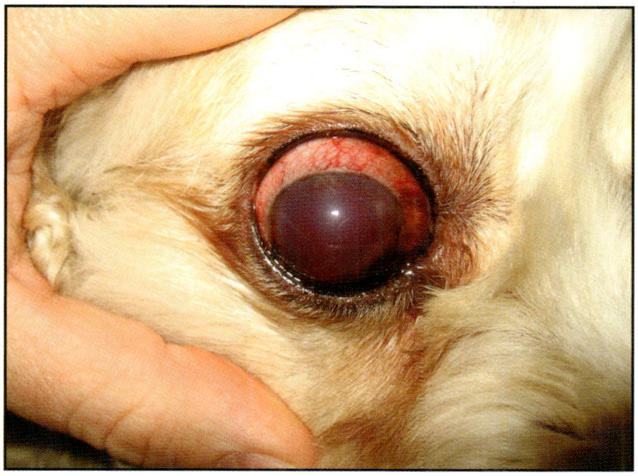

Figure 139.3 Clinical presentation associated with secondary glaucoma as a result of hyphema.

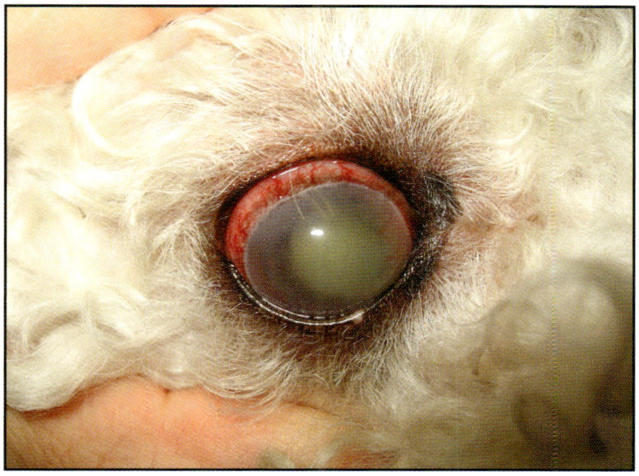

Figure 139.4 Clinical presentation associated with secondary glaucoma as a result of phacoclastic uveitis.

CHAPTER 140
FELINE AQUEOUS HUMOR MISDIRECTION SYNDROME (AHMS)

PRESENTATION

Feline aqueous humor misdirection syndrome (AHMS) represents a unique form of feline glaucoma, which occurs as a result of aqueous accumulation within the vitreous body, suspected to arise as a result of abnormalities associated with the anterior vitreous face. This condition has also been termed malignant glaucoma. Resultant changes include vitreous expansion, anterior displacement of the lens/iris diaphragm, anterior chamber shallowing, ciliary cleft collapse, and progressive intraocular pressure (IOP) elevation. Clinical symptoms may include mydriasis, anisocoria, discomfort, visual deficits, and/or blindness. Ultimately, bilateral involvement is most common. Any breed or crossed breed may be affected.

DIAGNOSIS AND TREATMENT

The diagnosis of AHMS is made on the basis of clinical findings (including tonometry), supported if necessary by B-mode ultrasonography. Management initially comprises medical therapy using topical carbonic anhydrase inhibitors (dorzolamide or brinzolamide) and/or miotic agents (demecarium bromide).

Potential Drug-Side-Effects

Potential complications associated with the use of demecarium bromide include ocular discomfort and gastrointestinal (GI) distress. Potential complications associated with the use of topical carbonic anhydrase-inhibitors include local irritation.

With time, progressive IOP elevation may dictate surgical intervention in the form of lensectomy, vitrectomy, and/or ciliary photocoagulation.

SELECTED REFERENCES

Blocker T, Van Der Woerdt A. The feline glaucomas: 82 cases (1995–1999). *Vet Ophthalmol* 2001;**4**(2):81–85.

Czederpiltz JM, La Croix NC, van der Woerdt A, Bentley E, Dubielzig RR, Murphy CJ, Miller PE. Putative aqueous humor misdirection syndrome as a cause of glaucoma in cats: 32 cases (1997–2003). *J Am Vet Med Assoc* 2005;**227**(9):1434–1441.

Wilcock BP, Peiffer RL Jr, Davidson MG. The causes of glaucoma in cats. *Vet Pathol* 1990;**27**(1):35–40.

Clinical Atlas of Canine and Feline Ophthalmic Disease, First Edition. Douglas Esson.

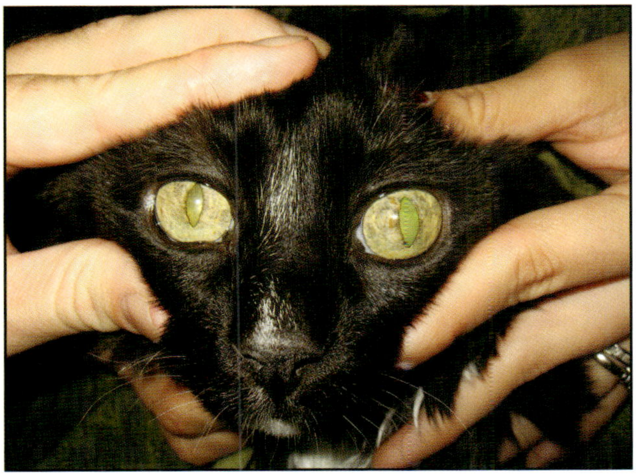

Figure 140.1 Clinical presentation associated with feline aqueous misdirection syndrome.

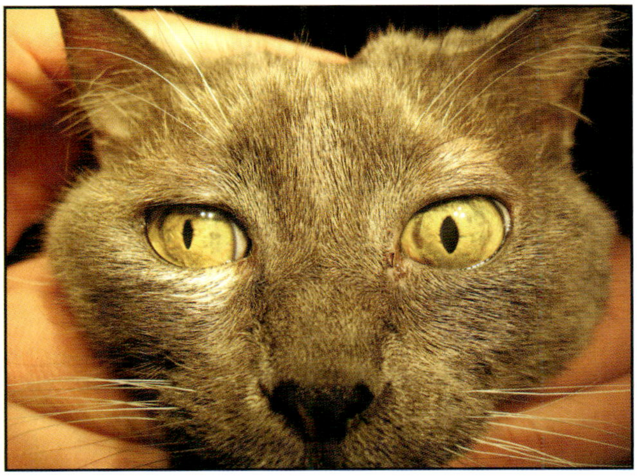

Figure 140.2 Clinical presentation associated with feline aqueous misdirection syndrome. Anisocoria and anterior chamber shallowing are notable.

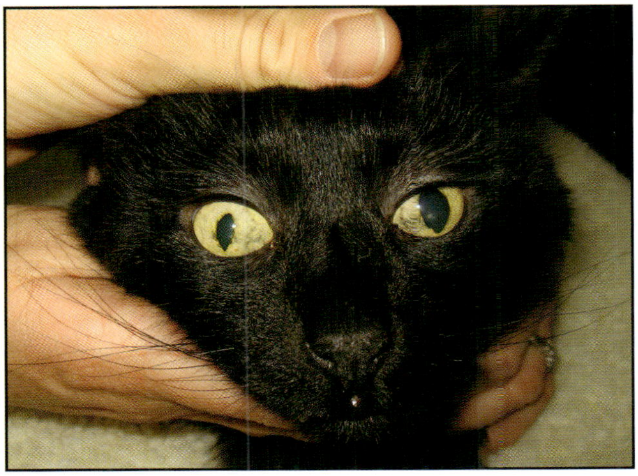

Figure 140.3 Clinical presentation associated with feline aqueous misdirection syndrome. Anisocoria is notable.

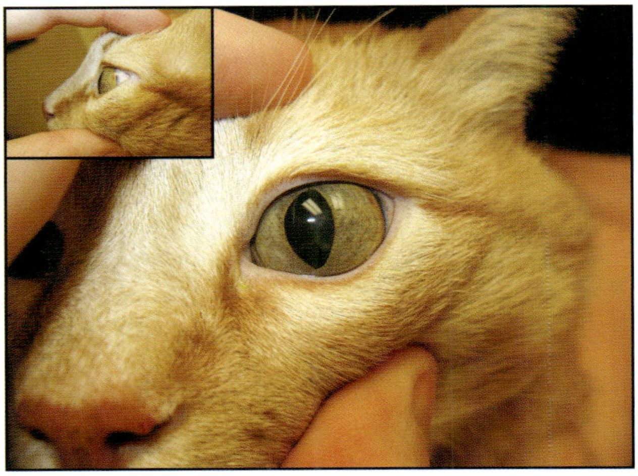

Figure 140.4 Clinical presentation associated with feline aqueous misdirection syndrome. Inset demonstrates anterior chamber shallowing.

CHAPTER 141
PIGMENTARY GLAUCOMA

PRESENTATION

Pigmentary glaucoma (also referred to as ocular melanosis) describes a pathological elevation in intraocular pressure (IOP), which occurs as a result of the proliferation and accumulation of cells containing melanin in the aqueous outflow tracts. Studies support a hereditary etiology. Symptoms are generally bilateral, although not always symmetrical and comprise the visible accumulation of pigment within the scleral/episcleral, corneal, and/or uveal tissues as well as any combination of corneal edema, blepharospasm, episcleral injection, visual deficits, blindness, and/or buphthalmos. Commonly affected breeds include the Cairn Terrier, Boxer, and Labrador Retriever.

DIAGNOSIS AND TREATMENT

The diagnosis of pigmentary glaucoma is made on the basis of clinical findings as well as evaluation of IOP using a tonometer. Typical changes include the irregular, dense pigmentation of scleral tissues, which overlie the ciliary body. Histopathological interpretation of enucleated tissues is confirmatory. Palliative management of affected patients comprises medical and/or surgical treatment of elevated IOP. Unfortunately, however, disease progression frequently means that a procedure of comfort is ultimately required (enucleation, cryoablation, intrascleral prosthesis placement, or chemical ciliary body ablation).

SELECTED REFERENCES

Petersen-Jones SM, Forcier J, Mentzer AL. Ocular melanosis in the Cairn Terrier: clinical description and investigation of mode of inheritance. *Vet Ophthalmol* 2007;**10**(Suppl 1):63–69.

van de Sandt RR, Boevé MH, Stades FC, Kik MJ. Abnormal ocular pigment deposition and glaucoma in the dog. *Vet Ophthalmol* 2003;**6**(4):273–278.

Clinical Atlas of Canine and Feline Ophthalmic Disease, First Edition. Douglas Esson.

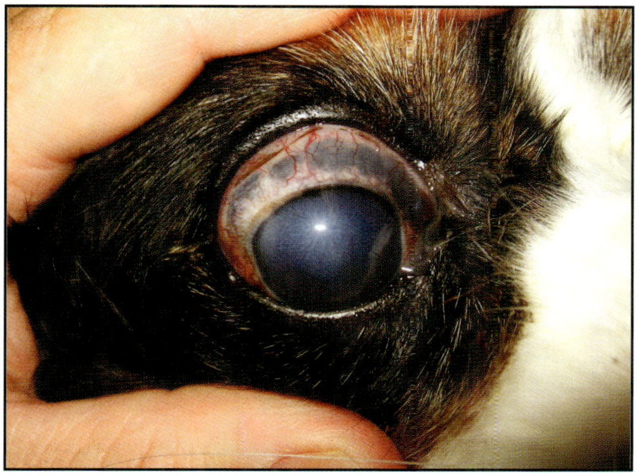

Figure 141.1 Clinical presentation associated with pigmentary glaucoma.

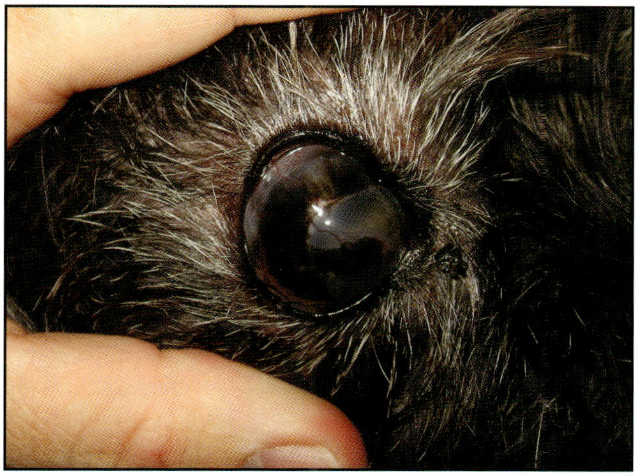

Figure 141.2 Clinical presentation associated with pigmentary glaucoma.

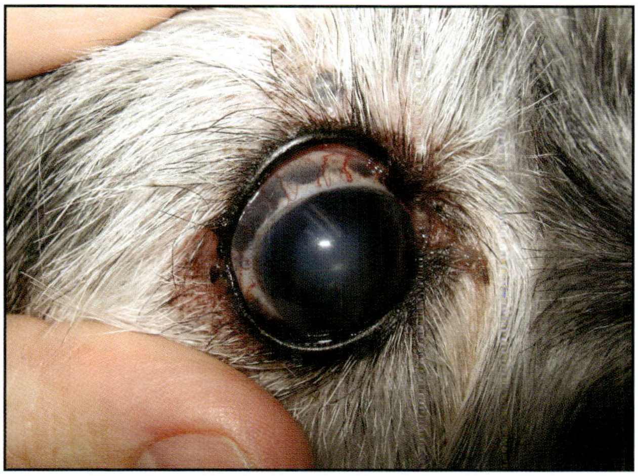

Figure 141.3 Clinical presentation associated with pigmentary glaucoma.

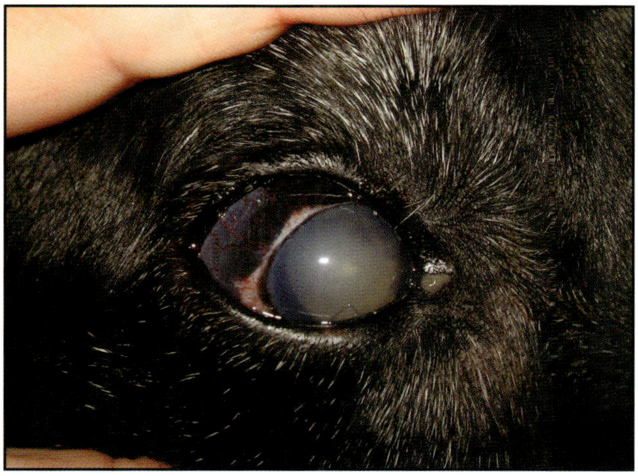

Figure 141.4 Clinical presentation associated with pigmentary glaucoma.

CHAPTER 142
GOLDEN RETRIEVER-ASSOCIATED UVEITIS AND GLAUCOMA

PRESENTATION

A syndrome comprising slowly progressive intraocular changes, typically culminating in secondary glaucoma, is well recognized within the Golden Retriever breed. This syndrome has been variably described as "pigmentary uveitis," "Golden Retriever uveitis," and "pigmentary and cystic glaucoma of Golden Retrievers." Findings may include any combination of conjunctival and/or episcleral hyperemia, corneal decompensation, thin-walled uveal cysts within the anterior or posterior chambers, proteinaceous exudation within the anterior chamber, anterior and/or posterior iridal adhesions, pigment dispersion within the anterior chamber and/or onto the anterior lens capsule, cataract formation, hyphema, and/or secondary glaucoma (see also Golden Retriever-Associated Uveitis). Uveal cysts may detach and move into the anterior chamber where they may rupture against corneal endothelial and/or iridal surfaces or collapse and rupture within the iridocorneal angle. The hallmark of this syndrome has been described as the appearance of pigment on the anterior lens capsule, typically distributed in a radial orientation. Initial symptoms are frequently noted in middle age and are usually bilateral, although not necessarily symmetrical. The etiology of this syndrome is poorly understood; however, genetic factors have been proposed on the basis of breed predilection as well as the absence of demonstrable infectious or neoplastic causes.

DIAGNOSIS AND TREATMENT

The diagnosis is made on the basis of a combination of signalment and clinical findings. Treatment is generally empirical, frequently comprising topical and/or systemic anti-inflammatory (either steroidal or nonsteroidal), immune-modulating (azathioprine or cyclosporine) and/or anti-glaucoma agents; however, secondary glaucoma is frequently the endpoint of this disease.

Potential Drug-Side-Effects

Potential adverse effects associated with the use of systemic corticosteroids include polyphagia, polydipsia, polyuria, hair coat changes, weight gain, pancreatitis, enteritis, muscular damage, hepatic impairment, and diabetes. Potential adverse effects associated with the use of azathioprine include gastrointestinal (GI) distress, pancreatitis, hepatotoxicity, and myelosuppression. Potential adverse affects associated with the use of cyclosporine include hypersensitivity and GI distress.

Patients affected by advanced disease, represent high-risk candidates for either cataract or glaucoma surgery based on the frequency and severity of complications encountered. Ultimately, a procedure of comfort (enucleation, cryosurgery, intrascleral prosthesis placement, or chemical ciliary body ablation) may be necessary in order to address blind and/or painful eyes.

SELECTED REFERENCES

Deehr AJ, Dubielzig RR. A histopathological study of iridociliary cysts and glaucoma in Golden Retrievers. *Vet Ophthalmol* 1998;**1**(2–3):153–158.

Esson D, Armour M, Mundy P, Schobert CS, Dubielzig RR. The histopathological and immunohistochemical characteristics of pigmentary and cystic glaucoma in the Golden Retriever. *Vet Ophthalmol* 2009;**12**(6):361–368.

Sapienza JS, Simó FJ, Prades-Sapienza A. Golden Retriever uveitis: 75 cases (1994–1999). *Vet Ophthalmol* 2000;**3**(4):241–246.

Townsend WM, Gornik KR. Prevalence of uveal cysts and pigmentary uveitis in Golden Retrievers in three Midwestern states. *J Am Vet Med Assoc* 2013;**243**(9):1298–1301. DOI: 10.2460/javma.243.9.1298.

Clinical Atlas of Canine and Feline Ophthalmic Disease, First Edition. Douglas Esson.

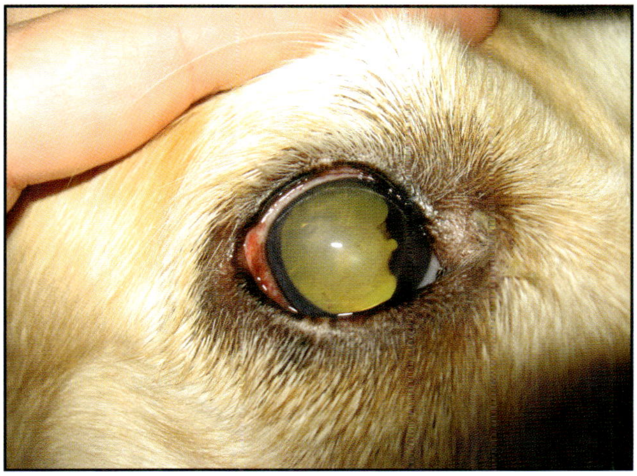

Figure 142.1 Glaucoma secondary to Golden Retriever-associated pigmentary uveitis.

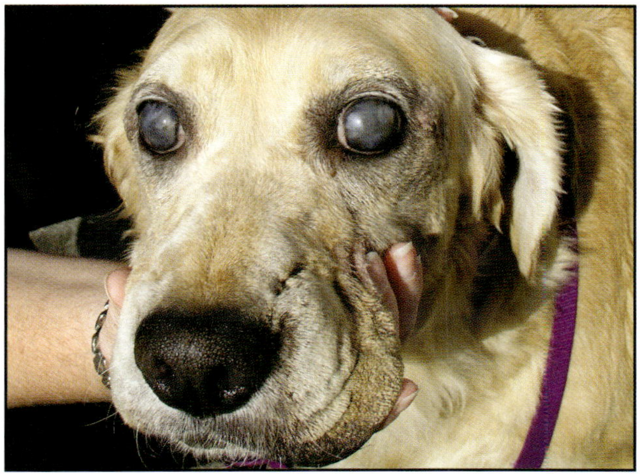

Figure 142.2 Glaucoma secondary to Golden Retriever-associated pigmentary uveitis. Changes are bilateral.

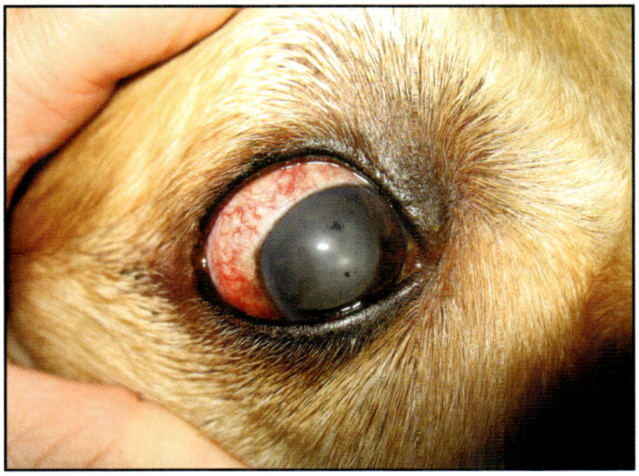

Figure 142.3 Glaucoma secondary to Golden Retriever-associated pigmentary uveitis.

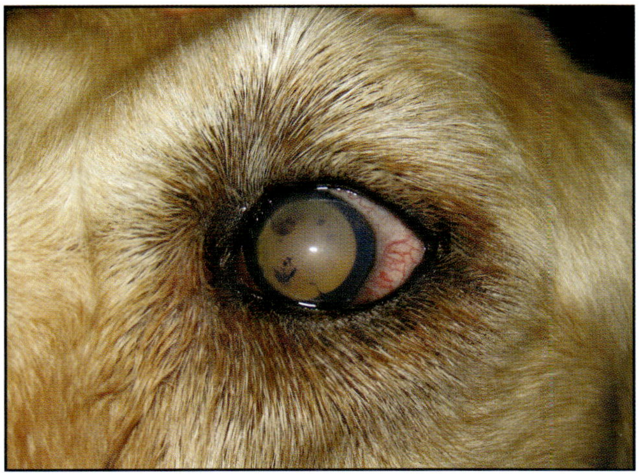

Figure 142.4 Glaucoma secondary to Golden Retriever-associated pigmentary uveitis.

CHAPTER 143
BUPHTHALMOS

PRESENTATION

Buphthalmos describes physical enlargement of the globe, resulting from severe elevations in intraocular pressure (IOP) of congenital, primary, or secondary etiology. Buphthalmos should not be confused with the following:

- Exophthalmos (anterior displacement of the globe within the obit),
- Proptosis (displacement of the globe from the orbit),
- Strabismus (deviation of the globe within the orbit),
- Non-bupthalmic glaucoma.

Typically, buphthalmos indicates chronically elevated IOP; however, young animals may develop these changes relatively rapidly as a result of juvenile scleral elasticity. Symptoms may include not only globe enlargement but also any combination of conjunctivitis, blepharospasm, visible tears within the corneal endothelium ("Haab's striae") corneal edema, keratopathy (including ulceration), lenticular (sub)luxation, and/or globe rupture.

DIAGNOSIS AND TREATMENT

Buphthalmos generally implies blindness secondary to chronic ocular changes and associated damage to the optic nerve; however, individuals may retain a degree of functional vision in spite of early buphthalmos—notably feline patients. Generally, a surgery comfort (enucleation, evisceration, cryotherapy, and/or chemical ciliary body ablation) of affected globes is indicated. Where possible, the underlying cause of glaucoma should be identified (most typically through histopathological interpretation of enucleated tissues), so that any predisposition to similar pathology within the contralateral eye can be addressed.

SELECTED REFERENCES

Brooks DE (1990) Glaucoma in the dog and cat. *Vet Clin North Am Small Anim Pract* **20**(3):775–797. Review.

McLaughlin SA, Render JA, Brightman AH 2nd, Whiteley HE, Helper LC, Shadduck JA. Intraocular findings in three dogs and one cat with chronic glaucoma. *J Am Vet Med Assoc* 1987;**191**(11):1443–1445.

Sandmeyer LS, Bauer BS, Grahn BH. Diagnostic ophthalmology. *Can Vet J* 2012;**53**(1):96–98.

Clinical Atlas of Canine and Feline Ophthalmic Disease, First Edition. Douglas Esson.

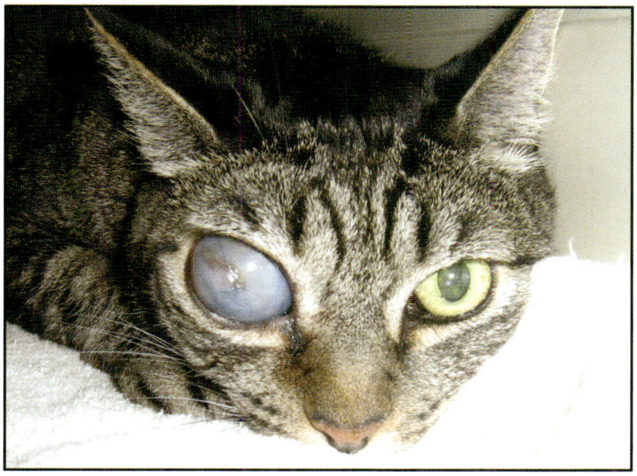

Figure 143.1 Clinical presentation associated with buphthalmos.

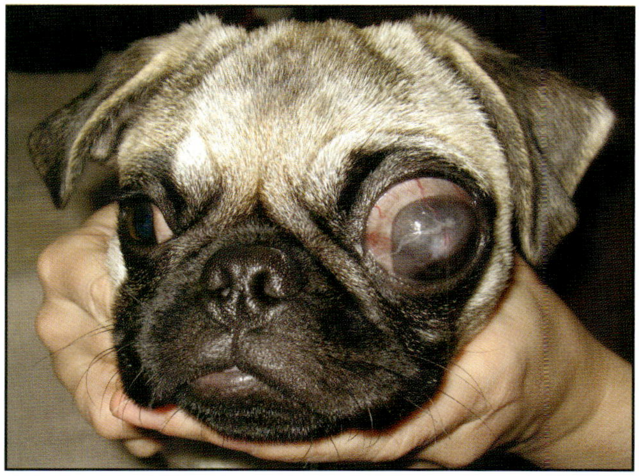

Figure 143.2 Clinical presentation associated with buphthalmos.

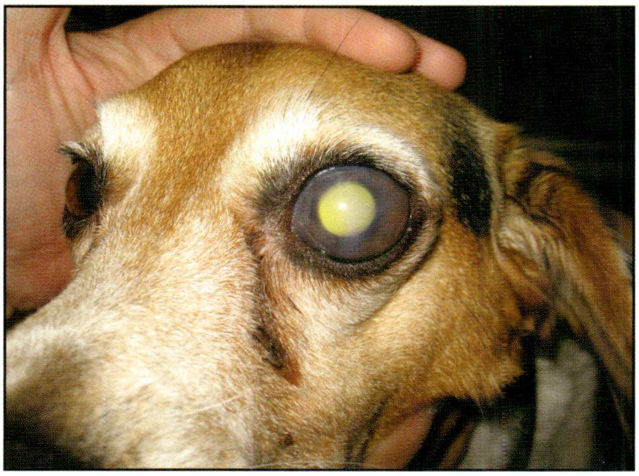

Figure 143.3 Clinical presentation associated with buphthalmos.

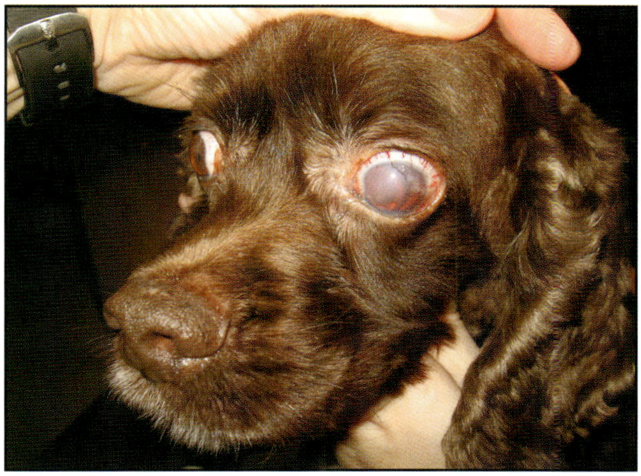

Figure 143.4 Clinical presentation associated with buphthalmos. Notable are corneal Haab's striae.

Section 10

Neuro-Ophthalmic Disease

CHAPTER 144
OPTIC NERVE HYPOPLASIA

PRESENTATION

Optic nerve hypoplasia (and, in rare cases, aplasia) results from a congenitally abnormal differentiation of these tissues. Clinically, affected patients display small, gray-colored and poorly myelinated optic nerve head tissue. Changes are typically bilateral; however, they may be unilateral and may be accompanied by other ocular abnormalities including anterior segment dysgenesis and/or vitreoretinal pathology. Associated visual deficits may vary from mild to complete blindness and are typically noted early in life (weeks to months). Commonly affected breeds include the German Shepherd and Shih Tzu.

DIAGNOSIS AND TREATMENT

The diagnosis of optic nerve hypoplasia is made on the basis of clinical examination including funduscopy, supported if necessary by adjunctive imaging (typically, B-mode ultrasonography). No treatment is available for affected animals.

SELECTED REFERENCES

Negishi H, Hoshiya T, Tsuda Y, Doi K, Kanemaki N. Unilateral optical nerve hypoplasia in a Beagle dog. *Lab Anim* 2008;**42**(3):383–388. DOI: 10.1258/la.2007.007033.

Rampazzo A, D'Angelo A, Capucchio MT, Sereno S, Peruccio C. Collie eye anomaly in a mixed-breed dog. *Vet Ophthalmol* 2005;**8**(5):357–360.

da Silva EG, Dubielzig R, Zarfoss MK, Anibal A. Distinctive histopathologic features of canine optic nerve hypoplasia and aplasia: a retrospective review of 13 cases. *Vet Ophthalmol* 2008;**11**(1):23–29. DOI: 10.1111/j.1463-5224.2007.00596.x.

Clinical Atlas of Canine and Feline Ophthalmic Disease, First Edition. Douglas Esson.

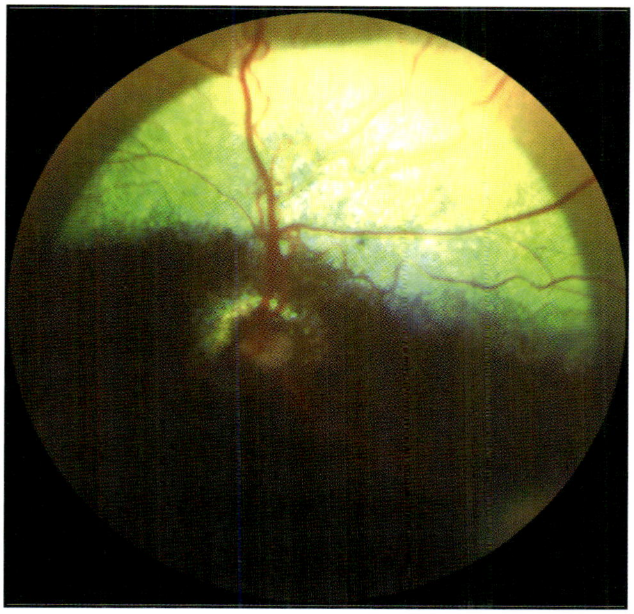

Figure 144.1 Funduscopic findings associated with optic nerve hypoplasia.

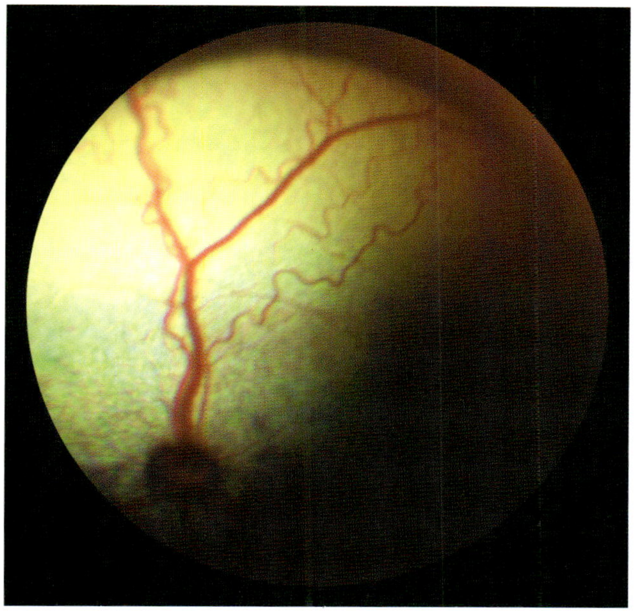

Figure 144.2 Funduscopic findings associated with optic nerve hypoplasia.

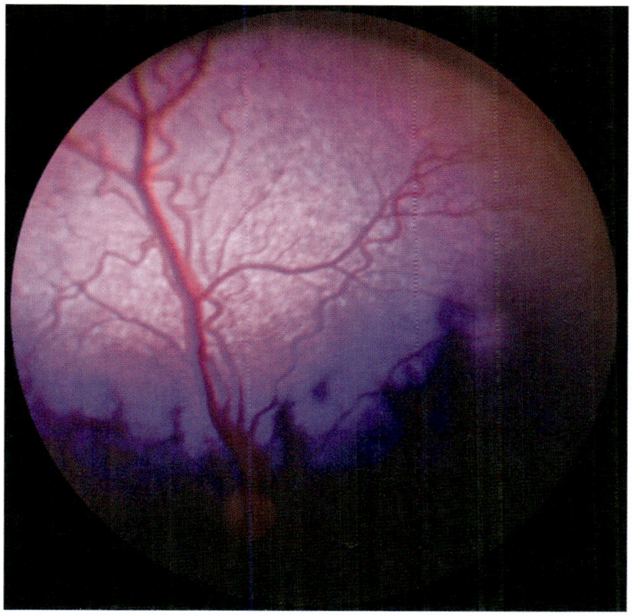

Figure 144.3 Funduscopic findings associated with optic nerve hypoplasia.

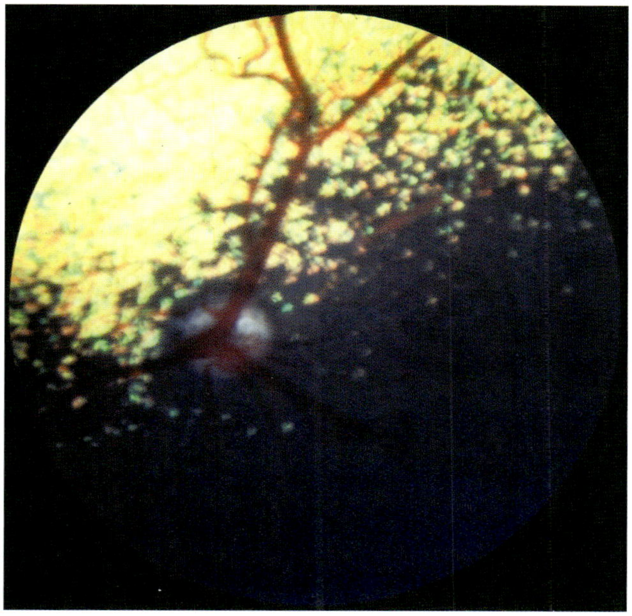

Figure 144.4 Funduscopic findings associated with optic nerve hypoplasia.

CHAPTER 145
LYSOSOMAL STORAGE DISEASE (LSD)

PRESENTATION

The lysosomal storage diseases (LSDs) represent a group of relatively uncommon, hereditary, inborn errors of metabolism, which result in the pathological accumulation of metabolic products within cellular lysosomes. Major diseases within this group include the following:

- (The) neuronal ceroid lipofuscinoses
- Globoid cell leukodystrophy
- (The) mucolipidoses
- (The) gangliosidoses
- Alpha-mannosidosis
- Fucosidosis
- (The) mucopolysaccharidoses.

Clinical symptoms frequently become apparent early in life, generally by 6–12 months of age; however, may vary in severity based both on disease subtype as well as degree of metabolic pathology present. Symptoms may include any combination of lethargy, weakness, dysphagia, "failure to thrive," facial dysmorphism, musculoskeletal malformation, renal/cardiac/hepatic insufficiency, corneal dystrophy, retinopathy, decreased visual function/blindness, and/or neurologic dysfunction. Affected dog breeds may include the Beagle, Springer Spaniel, Siberian Husky, German Shorthaired Pointer, Cairn Terrier, West Highland White Terrier, Miniature Pinscher, English Setter, Golden Retriever, Dachshund, and Miniature Schnauzer. Affected cat breeds may include the Siamese, Persian, and Korat.

DIAGNOSIS AND TREATMENT

The diagnosis of LSD can be challenging and is based on clinical findings, serum chemistry values, and specific genetic testing where available (http://research.vet.upenn.edu/WSAVA-LabSearch). The long-term prognosis for affected animals is generally poor; however, experimental therapy including emerging pharmaceutical agents, enzyme therapy, bone marrow transplantation, and gene therapy may be possible in selected cases.

SELECTED REFERENCES

Haskins ME. Animal models for mucopolysaccharidosis disorders and their clinical relevance. *Acta Paediatr Suppl* 2007;**96**(455):56–62.

Jolly RD, Walkley SU. Lysosomal storage diseases of animals: an essay in comparative pathology. *Vet Pathol* 1997;**34**(6):527–548.

Narfström K. Hereditary and congenital ocular disease in the cat. *J Feline Med Surg.* 1999;**1**(3):135–141.

Skelly BJ, Franklin RJ (2002)Recognition and diagnosis of lysosomal storage diseases in the cat and dog. *J Vet Intern Med* **16**(2):133–141. Review.

Slutsky J, Raj K, Yuhnke S, Bell J, Fretwell N, Hedhammar A, Wade C, Giger U. A web resource on DNA tests for canine and feline hereditary diseases. *Vet J.* 2013;**197**(2):182–187. DOI: 10.1016/j.tvjl.2013.02.021. Epub 2013 Apr 11.

Clinical Atlas of Canine and Feline Ophthalmic Disease, First Edition. Douglas Esson.

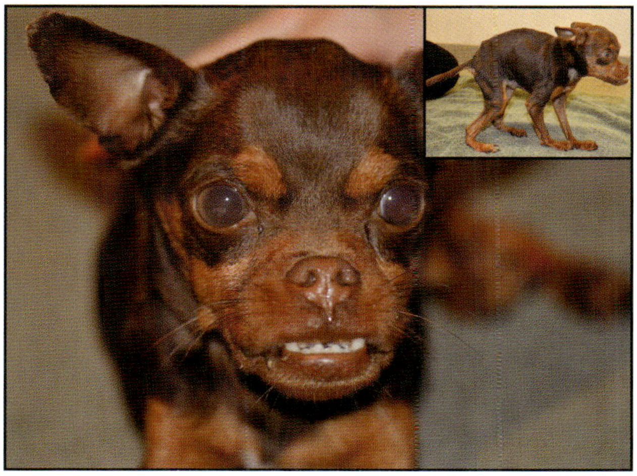

Figure 145.1 Clinical presentation associated with mucopolysaccharidosis. Notable is facial dysmorphism and corneal dystrophy. Inset demonstrates musculoskeletal malformation.

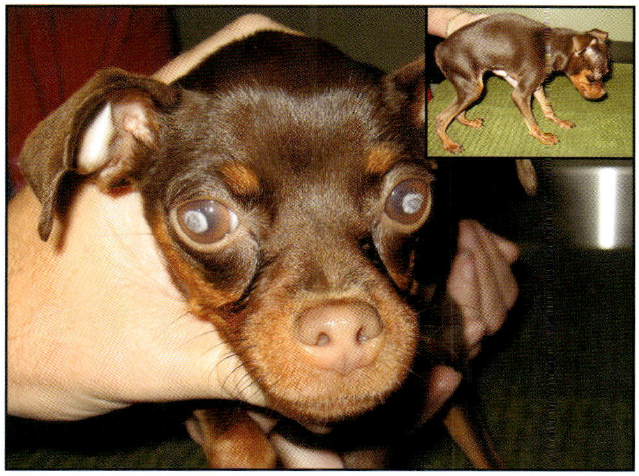

Figure 145.2 Clinical presentation associated with mucopolysaccharidosis. Notable is facial dysmorphism and corneal dystrophy. Inset demonstrates musculoskeletal malformation.

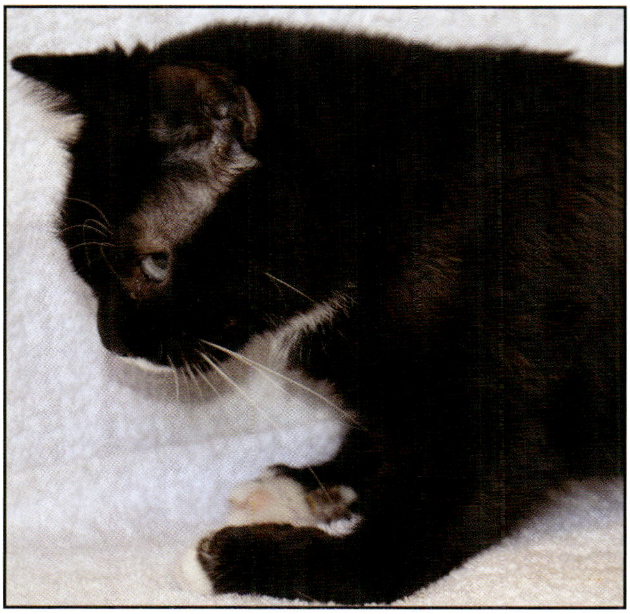

Figure 145.3 Clinical presentation associated with mucolipidosis. Notable is facial dysmorphism and musculoskeletal malformation.

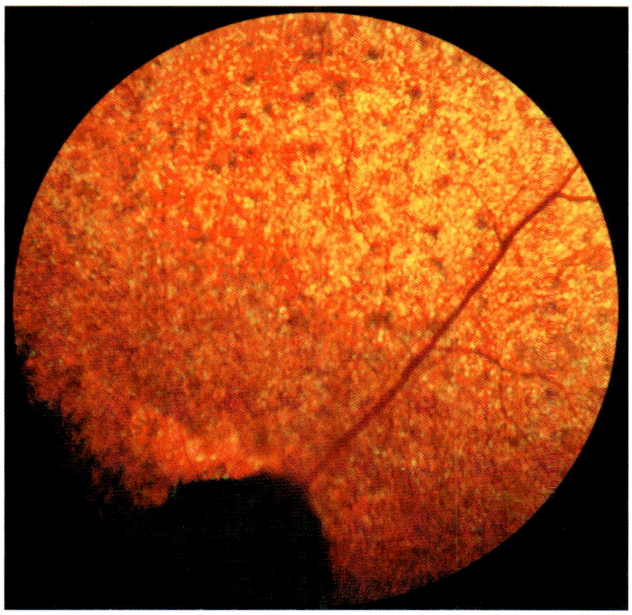

Figure 145.4 Funduscopic changes associated with neuronal ceroid lipofuscinosis. Multifocal tapetal discoloration is the result of pathological protein accumulation.

CHAPTER 146
SYMPATHETIC DENERVATION (HORNER'S SYNDROME)

PRESENTATION

Sympathetic innervation to the eye mediates the action of the iris dilator and contractor muscles (via "double-reciprocal innervation"), the smooth muscle of the orbit, and the Muller's muscles of the upper and lower eyelids. This pathway originates in the hypothalamus, exits the spinal cord with the ventral thoracic roots and synapses in the cranial cervical ganglion, adjacent to the tympanic bullae. Post-ganglionic fibers follow the ophthalmic division of the trigeminal nerve before entering the eye via the long ciliary nerves. Partial or complete interruption of sympathetic innervation to the ocular structures results in a group of symptoms referred to as Horner's syndrome, comprising variable combinations of pupillary miosis, third eyelid protrusion, enophthalmos, and/or upper lid ptosis.

DIAGNOSIS AND TREATMENT

The diagnosis of Horner's syndrome is confirmed via pharmacological testing using topical phenylephrine, which results in the resolution of symptoms in a timeframe consistent with the location of the lesion (typically less than 30 min). Horner's syndrome symptoms may be idiopathic in etiology, or associated with inflammation at any point along the sympathetic tract, notably at the level of the ear canal/tympanic bullae. As a result, underlying inflammatory or neoplastic disease and/or neuropathy should be specifically addressed. Systemic anti-inflammatory therapy using corticosteroids may be beneficial in selected cases; however, most cases of Horner's syndrome display spontaneous resolution of symptoms. Resolution may take weeks to months.

Potential Drug-Side-Effects

Potential adverse effects associated with the use of systemic prednisone include polyphagia, polydipsia, polyuria, hair coat changes, weight gain, pancreatitis, gastrointestinal (GI) distress, muscle damage, hepatic impairment, and diabetes.

SELECTED REFERENCES

Boydell P. Idiopathic horner syndrome in the golden retriever. *J Neuroophthalmol* 2000;**20**(4):288–290.

Kern TJ, Aromando MC, Erb HN. Horner's syndrome in dogs and cats: 100 cases (1975–1985). *J Am Vet Med Assoc* 1989;**195**(3):369–373.

Simpson KM, Williams DL, Cherubini GB. Neuropharmacological lesion localization in idiopathic Horner's syndrome in golden retrievers and dogs of other breeds. *Vet Ophthalmol* 2013. DOI: 10.1111/vop.12096.

Clinical Atlas of Canine and Feline Ophthalmic Disease, First Edition. Douglas Esson.

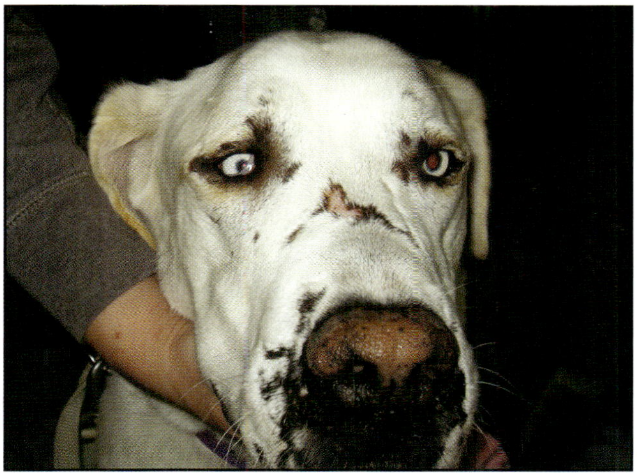

Figure 146.1 Clinical presentation associated with Horner's syndrome. Notable are enophthalmos, upper eyelid ptosis, third eyelid elevation, and pupillary miosis.

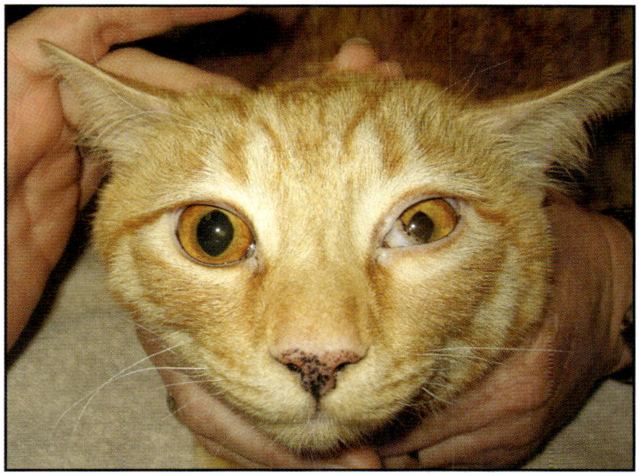

Figure 146.2 Clinical presentation associated with Horner's syndrome. Notable are enophthalmos, upper eyelid ptosis, third eyelid elevation, and pupillary miosis.

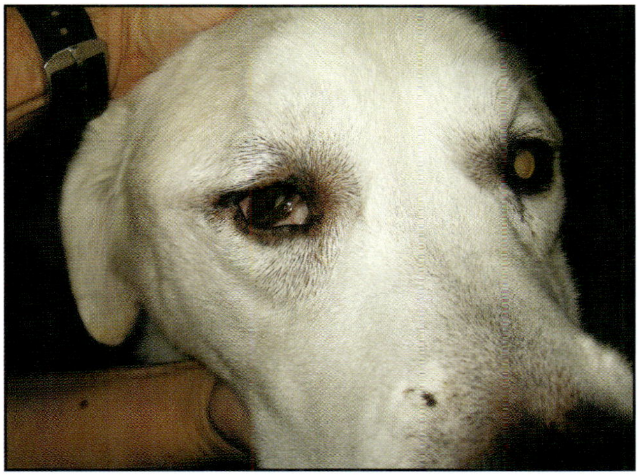

Figure 146.3 Clinical presentation associated with Horner's syndrome. Notable are enophthalmos, upper eyelid ptosis, third eyelid elevation, and pupillary miosis.

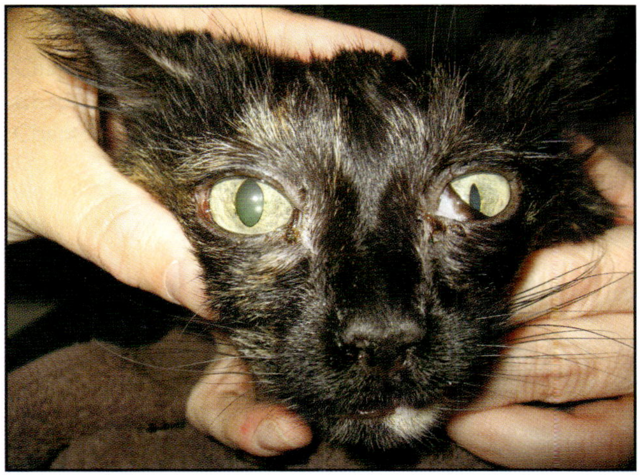

Figure 146.4 Clinical presentation associated with Horner's syndrome. Notable are enophthalmos, upper eyelid ptosis, third eyelid elevation, and pupillary miosis.

CHAPTER 147
OPHTHALMOPLEGIA

PRESENTATION

The term ophthalmoplegia describes a syndrome of neurological deficits arising as a result of damage to the oculomotor nerve (CN III) and/or its nucleus. CN III normally provides somatic efferent innervation to the dorsal, medial, and ventral rectus and ventral oblique muscles of the eye, as well as the levator palpebral muscle. This nerve also contains the parasympathetic fibers, which innervate the pupillary muscles (through "double reciprocal innervation"). As a result, lesions affecting CN III may result in:

- internal ophthalmoplegia (dilated nonresponsive pupil, without visual deficits)
- external ophthalmoplegia (ventrolateral strabismus and/or upper lid ptosis)
- complete ophthalmoplegia (combined internal and external ophthalmoplegia).

The superficial location of the parasympathetic fibers results in internal ophthalmoplegia being the most common clinical presentation. Ophthalmoplegia frequently results from a lesion affecting CN III at the level of the cavernous venous sinus (so-called "cavernous sinus syndrome"). Additional symptoms, depending on the site of the lesion may include reduced corneal and/or facial sensation as a result of impaired trigeminal nerve function and/or neurogenic keratoconjunctivitis sicca (KCS) (see also Neurogenic KCS and Xeromycteria).

DIAGNOSIS AND TREATMENT

The diagnosis of ophthalmoplegia is made on the basis of clinical findings as well as pharmacologic testing using topical pilocarpine, which will result in the resolution of mydriasis within 30 min. Cranial soft tissue imaging (magnetic resonance imaging (MRI)) is generally indicated in order to visualize affected structures. The treatment of ophthalmoplegia comprises treating the underlying lesion, typically encompassing the management of neoplastic lesions using targeted radiotherapy and/or chemotherapy. Secondary symptoms including ulcerative keratitis and/or KCS should also be managed if present.

SELECTED REFERENCES

Guevar J, Gutierrez-Quintana R, Peplinski G, Helm JR, Penderis J. Cavernous sinus syndrome secondary to intracranial lymphoma in a cat. *J Feline Med Surg* 2013;**16**(6):513–516. Epub ahead of print.

Murphy CJ, Koblik P, Bellhorn RW, Pino M, Hacker D, Burling T. Squamous cell carcinoma causing blindness and ophthalmoplegia in a cat. *J Am Vet Med Assoc* 1989;**195**(7):965–968.

Theisen SK, Podell M, Schneider T, Wilkie DA, Fenner WR. A retrospective study of cavernous sinus syndrome in 4 dogs and 8 cats. *J Vet Intern Med* 1996;**10**(2):65–71. Erratum in: J Vet Intern Med 1996 May–Jun;10(3):197.

Webb AA, Cullen CL, Rose P, Eisenbart D, Gabor L, Martinson S. Intracranial meningioma causing internal ophthalmoparesis in a dog. *Vet Ophthalmol* 2005;**8**(6):421–425.

Clinical Atlas of Canine and Feline Ophthalmic Disease, First Edition. Douglas Esson.

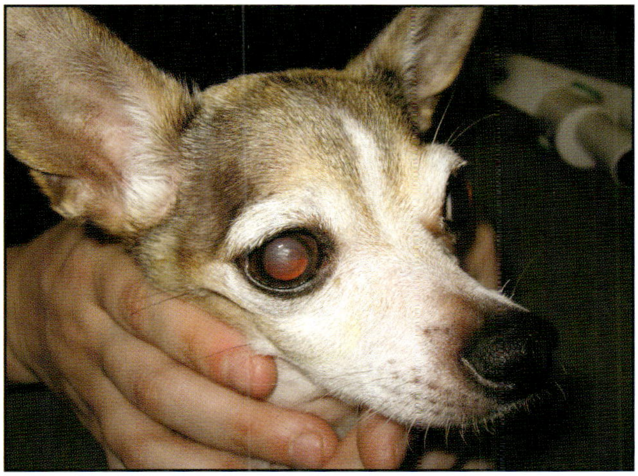

Figure 147.1 Clinical presentation associated with ophthalmoplegia. The characteristic finding is a dilated, non-responsive pupil without visual deficits. This figure displays concurrent corneal disease as a result of trigeminal pathology.

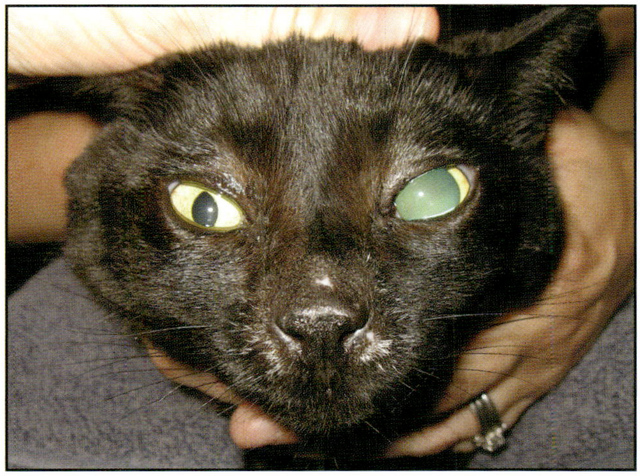

Figure 147.2 Clinical presentation associated with ophthalmoplegia. The characteristic finding is a dilated, non-responsive pupil without visual deficits.

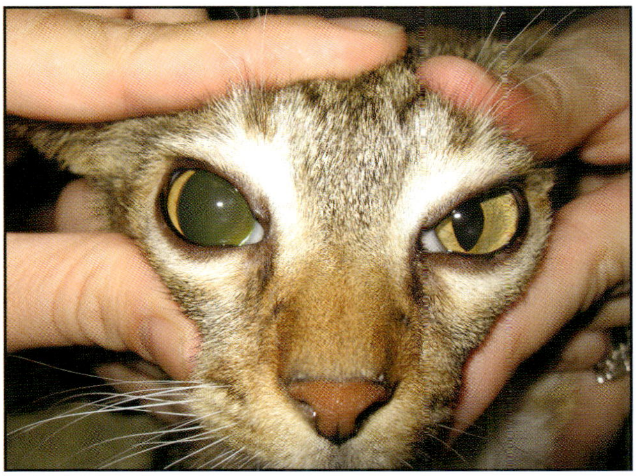

Figure 147.3 Clinical presentation associated with ophthalmoplegia. The characteristic finding is a dilated, non-responsive pupil without visual deficits.

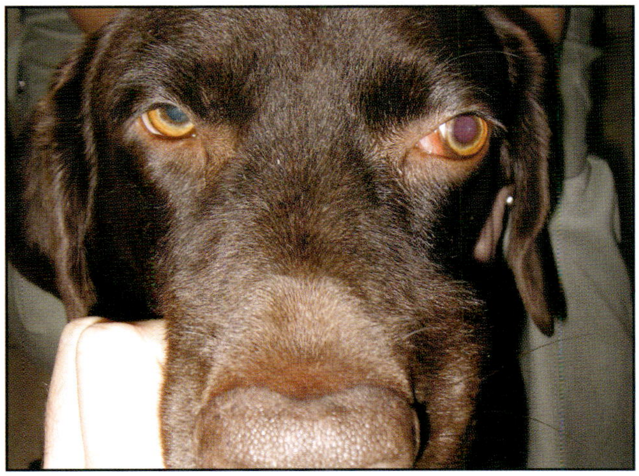

Figure 147.4 Clinical presentation associated with ophthalmoplegia. The characteristic finding is a dilated, non-responsive pupil without visual deficits. This figure displays concurrent ventrolateral strabismus.

CHAPTER 148
NEUROPARALYTIC KERATITIS/HEMIFACIAL PARALYSIS

PRESENTATION

The facial nerve (CN VII) provides somatic innervation to the facial and periocular muscles, notably to the orbicularis oculi muscle (which mediates eyelid closure) via its auriculopalpebral branch. Interruption of innervation may result in any combination of a widened palpebral fissure, a diminished or absent palpebral reflex, deviation of the nasal planum, and/or drooping of the upper and/or lower lips. Symptoms are more commonly unilateral. Inability to effectively close the eyelids, results in exposure keratopathy, which may progress to ulcerative and/or perforating keratitis. Associated damage to (parasympathetic) lacrimal innervation may result in concurrent keratoconjunctivitis sicca (KCS) and/or xeromycteria (see also Neurogenic KCS and Xeromycteria). Commonly affected breeds include the Cocker Spaniel and the Pug.

DIAGNOSIS AND TREATMENT

Cases of facial paralysis are commonly idiopathic in etiology; however, potential causes include trauma (notably to the auriculopalpebral branch of the facial nerve where it crosses the zygomatic arch), neoplasia, otitis, vascular infarcts, and/or endocrine-associated neuropathy. Treatment comprises addressing an underlying cause where identified, as well as the administration of systemic anti-inflammatory therapy, typically corticosteroids unless contraindicated. The prognosis for the recovery of neurologic function is variable. Lacrimal function, if impaired/absent, can sometimes be reestablished using a combination of anti-inflammatory therapy and orally administered pilocarpine. Pilocarpine is dosed in an increasing incremental manner in order to minimize the risk of unwanted side effects. Frequent corneal lubrication using an ophthalmic visco-gel is recommended. In addition, partial tarsorrhaphy (temporary or permanent) may be indicated in order to afford improved corneal protection. If lacrimal function cannot be reestablished, affected patients may be managed using either topical lubrication or, where indicated, parotid duct transposition surgery.

Potential Drug-Side-Effects

Potential adverse effects associated with the use of systemic pilocarpine include gastrointestinal (GI) distress. Potential adverse effects associated with the use of systemic prednisone include polyphagia, polydipsia, polyuria, hair coat changes, weight gain, pancreatitis, GI distress, muscle damage, hepatic impairment, and diabetes.

SELECTED REFERENCES

Garosi LS, Lowrie ML, Swinbourne NF. Neurological manifestations of ear disease in dogs and cats. *Vet Clin North Am Small Anim Pract* 2012;**42**(6):1143–1160. DOI: 10.1016/j.cvsm.2012.08.006. Epub 2012 Oct 10. Review.

Spivack RE, Elkins AD, Moore GE, Lantz GC. Postoperative complications following TECA-LBO in the dog and cat. *J Am Anim Hosp Assoc* 2013;**49**(3):160–168. DOI: 10.5326/JAAHA-MS-5738. Epub 2013 Mar 27.

Varejão AS, Muñoz A, Lorenzo V. Magnetic resonance imaging of the intratemporal facial nerve in idiopathic facial paralysis in the dog. *Vet Radiol Ultrasound* 2006;**47**(4):328–333.

Wright JA. Ultrastructural findings in idiopathic facial paralysis in the dog. *J Comp Pathol* 1988;**98**(1):111–115.

Clinical Atlas of Canine and Feline Ophthalmic Disease, First Edition. Douglas Esson.

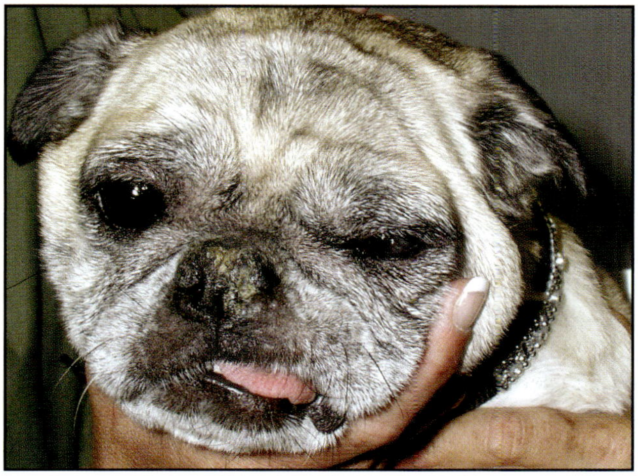

Figure 148.1 Clinical presentation associated with facial nerve damage. Xeromycteria, marked by a dry, crusted ipsilateral nostril is notable.

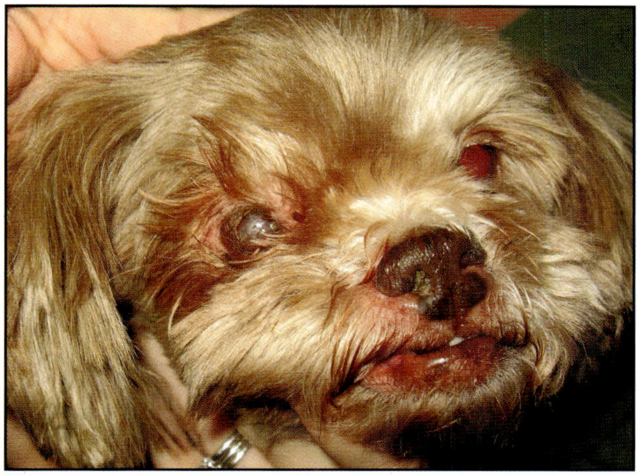

Figure 148.2 Clinical presentation associated with facial nerve damage. Xeromycteria, marked by a dry, crusted ipsilateral nostril is notable.

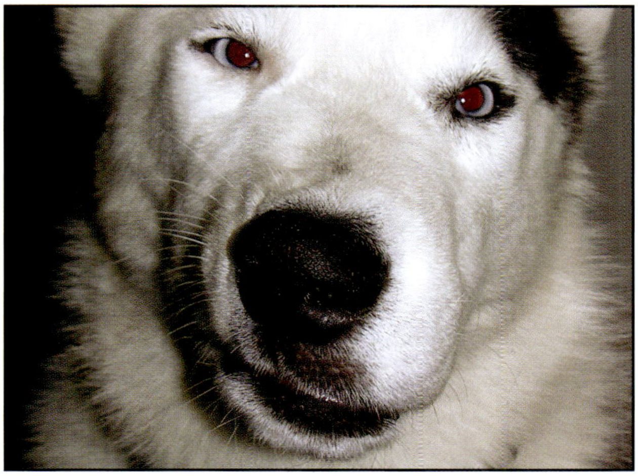

Figure 148.3 Clinical presentation associated with facial nerve damage. Deviation of the nasal planum is notable.

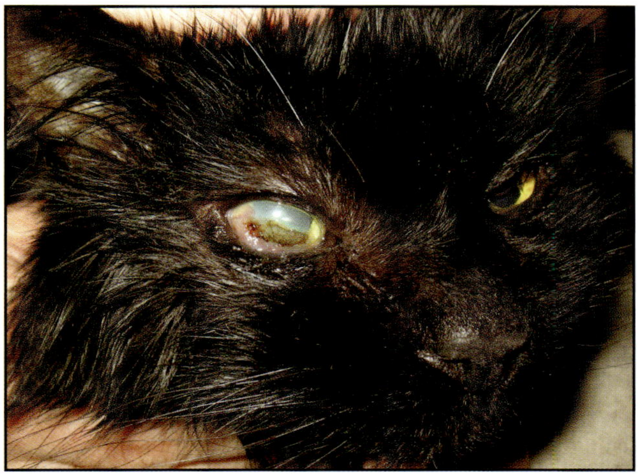

Figure 148.4 Clinical presentation associated with facial nerve damage. Exposure keratopathy is notable.

CHAPTER 149
NEUROGENIC KCS AND XEROMYCTERIA

PRESENTATION

Parasympathetic innervation to the lacrimal glands originates in the parasympathetic nucleus of the facial nerve. Fibers extend rostrally with the facial nerve and synapse within the pterygopalatine ganglion before reaching the lacrimal structures via the zygomatic branch of the trigeminal nerve. Damage anywhere along this pathway may result in partial or complete loss of innervation to the lacrimal glands and resultant "neurogenic keratoconjunctivitis sicca (KCS)." Neurogenic KCS is frequently characterized by an associated dry/crusted ipsilateral nostril (termed "xeromycteria") as a result of impaired innervation of the nasal gland. Potential etiologies include inflammatory, traumatic, and/or neoplastic processes. Additional symptoms, depending on the site of the lesion may include reduced corneal and/or facial sensation as a result of impaired trigeminal nerve function and/or Horner's syndrome.

DIAGNOSIS AND TREATMENT

The diagnosis of neurogenic KCS is made on the basis of clinical findings. In many cases of neurogenic KCS, lacrimomimetic function is completely absent, marked by Schirmer tear test values of 0 mm/wetting per minute (termed "absolute KCS"). Treatment of neurogenic KCS comprises identification and treatment of the underlying lesion where possible. This may encompass cranial imaging (magnetic resonance imaging (MRI)). Lacrimal function can sometimes be reestablished using a combination of anti-inflammatory therapy and orally administered pilocarpine. Pilocarpine is dosed in an increasing incremental manner in order to minimize the risk of unwanted side effects. Frequent corneal lubrication using an ophthalmic visco-gel is recommended. In addition, partial (temporary or permanent) tarsorrhaphy may be indicated in order to afford improved corneal protection. If lacrimal function cannot be reestablished, affected patients may be managed using either topical lubrication or, where indicated, parotid duct transposition surgery.

Potential Drug-Side-Effects

Potential adverse effects associated with the use of systemic pilocarpine include gastrointestinal (GI) distress. Potential adverse effects associated with the use of systemic prednisone include polyphagia, polydipsia, polyuria, hair coat changes, weight gain, pancreatitis, GI distress, muscle damage, hepatic impairment, and diabetes.

SELECTED REFERENCES

Matheis FL, Walser-Reinhardt L, Spiess BM. Canine neurogenic Keratoconjunctivitis sicca: 11 cases (2006–2010). *Vet Ophthalmol* 2012;**15**(4):288–290. DOI: 10.1111/j.1463-5224.2011.00968.x. Epub 2011 Oct 31.

Rhodes M, Heinrich C, Featherstone H, Braus B, Manning S, Cripps PJ, Renwick P. Parotid duct transposition in dogs: a retrospective review of 92 eyes from 1999 to 2009. *Vet Ophthalmol* 2012;**15**(4):213–222. DOI: 10.1111/j.1463-5224.2011.00972.x. Epub 2011 Nov 24.

Slatter D, Severin GA. Use of pilocarpine for treatment of keratoconjunctivitis sicca. *J Am Vet Med Assoc* 1995;**206**(3):287–289.

Clinical Atlas of Canine and Feline Ophthalmic Disease, First Edition. Douglas Esson.

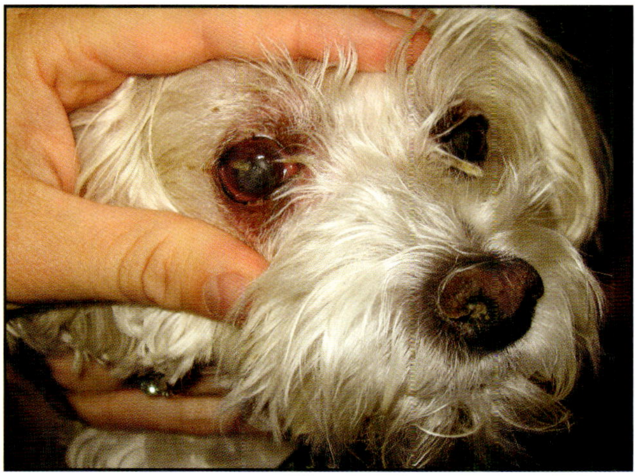

Figure 149.1 Clinical presentation associated with neurogenic KCS. Xeromycteria, marked by a dry, crusted, ipsilateral nostril is notable.

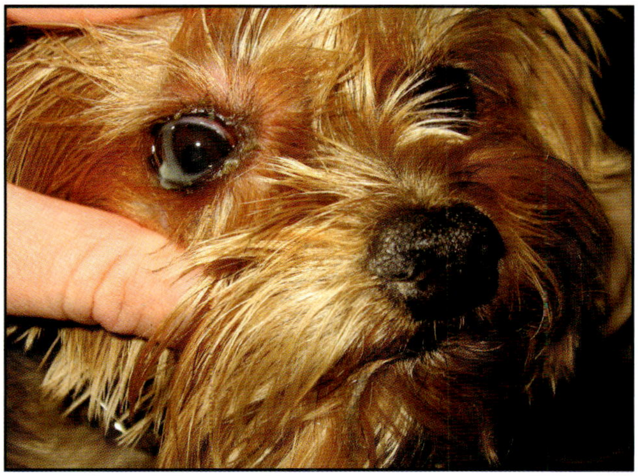

Figure 149.2 Clinical presentation associated with neurogenic KCS. Xeromycteria, marked by a dry, crusted, ipsilateral nostril is notable.

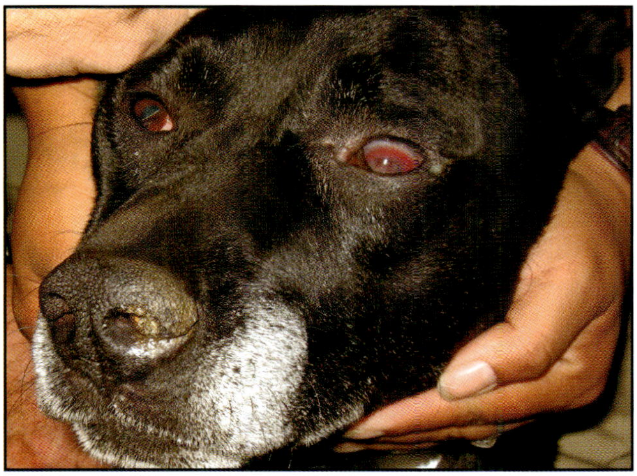

Figure 149.3 Clinical presentation associated with neurogenic KCS. Xeromycteria, marked by a dry, crusted, ipsilateral nostril is notable.

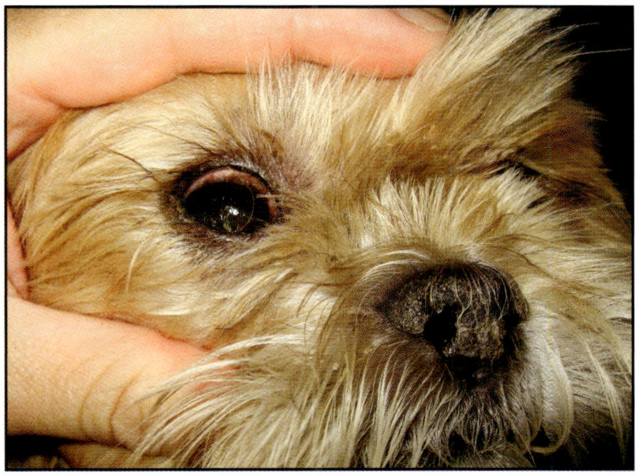

Figure 149.4 Clinical presentation associated with neurogenic KCS. Xeromycteria, marked by a dry, crusted, ipsilateral nostril is notable.

CHAPTER 150
OPTIC NEURITIS/MENINGITIS

PRESENTATION

The post-retinal visual pathways comprise the retrobulbar optic nerves (ONs), optic chiasm, optic tracts, lateral geniculate nuclei, optic radiations, and visual cortices. Optic neuritis describes inflammation of any portion of the ON(s) with or without concurrent evidence of more generalized central nervous system (CNS) inflammation. Presenting signs typically include blindness in association with dilated, nonresponsive or poorly responsive pupils. Symptoms may be unilateral or bilateral and are generally acute in onset. Additional ophthalmic findings may include any combination of chorioretinitis, papilledema, and/or hemorrhage of the ON head and surrounding neuroretina. Symptoms of more generalized CNS involvement may include altered mentation, lethargy, ataxia, and or seizure-like activity. Optic neuritis occurs most commonly in association with granulomatous meningoencephalitis (GME); however, other potential etiologies include necrotizing leukoencephalitis/meningoencephalitis, infectious encephalomyelitis (associated with viral, bacterial, fungal, rickettsial, protozoal, or parasitic organisms). or neoplasia. The underlying cause of GME frequently remains unclear; however, an autoimmune mechanism is suspected. Canine and feline patients of any breed may develop optic neuritis; however, small-breed dogs are more commonly affected, notably the Chihuahua and Dachshund.

DIAGNOSIS AND TREATMENT

The diagnosis of optic neuritis is made on the basis of a combination of clinical findings (including funduscopy) as well as adjunctive diagnostics including complete blood count (CBC)/chemistry analysis, infectious titer testing, cerebrospinal fluid (CSF) evaluation, and/or cranial magnetic resonance imaging (MRI). CSF analysis may reveal increased protein levels with or without a leukocytosis. MRI findings typically include subtle, patchy hyperintensity affecting multiple areas of the brain and meninges. Hyperintensity of the ONs may or may not be noted. Electroretinography may additionally be employed in order to rule out primary retinal disease (see SARDs/IMR). Differentials include inherited lysosomal storage diseases (notably, the gangliosidoses and neuronal ceroid lipofuscinoses), hydrocephalus, trauma, hypoxia (notably, as a result of anesthetic complication), metabolic disease, vascular pathology, or central neoplasia (notably, pituitary adenomas, lymphoma and meningioma). Treatment comprises immunomodulation using varying combinations of systemic prednisone, azathioprine, and/or cyclosporine. When successful, treatment should be tapered with caution over a significantly extended timeframe (typically months), and long-term therapy may be required in order to prevent recurrence of symptoms.

SELECTED REFERENCES

Armour MD, Broome M, Dell'Anna G, Blades NJ, Esson DW. A review of orbital and intracranial magnetic resonance imaging in 79 canine and 13 feline patients (2004–2010). *Vet Ophthalmol* 2011;**14**(4):215–226. DOI: 10.1111/j.1463-5224.2010.00865.x. Epub 2011 Apr 18.

Nell B. Optic neuritis in dogs and cats. *Vet Clin North Am Small Anim Pract* 2008;**38**(2):403–415, viii. DOI: 10.1016/j.cvsm.2007.11.005. Review.

Seruca C, Ródenas S, Leiva M, Peña T, Añor S. Acute postretinal blindness: ophthalmologic, neurologic, and magnetic resonance imaging findings in dogs and cats (seven cases). *Vet Ophthalmol* 2010;**13**(5):307–314. DOI: 10.1111/j.1463-5224.2010.00814.x.

Clinical Atlas of Canine and Feline Ophthalmic Disease, First Edition. Douglas Esson.

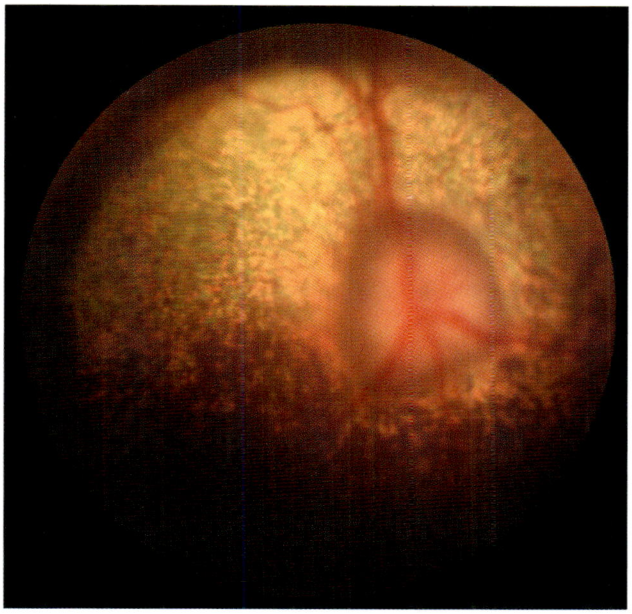

Figure 150.1 Funduscopic findings associated with optic neuritis. Optic nerve head swelling ("papilledema") is notable.

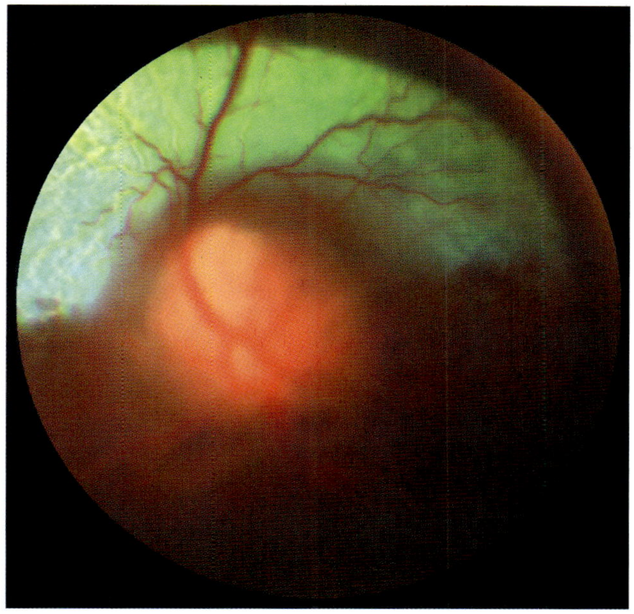

Figure 150.2 Funduscopic findings associated with optic neuritis. Optic nerve head swelling ("papilledema") is notable.

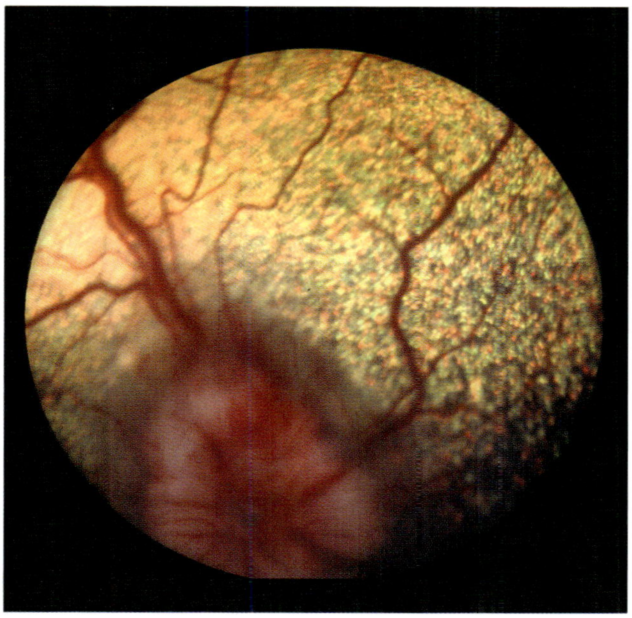

Figure 150.3 Funduscopic findings associated with optic neuritis. Peripapillary edema and hemorrhage are notable.

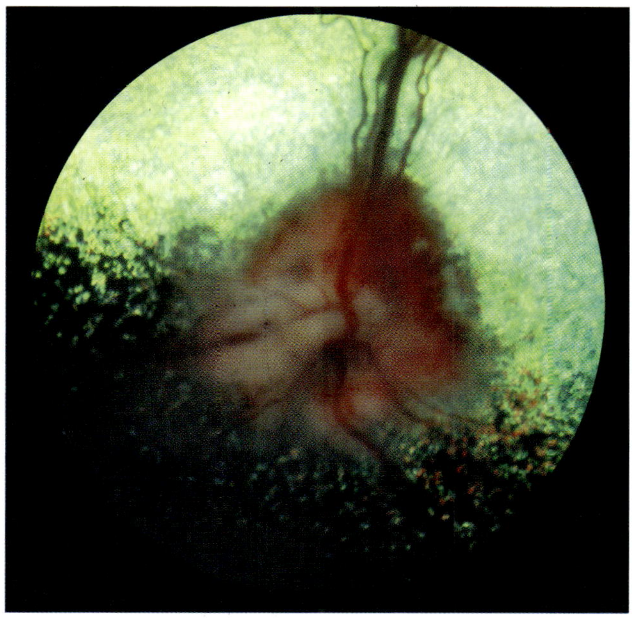

Figure 150.4 Funduscopic findings associated with optic neuritis. Peripapillary edema and hemorrhage are notable.

Potential Drug-Side-Effects

Potential adverse effects associated with the use of systemic corticosteroids include polyphagia, polydipsia, polyuria, hair coat changes, weight gain, pancreatitis, gastrointestinal (GI) distress, muscle damage, hepatic impairment, and diabetes. Potential adverse effects associated with the use of azathioprine include GI distress, pancreatitis, hepatotoxicity, and myelosuppression. Potential adverse effects associated with the use of cyclophosphamide include GI distress, pancreatitis, hepatotoxicity, and myelosuppression.

INDEX

Clinical Atlas of Canine and Feline Ophthalmic Disease, First Edition. Douglas Esson.